POCKET
GUIDE
TO
THE
OPERATING
ROOM

POCKET GUIDE TO THE OPERATING ROOM

Maxine A. Goldman, B.S., R.N.
Clinical Nurse IV
Formerly, Operating Room Clinical Education
Instructor
Tarzana Regional Medical Center
Tarzana, California

 F. A. DAVIS COMPANY ● Philadelphia

Copyright © 1988 by F. A. Davis Company

Printed in the United States of America

Last digit indicates print number:

10 9 8 7 6 5

Library of Congress Cataloging-in-Publication Data

Goldman, Maxine A., 1947–
    Pocket guide to the operating room.

    Bibliography: p.
    Includes index.
    1. Surgery, Operative—Handbooks, manuals, etc.
  2. Surgical instruments and apparatus—Handbooks, manuals, etc.   3. Operating rooms—Equipment and supplies—Handbooks, manuals, etc.   I. Title.
[DNLM: 1. Operating Rooms—handbooks.   2. Surgery, Operative—handbooks.   WO 39 G6193p)
RD32.3.G65 1988   617'.91   88-7165
ISBN 0-8036-4174-5

PREFACE

This guide is intended for the practitioner, as well as the student surgical technologist or nurse who requires a concise, yet comprehensive, reference regarding the technological aspects of patient care in the operating room. The material is presented in a systematic manner to encourage the reader to follow a logical sequence of events as they actually occur when a patient enters the operating room. Background clinical information is provided in order to enhance the reader's perspective.

For optimal utilization of this guide, a basic understanding of anatomy, physiology, microbiology, and asepsis is presupposed. Over 300 surgical procedures are described, and they are arranged in chapters according to anatomical site and/or surgical specialty. The format for every procedure includes a definition, a discussion, notes on preparation of the patient and draping techniques, and necessary equipment, instrumentation, supplies, and step-by-step description of the procedure. Special notes particular to each surgery are also provided. Chapters on anesthesia, patient safety and psychological care of the patient depart from the standardized format. A discussion of laser technology is included in the Appendix.

The conduction of a surgical procedure varies from institution to institution, among different sections of the country, and according to the preference of the surgeon. Consequently, the suggested instrument trays are not meant to imply that these instruments must be used, but rather that these trays include the basics; various instruments can be added or deleted according to preference. Likewise, instrument nomenclature, availability of supplies, techniques for draping, and so forth will also vary. Precise details regarding certain items, e.g., suture material, have been omitted due to the myriad of products available.

In an attempt to limit its physical size, this work is confined to the operative phase of patient care; perioperative care outside of the surgical department has been omitted. Recognizing that one must understand a surgical procedure before optimal care of the individual patient can be implemented, it is hoped that the information base presented here will serve as a generally applicable foundation upon which the reader can build.

M.A.G.

ACKNOWLEDGMENTS

In undertaking the writing of this pocket guide as a single author, I am appreciative of the assistance of a number of persons.

I would like to thank the following instructors who so diligently reviewed the many drafts of the manscript: Merle Curtis, M.Ed., R.N., Boise State University; Florence C. Elmore, R.N., M.S., Indiana Vocational and Technical College; Jane Johnson, M.S.N., R.N., CNOR, Delaware County Community College; Janet R. Miller, R.N., Milwaukee Area Technical College; Jane C. Rothrock, DNSc, R.N., CNOR, Delaware County Community College; Dianne Sharp, R.N., CNOR, Des Moines Area Community College; Mildred Simmons, CST, Sheridan Valley Vo-Tech Center; Darlette Stanley, CST, York Technical Education Center; and Gerald W. Young, CST, BLS, St. Louis Community College.

My sincere thanks also go to the several typists who transcribed the original notes, and to Mrs. Francine Stockser who worked tirelessly to commit these notes to computer disks. I also thank my colleagues who urged me to complete this work, and who on occasion shared with me their expertise pertaining to their specialties. To Mrs. Francine Kubrin, medical librarian at Valley Presbyterian Hospital, Van Nuys, California, who patiently assisted me in obtaining multiple references, I am grateful. I am likewise grateful to my editor, Mr. Jean-François Vilain, who maintained at all times a friendly and open line of communication. I would also like to extend my gratitude to my children and friends, who offered me continuous encouragement and support despite my neglect of them during the preparation of this work. Finally, I wish to thank my husband Harris, my partner in all endeavors, whose knowledge and love sustained me through the completion of this pocket guide.

M.A.G.

CONTENTS

PART IV. INSTRUMENT TRAYS   **507**

Part I

PERIOPERATIVE CONSIDERATIONS

Chapter 1

PSYCHOLOGIC SUPPORT OF THE SURGICAL PATIENT

Surgical procedures are classified as major or minor. These distinctions do not take into consideration the degree of anxiety the patient may experience regarding his or her surgery. The operating room personnel may allay a patient's fears by conducting themselves in a kind, reassuring, and confident manner.

The process of psychologic support for the surgical patient actually begins well before the patient enters the operating room suite. The patient's physician and surgeon will have initiated this process at the time the surgery is scheduled. The demeanor of the hospital (or surgicenter) admitting office personnel may also help to reassure the patient. The reception of the patient to the floor (or holding areas of the surgicenters) likewise must serve to reassure the patient.

In some institutions the patient's first contact with the operating room staff might occur the day before surgery or in the case of same-day admissions, several hours before the procedure. An orientation (teaching) session may be offered directly by operating room personnel or by closed circuit television or videocassette that describes to some extent the surgical preliminaries and immediate postoperative considerations so that fewer unanticipated events will be experienced. An opportunity may be given the patient to express anxieties or ask questions.

Perhaps the most significant of the events in this chain occurs when the patient, although often partially sedated, is transported to the operating room suite. There the circulator will make certain of the patient's identity, the type of surgery to be performed, and the name of the surgeon. A checklist concerning the patient's fasting status, possible prosthetic devices, special physical conditions, and possible drug intolerances are again discussed with the patient and reviewed in the chart. The chart is checked with respect to consent forms and medical and laboratory data; see Surgical Checklist, p. 16. During this review the circulator will reassure the patient that every effort will be made to maintain the patient's well-being and safety during the procedure. These measures of psychologic support are continued until the patient is totally anesthetized or they may be continued throughout the procedure when there are varying degrees of consciousness.

Postoperatively these measures are continued, but are now in the hands of the recovery room staff or other appropriate nursing personnel.

In no small way do these considerations affect the ultimate outcome of the patient's surgery. The importance of these measures must be anticipated by all those concerned.

PROTECTION OF THE PATIENT IN SURGERY

ADMISSION PROCEDURE

On admission of the patient to the operating room, the circulator verifies the patient's name, the name of the patient's surgeon, and the surgery to be performed verbally with the patient, and by inspection of the patient's armband and the chart.

Evidence of the preoperative preparation of the patient as required by hospital protocol should be complete and recorded on the chart. Mandatory requirements include a valid signed and dated informed consent form and a record (recent) of the patient's health history and physical examination. A special permit may be required to perform operations such as sterilization, therapeutic abortion, or the amputation of a body part. Other requirements may include laboratory data, a chest x-ray examination record, etc. Most institutions have a preoperative checklist that is vital in preventing oversights in preparing the patient for surgery. See example of Surgical Checklist at the end of this chapter.

TRANSFER PROCEDURE

The patient is transferred to the operating table by two persons in order to prevent injury. One person stabilizes the gurney (stretcher) as close to the operating table as possible and locks the wheels. The patient is instructed how to move (if alert and physically capable). Care is taken to protect all catheters and tubings (e.g., intravenous lines and Foley catheter), etc. while moving the patient. The second person stands on the opposite side of the operating room table to receive the patient and prevent falls. The restraint (safety) strap is fastened above the patient's knees. Adequate help should be obtained to safely move the patient to the operating table when the patient cannot move without assistance.

POSITIONING

The patient's position is determined according to the procedure to be performed, the physical condition of the patient, and the surgeon's preference in consultation with the anesthetist. Proper body alignment must be maintained. Adequate assistance should be obtained when lifting patients. The anesthetized patient is *never* moved without the anesthetist's permission. Care is taken to avoid interference with respiration (e.g., by use of chest rolls when the patient is prone). Extremities and bony prominences must be adequately padded and supported to avoid damage to the skin and nerves. There should be no interference with the circulation (e.g., crossed legs, restraints too tightly applied), and position changes (e.g., lowering the legs from lithotomy) should be made slowly to allow the circulatory system to adjust, thereby preventing a drop in blood pressure. The physical condition (e.g., arthritis) of the patient may place limitations on the desired position and should be taken into account. Special equipment and table attachments are designed to help maintain the patient's position. For descriptions of the position(s) employed and the equipment necessary, see the specific procedure.

ENVIRONMENTAL CONTROLS

In light of the present knowledge on the transmission of infection, hospitals establish policies and procedures to curtail contamination. Various regulatory agencies mandate that health facilities adhere to these policies and conduct ongoing surveillance studies. The cleansing and disinfection of each individual operating room including furnishings and equipment should be performed after each procedure. In addition, the entire surgical department including its corridors, storage rooms, and other auxiliary areas are cleaned according to an established schedule. Traffic patterns are developed to minimize intrusion into restricted areas. Airborne contaminants are reduced by traffic restriction, air-conditioning (using high-efficiency particulate air filters), and laminar airflow systems (e.g., used during joint replacement procedures). Through the use of barriers (i.e., restricted areas of the surgery department), the wearing of masks, head and shoe coverings, and specially laundered clothing, the number of microorganisms in the surgical environment is reduced. By strict attention to "scrubbing" technique by personnel involved in the sterile field, adequate skin preparation of the surgical site, and the constant implementation of aseptic technique, the number of contaminants present about the surgical field is also reduced. Careful attention to the controlled sterilization of instrumentation and proper opening of packaged sterile supplies must be observed. The disposal of waste and the removal of laundry in specially labeled plastic bags or containers is mandatory. Frequent handwashing and the observance of restrictions regarding the changing of clothing and use of protective head and shoe coverings is incumbent upon all members of the surgical department.

ELECTRICAL AND FIRE HAZARDS

Electrical and fire safety precautions are set forth in hospital policy and are carried out by the operating room staff. Safety measures include restricted areas for smoking, determination of the safety of equipment before permitting its use in the operating room (by the engineering department), and the ongoing inspection of equipment prior to each use. Personnel must receive instruction for the safe operation of electrical equipment and then demonstrate their ability to use the equipment safely. All personnel should receive special instruction regarding their responsibilities in case of fire. Flammable anesthetic agents are rarely employed today. The electrosurgical unit should not be used in the mouth or pleural cavity during the administration of high concentrations of oxygen. Disposable drapes, gowns, head and shoe coverings, etc. are treated with flame retardant chemicals. Flammable antiseptic solutions should not be used to prepare the skin when the electrosurgical unit is used.

ELECTROSURGERY

The electrosurgical unit is commonly employed in all the surgical specialties for the purpose of coagulating or cutting tissue. The current flows from the generator (electrosurgical unit) to an active electrode through tissue and returns to the unit through an inactive electrode. In the monopolar electrosurgical unit the active electrode is usually an "electrosurgical pencil" and the inactive electrode is the dispersive (grounding) pad. In the bipolar unit the active electrode is one side of the forceps and the inactive electrode is the other side of the forceps; therefore, no dispersive pad is necessary.

Precautions must be taken when employing electrosurgery in order to prevent injury to the patient. These include

1. All connections must be secure.
2. The inactive electrode should cover a sufficiently large area of skin (relatively free of hair, which acts as an insulator) and be as close as possible to the site of application of the active electrode (in order to minimize the pathway of the current through the body).
3. The patient's body should *not* make direct contact with metal surfaces. If the return circuit is faulty, the ground circuit could be completed through the contact area thus creating an inadvertent burn injury.
4. Electrocardiogram electrodes should be placed as far away from the operative site as possible.

Repeated requests to increase the current should be thoroughly investigated by the circulator. Check all connections and the dispersive pad; if no problem is found the unit may be faulty. Turn the unit off and unplug it.

Special notes

If the patient has an implanted pacemaker the electrosurgical unit could cause malfunction. The patient needs to be continuously monitored. The cardiac arrest cart (complete with defibrillator and paddles) should be in close proximity.

OPERATIVE RECORD

The legal rights of the patient as well as those of operating room personnel are protected by the documentation in the patient's operative record. The Joint Commission on Accreditation of Health Care Organizations (JC) requires that the operative procedure report include the preoperative diagnosis, the procedure performed, the postoperative diagnosis, specimens obtained, and the names of the surgical team providing intraoperative care. The documentation of other information such as the taking of counts (e.g., sponge, sharps, and instrument), placement of catheters, intravenous lines, wound packing, and use of equipment (e.g., electrosurgical unit, tourniquets, etc.) is invaluable. An example of the suggested format for the Operative Record is shown on p. 11.

In addition, the JC requires an anesthesia record for each operative procedure, completed by the anesthetist. According to hospital policy, when an anesthetist is not present during the procedure, the circulator documents the patient's vital signs, blood pressure, the names and amounts of drugs and anesthetics administered by or at the direction of the surgeon, and records all pertinent times.

COUNTING PROCEDURE

Each institution should have its own written policy and procedure regarding the counting of sponges, sharps, and instruments. The following guidelines should be observed when counting all objects potentially subject to inadvertent seclusion in a wound:

1. All items are counted initially by the circulator and the scrub person together (aloud) as the scrub person touches each item.
2. The number (count) of each type of item is immediately recorded by the circulator.
3. If there is any uncertainty regarding the initial count it is repeated.
4. As additional items (e.g., sponges, needles) are added to the sterile field during the procedure the scrub person counts the item(s) with the circulator, who adds the count to the record and initials it.

OPERATIVE RECORD

DATE _____ PT. ROOM NO. _____ O.R. No. _____
Preoperative Diagnosis _____
Procedure _____
Postoperative Diagnosis _____
Surgeon _____ Circulator _____
Assistant _____ Scrub Person _____
Anesthetist _____ Type Anesthesia _____
   Drugs used _____ Intubation _____
_____
Time Patient arrived in OR _____
   Anesthesia began _____ Operation began _____
   Anesthesia ended _____ Operation ended _____
Position _____
Comments _____
Prep solution _____ Area prepped _____ Prep by _____

ESU Dispersive pad used _____ _____
                                   location   plate no.
Skin condition Preop _____ Postop _____
Tourniquet used _____ Location _____
   Time began _____ Ended _____
Prosthesis used _____
   Location _____ Manufacturer _____
   Type, size, serial no. _____
Irrigation solutions _____
Medications _____
Invasive lines _____
Blood given _____ No. of units _____
Blood unit(s) No. _____
Cell Saver used _____ No. of units _____
X-rays taken _____ Fluoroscopy _____
Drains _____ Type _____ Location _____ Placed by_____
Packs _____ Type _____ Location _____
Specimens _____ Number _____
Cultures _____
Intraoperative Notes
_____
_____
_____
_____

Sponge, sharps, instrument counts correct
   (1st) _____ (2nd) _____
Signatures _____ _____
               Scrub person   Circulator

5. Nothing (including laundry, trash, instruments, sponges) may be removed from an operating room while a procedure is in progress until the final count is acknowledged to be correct.
6. Whenever there is a change of team members a count is taken.
7. When an incorrectly numbered package of items is dispensed the items should be bagged, labeled accordingly, set aside, and not recorded in the count.
8. Counts are taken before beginning the procedure, before wound closure begins, and when skin closure is initiated.
9. An additional count is taken prior to the closure of an organ within a cavity (e.g., uterus, bladder).

Incorrect closure counts must be repeated immediately. If the count remains incorrect, the circulator alerts the surgeon, who will inspect the patient's wound for the missing item. If the item is not located, hospital policy must be followed (usually to include immediate x-ray examination) and an incident report filed.

Sponge counts

All sponges, neurologic sponges (cottonoids), and soft goods (e.g., umbilical tapes) are counted. Each type and size sponge is kept separate. All sponges used within the wound must be x-ray detectable. X-ray detectable sponges are never used for dressings, and dressing sponges are never used to dry the surgical field. Sponges are discarded following use in a plastic lined receptacle. Soiled sponges are counted by the scrub person and the circulator together and then bagged in impervious plastic bags according to a predetermined number (usually in sets of five or ten). When the counts are taken the scrub nurse counts the sponges according to type, beginning with the sponges on the field and proceeding to the sponges on the back table and then those off the field. The circulator informs the surgeon of the results of the counts.

Sharp counts

All needles, knife blades, electrosurgical blades, and any other sharps are counted. Needles in multiple suture packs may be counted according to the number on the package; some hospitals require each package to be opened and each needle counted individually. Used needles, blades, and other sharps should be retained on a needle magnet or counter pad to facilitate counting. All parts of any needle broken during a procedure must be accounted for. Closure counts for sharps follow the same format as those for sponges.

Instrument counts

Instruments should be counted for all surgical procedures. All parts of disassembled or broken instruments must be accounted for in their entirety. Closure counts for instruments follow the format for other counts.

STERILIZATION

All items (instruments, supplies, equipment, etc.) that come in contact with the sterile field and the wound must be sterile. As soon as possible following use, soiled instruments are cleaned in the washer-sterilizer. Following terminal decontamination in the washer-sterilizer, the instruments are cleaned in an ultrasonic cleaner to remove any remaining soil.

The three most commonly used methods of sterilization employed in the operating room (or central supply) include:

1. Saturated steam under pressure
2. Gas chemical sterilization
3. Liquid chemical sterilization

Discussion of other methods of sterilization such as ionizing radiation (e.g., Cobalt-60) used by manufacturers for prepackaged items is beyond the scope of this guide.

Saturated steam under pressure

The *flash sterilizer* is frequently used in the operating room for urgently needed unwrapped instruments. Customarily the temperature is set at 270°F (132°C) for a 3-minute or 10-minute cycle. The length of the cycle is determined by the density of the item(s) to be sterilized. The recommendation of the manufacturer of the item regarding the temperature and length of exposure time at that temperature must be followed. The recording device on the sterilizer should be checked to confirm that the instrument(s) to be sterilized has (have) been exposed to the proper temperature for the desired length of time. Heat-sensitive indicators should accompany the instrument(s). Trays with mesh bottoms are recommended.

Wrapped instruments, trays, basins, etc. are usually sterilized in a prevacuum, high-temperature steam sterilizer. Proper wrapping of trays and packages is mandatory, as is the proper loading of the sterilizer. The Bowie-Dick test is used to verify that there were no air pockets, which would negate the sterilization conditions. A heat-sensitive indicator is placed within each wrapped tray (or package) and each package is secured with heat-sensitive tape.

Gas chemical sterilization

Ethylene oxide gas is used to sterilize items that are vulnerable to heat or moisture. Any item that can withstand sterilization by steam under pressure should not be gas-sterilized. Ethylene oxide sterilization depends on concentration of gas, temperature, humidity, and exposure time. The ethylene oxide sterilizer must be operated exactly according to the manufacturer's instructions to ensure that the requirements for sterilization are met. Type of item, arrangement of the load, and rate of penetration influence the amount of exposure time required. Penetration of the gas is aided by an initial vacuum within the sterilizer. Usually cycles of 3 to 7 hours are employed. An ethylene oxide chemically sensitive indicator that is placed inside the wrapped package indicates that the item was exposed to ethylene oxide but does not necessarily indicate that sterilization has occurred; therefore, the sterilization process must conform to manufacturer's specifications.

Inhalation of ethylene oxide is to be avoided, as is direct contact with the sterilized items prior to aeration. The length of aeration time required depends on the composition of the items, the type of wrapper used, the concentration of the ethylene oxide used, the airflow rate, and the temperature during aeration. When items are aerated in a mechanical aerator the air is automatically changed a minimum of four times an hour. The temperature is controlled at 122°F (50°C) to 140°F (60°C) for 8 to 12 hours. If a mechanical aerator is unavailable, items should be aerated in a well-ventilated room at a controlled temperature of 65°F (18°C) to 72°F (22°C) for 7 days.

Liquid chemical sterilization

When items cannot tolerate sterilization by saturated steam under pressure and when the time required for gas sterilization is impractical, liquid chemical sterilization is employed. A 2% activated aqueous glutaraldehyde solution (e.g., Cidex) is the agent often employed when liquid chemosterilization is desired. Instruments and other items must be completely immersed in the solution for 10 hours to achieve sterilization. Disinfection is effected if the instrument is submerged for 10 minutes. All items must be thoroughly rinsed in sterile distilled water before use.

Patient Identification Plate
Patient's Name, age
Hospital Number
Admitting Physician

SURGICAL CHECKLIST

Nursing Unit

Surgical procedure _____
Consent signed _____
Special Consent signed _____
Prep done by _____
History & Physical charted _____
Allergies _____
Blood ordered _____ No. units available _____
Preoperative instructions _____
NPO time _____
Height _____ Weight _____
BP _____ TPR _____
Laboratory charted
 CBC _____ PTT _____
 UA _____ K+ _____
 Other _____
Drains, catheters, intravenous lines _____
Preop medication type _____ time _____ by _____

Operating Room

Check	Comments

Prosthesis	None	Removed	Disposition	In	
Retainers, bridges, plates					
Artificial limb					
Artificial eye					
Contact lenses					
Hearing aid					
Valuables					
Glasses					
Wallet					
Jewelry					
Radio					

Electric shaver

Identification band checked with chart _____

Special considerations (artificial joints, pacemaker, etc.) _____

_____	_____		_____	_____
Signature	date		Signature	date

17

EMERGENCIES AND DISASTERS

Most operating rooms are equipped with a special emergency signal that can be operated from within each separate operating room to alert others to the emergency.

In the event a patient suffers a cardiopulmonary arrest the anesthetist and surgeon administer cardiopulmonary resuscitation (CPR). Health care providers are required to know CPR. In the absence of an anesthetist or surgeon, nursing personnel must administer CPR. An emergency cardiopulmonary arrest cart should be available in the surgery department at all times. Included on this well-stocked cart are in-date emergency drugs, needles and syringes, infusion equipment, a defibrillator, and monitoring equipment. Nursing personnel responding to the emergency signal should bring the cardiopulmonary arrest cart into the room. Documentation of all medications and procedures administered is made.

Hospitals are equipped with an alternative power source that takes over if a power failure occurs. All team members are required to know the location of high-intensity flashlights kept in the department for use during the time lapse until the alternate power source begins functioning.

Malignant hyperthermia is a rare, dangerous condition thought to be associated with the use of some general anesthetics. Proper treatment initiated immediately by the administration of dantrolene (Dantrium), iced intravenous solutions, and steroids, and by cooling the patient with ice packs can significantly reduce mortality. In preparation to meet this emergency situation, operating room personnel need to be informed of the protocol set up by the anesthesia department.

Should death occur in the operating room, individual state law and hospital policy must be adhered to regarding handling of the deceased patient. An incident report is submitted detailing the events leading to the patient's death.

Chapter 3

SAFETY FOR OPERATING ROOM PERSONNEL

The operating room staff needs to be aware of the hazards related to working in surgery. By strict adherence to departmental policy regarding safety measures, potential problems can be avoided. Many factors that apply to patient safety in the operating room also apply to personnel safety (see Chapter 2).

IN-SERVICE EDUCATION

Most hospitals have in-service orientation programs for new employees to inform them of the hospital's policies and procedures including the subjects of fire prevention and individual responsibilities in case of fire and disasters. In addition to this general orientation most operating rooms have a departmental orientation program for new personnel, and a scheduled monthly in-service education program for all personnel. These programs serve not only to keep the operating room staff abreast of new technology, procedures, instrumentation, and nursing care in general, but also serve to reiterate departmental safety measures.

BODY MECHANICS

Through the application of good body mechanics, particularly when lifting or moving patients, heavy instrument trays, or equipment, strains and other injuries can be prevented. Lifting should be done by bending the knees, positioning one's body under the load, and then straightening the legs allowing the lower extremity muscles to do the lifting. A roller (e.g., Davis) can be of significant value in preventing strains when moving unconscious or obese patients.

FATIGUE FACTORS

Fatigue can be minimized through working quickly and efficiently. Wasted motions not only increase the patient's anesthesia and operating room time, but are also tiring for the staff member. Integration of individual motions and thoughtful organization of the day's total workload can greatly influence one's job performance and endurance.

RADIATION SAFETY

Operating room personnel may be exposed to radiation when intraoperative x-rays are taken and when radioactive implant procedures are performed. To reduce the deleterious effects of radiation exposure, hospital policy must be strictly followed.

The effect of radiation exposure depends on the amount of radiation, the proximity of the radiation source, and the length of time of the exposure. Hospital protective measures should include

1. All nonsterile team members should leave the room (whenever possible) or wear a lead apron.
2. Sterile team members should either stand behind a lead screen or wall or wear a lead apron.
3. Monitoring devices (e.g., dosimeters) should be worn by personnel routinely exposed to radiation; readings should be computed weekly.
4. Pregnant personnel should avoid all exposure to radiation.
5. Personnel holding x-ray cassettes during radiography should wear lead gloves in addition to a lead apron.

INFECTION CONTROL

Acquired immune deficiency syndrome (AIDS), hepatitis, and pyogenic infection can be transmitted by puncture wounds. Hospital procedure must be followed regarding the disposal of sharps. A needle magnet is available encased in a flat plastic compact, the lid of which can be closed for the safe disposal of its contents. A rigid plastic container is used for the disposal of needles and plastic syringes; an attached device is employed to separate the hub and shaft of the needle and break the syringe tip prior to discarding them.

All personnel should wear gloves when handling potentially contaminated articles such as soiled sponges, instruments, blood transfusion pouches, etc. that might cause infection through a break in the skin. Some authorities advocate double gloving when virulent infections are present or suspect.

Similarly, during endoscopy procedures or procedures in which drills or saws are employed, personnel may be spattered or sprayed by potentially contaminated tissue fragments, saliva, irrigation fluid, and so on, and safety goggles or glasses should be worn.

CHEMICAL HAZARDS

The National Institute of Occupational Safety and Health has established guidelines regarding safe levels of waste anesthetic gases in the operating room. The removal of waste gases in the operating room is accomplished with scavenging systems that require careful maintenance. By employing well-maintained scavenging systems, air-conditioning systems (using high-efficiency particulate air filters), and nitrous oxide leak detectors, the exposure to hazardous gases in the operating room can be min-imized.

Part II

ANESTHESIA

Chapter 4

GENERAL INFORMATION

Anesthesia is loss of sensation. In the operating room anesthesia is administered by a physician (anesthesiologist) or a certified registered nurse anesthetist (CRNA). In addition, local or regional anesthetics may be administered by the surgeon. In this guide, the term anesthetist will apply to the anesthesiologist as well as the CRNA.

The most common techniques used in the operating room include

1. *General anesthesia.* The patient is made unconscious.
2. *Conduction anesthesia.* Anatomic areas of the patient are anesthetized by infiltration or topical application of various agents. Nerve blocks are produced at central or peripheral sites. *Local anesthesia,* and *topical anesthesia,* are established immediately about the area to be treated.

Prior to the administration of anesthesia, premedication, as a single drug or a combination of various drugs, is often given. The purpose of the premedication is to allay anxiety, to help the patient relax, and to diminish secretions. Premedication is usually given by intramuscular injection about 30 to 60 minutes before surgery. In emergency surgery premedication may be given intravenously or may be omitted. These drugs are selected according to the patient's general condition and the extent and nature of the surgery to be performed. Outpatients or surgicenter patients are given less premedication or none at all.

Specialized equipment is required to implement anesthesia. For general anesthesia an anesthesia machine delivers an anesthetic gas mixture to the patient at a specific rate and concentration as determined by the anesthetist. The most simple machine might consist of a cart with attached tanks of nitrous oxide (or other agent) and oxygen with flow meters and pressure gauges. Usually expired "air" from the patient passes through a carbon dioxide absorbing tank or cartridge. In the modern operating room a very sophisticated machine able to store and deliver several compressed gaseous and highly volatile liquid anesthetic agents is employed. In addition, the compact anesthesia cart contains a variety of monitoring devices, oxygen depletion alarm, and special equipment that includes masks, laryngoscopes with interchangeable blades, McGill forceps, endotracheal tubes and obturators, etc. as well as a source of suction. An additional cart of drawers is required for drugs and supplies. Equipment and prepackaged kits for various procedures (e.g., insertion of arterial and central venous catheters) must be stored nearby. A variety of intravenous fluids, administration sets, and stands for these items must be provided.

The role of the circulator with respect to anesthesia is to provide an "extra hand" for the anesthetist. In some institutions an anesthesia technologist may perform this role. Prior to the induction of anesthesia the circulator is responsible for maintaining the patient's immediate safety, allaying anxiety, and being attentive to special needs of the patient.

GENERAL ANESTHESIA

For the administration of general anesthesia, the patient is initially in the supine position. An intravenous line is inserted, an (automatic) blood pressure cuff and sensor, and electrocardiograph (ECG) monitoring electrodes are placed. Induction is usually begun by injecting a rapidly acting intravenous agent (e.g., thiopental (Pentothal) or methohexital (Brevital)). As the patient loses consciousness oxygen and gaseous agents are gradually introduced by mask. If an endotracheal tube is to be inserted (transnasally or transorally) a fast-acting muscle relaxant, succinylcholine (or curare-like drug), is given after which the endotracheal tube is inserted under direct vision with the aid of a laryngoscope and McGill forceps, if needed. Several milliliters of lidocaine 4% solution may be instilled into the larynx prior to placing the endotracheal tube, which has been lubricated with anesthetic ointment. The tube is inflated and secured with tape, monitoring devices are attached, and the patient's position changed as necessary. The circulator may be required to assist the anesthetist by providing easy access to the equipment, giving additional premeasured drugs, manipulating the trachea, etc. at the instruction of the anesthetist. A wide variety of drugs and inhalation agents are available; see Table 4–1.

CONDUCTION ANESTHESIA

A *central block* refers to spinal, epidural, or caudal anesthesia. Appropriate supplies for their administration are available in most hospitals in disposable prepackaged trays. Additional drugs may be requested. If a longer procedure is contemplated, or postoperative analgesia is to be prolonged, a catheter is placed by the anesthetist to

TABLE 4–1. General Anesthetics

Agent	Route of Administration	Form	Comments
Nitrous oxide	Inhalation	Compressed gas	Most commonly used; not used alone for deep anesthesia; used to potentiate the effects of other agents
Thiopental (Pentothal)	Intravenous	Stable liquid	Rapid induction; short duration; respiratory depressant; can cause laryngospasm and hypotension
Methohexital (Brevital)	Intravenous	Stable liquid	Rapid; ultra-short-acting; for induction, occasionally for maintenance; fast recovery; hiccoughs
Halothane (Fluothane)	Inhalation	Volatile liquid	Slow, smooth induction; maintenance; may cause bradycardia; increased sensitivity if used with epinephrine; good with burn patients and children; may cause liver damage
Enflurane (Ethrane)	Inhalation	Volatile liquid	Rapid induction; occasionally used for maintenance; rapid recovery; may cause hypotension; may cause convulsions in children
Isoflurane (Forane)	Inhalation	Volatile liquid	Maintenance; good muscular relaxation; cardiovascular stability, useful in cardiac patients
Ketamine (Ketaject, Ketalar)	Intravenous; intramuscular	Stable liquid	Induction; short-acting anesthetic; long-acting analgesic; good

TABLE 4-1. General Anesthetics (Continued)

Agent	Route of Administration	Form	Comments
			for children; may cause hallucinations if given in larger doses

deliver increments of anesthetic agent, as in continuous epidural or continuous caudal anesthesia. Postoperatively, morphine (Duramorph) specially prepared for this purpose may be similarly injected for pain relief. For these blocks the patient, with intravenous line already established, is positioned by the anesthetist; the circulator helps the patient maintain this position while the block is administered. When an anesthetic catheter is placed it must be secured with tape. The patient may then be placed in a temporary position to allow the block to take effect, or moved to the position of surgery at the direction of the anesthetist. A central block can be supplemented by heavy sedation. Oxygen and inhalation anesthetics may be administered by mask.

There are numerous types of *regional blocks*. Often, the surgeon will administer these anesthetics. Examples include brachial plexus blocks, retrograde intravenous blocks (for surgery upon the extremities), pudendal blocks (for gynecologic surgery), perianal blocks (for anorectal surgery), and "field" blocks (as for inguinal hernia repair). These blocks may be supplemented by heavy sedation or inhalation anesthetics.

Local anesthesia

Local anesthesia is frequently used for lesser procedures, and many plastic surgeries, ophthalmic procedures, anorectal procedures, etc; the surgeon administers the anesthetic. With few exceptions an intravenous line is inserted. When "anesthesia standby" is requested, the anesthetist will monitor the patient and administer supplemental sedation or even general anesthesia as required.

TABLE 4–2. Commonly Used Conduction Anesthetics*

Method of Adminis-tration	Agent	Concen-tration/ Dose	Comments
Spinal	Lidocaine (Xylocaine)	5%	Rapid onset; shorter acting
Spinal	Bupivacaine (Marcaine, Sensor-caine)	0.75%	Longer acting; longer lasting analgesia after return of sensation
Spinal	Tetracaine (Ponto-caine)	0.5–1.0%/ 5–12 mg	Rapid onset; longer with higher dosage and/or added ephedrine or epinephrine
Epidural/ Caudal	Lidocaine (Xylocaine)	1–2%/ 500 mg	Rapid onset; shorter duration
Epidural/ Caudal	Bupivacaine (Marcaine, Sensor-caine)	0.25–0.75%/ 150 mg	Longer acting; obstetrics
Nerve block (regional)	Lidocaine (Xylocaine)	1–2%/ 500 mg	Rapid onset
		0.33%/ 100–150 mg	Retrograde intravenous block
Nerve block (regional)	Bupivacaine (Marcaine, Sensor-caine)	0.25–0.5%	Long acting
Local	Lidocaine (Xylocaine)	0.5–2.0%/ 500 mg	Commonly used
Local	Bupivacaine (Marcaine, Sensor-caine)	0.25–5.0%/ 300 mg	Long acting; may result in less need for analgesics postoperatively
Topical	Lidocaine (Xylocaine)	2–4%/ 200 mg	Low toxicity; short acting
	Liquid Jelly Ointment	2%/ 15–30 ml 4%/15 ml	Cystoscopy; other endoscopies

TABLE 4–2. Commonly Used Conduction Anesthetics* *(Continued)*

Method of Adminis- tration	Agent	Concen- tration/ Dose	Comments
Topical	Cocaine	2–10%/ 200 mg	High potency; rapid absorption through mucous membranes
Topical	Tetracaine (Ponto- caine)	0.5%/drops	Ophthalmic use; rapid onset

*All conduction anesthetic agents when administered in greater than recommended dosages or if accidentally given intravenously (or by idiosyncratic reaction) may cause extreme agitation, convulsions, cardiac arrest, and death. Resuscitative equipment and drugs must be immediately available whenever these agents are employed.

The preceding chart lists only several of the most commonly used anesthetic agents primarily for adult patients. Additional agents are employed particularly for pediatric surgeries. Numerous ancillary drugs including muscle relaxants, tranquilizers, narcotics, and amnestic agents likewise have not been listed since use of these agents varies widely between anesthetists and institutions.

When an anesthetist is not present the circulator will insert an intravenous line (as per hospital policy), place ECG electrodes, monitor the patient's vital signs, blood pressure, and ECG, and administer supplementary drugs at the direction of the surgeon. The circulator also completes the anesthetic record including documenting the times of the beginning and the termination of the procedure, vital signs and blood pressure at appropriate intervals, and the times and amounts of anesthetic agents or any other drugs administered.

Topical anesthesia

Topical anesthesia is the direct application of anesthetic agent such as a liquid solution, eyedrops, jelly, ointment, and/or spray to the site of the surgery; see Table 4–2. Local or general anesthesia may be required to supplement these anesthetics.

The preceding charts list only several of the more commonly employed agents for adult patients. Numerous other agents can be used including those reserved for pediatric patients. In addition, a wide array of ancillary agents including muscle relaxants, tranquilizers, narcotics, amnestic agents, etc. have not been listed because their use varies widely between anesthetists and institutions.

On completion of the surgical procedure and placement of dressings, etc. the circulator accompanies the patient to the recovery room. While the patient is repositioned (as necessary) for movement onto the gurney (or special bed or frame), intravascular lines, urinary catheter, splinted extremities, etc. are protected. The security of the airway is the responsibility of the anesthetist. When the patient has been expeditously transported to the recovery room the anesthesia and operative records, special appliances, etc. are given to the recovery room nurse. The circulator reports to the recovery room nurse any significant intraoperative events such as a severe fluctuation in cardiovascular or pulmonary functions, any untoward reaction to drugs, and/or the need for multiple transfusions or special medications. The chart may be temporarily retained by the surgeon to complete operative notes, postoperative orders, or dictation. If the chart is not immediately available, the circulator will advise the recovery room nurse of any postoperative orders requiring immediate attention such as the application of an ice pack or the connection of drainage systems to a suction source. etc. When the anesthetist is satisfied that the patient has been transferred safely, the operating room personnel resume their other assignments.

Chapter 5

GENERAL ANESTHESIA

Definition

Administration of agents by intravenous injection or inhalation that render the patient unconscious or extremely obtunded; intramuscular injection and rectal installation are rarely used.

Discussion

This anesthetic method is commonly employed. The depth and duration of the anesthetic is regulated by type and amount of agent(s) given. In addition to numerous intravenous and inhalation anesthetics, a large number of other agents including muscle relaxants, tranquilizers, and narcotics are employed. Rarely is a single drug used, but for limited procedures a single agent (e.g., ketamine) may be employed. During all general anesthetics the patient must be well oxygenated and the patency of the airway maintained. The anesthetist must also support the patient's cardiovascular system and other vital functions.

Preparation of the patient

The patient is supine with safety strap in place. Following induction the airway is maintained by insertion of an endotracheal tube if the patient's position for surgery is other than supine or lithotomy, for a prolonged procedure in the supine position, for surgeries that affect respiration, or when profound muscular relaxation is needed. A variety of types and sizes of these tubes are available. Most often the endotracheal tube is placed transorally, but may also be inserted transnasally or via an established tracheostomy. Prior to any change from the supine position, the anesthetist must state that the airway is secure, and will then control the airway and protect the head and neck as the patient is repositioned. The patient's eyes are protected by instillation of ophthalmic ointment and/or taping the lids. For positions other than supine, refer to specific surgeries.

Draping

None

Equipment

As selected by the anesthetist according to the needs of the individual patient. May include
Suction source, preferably a separate unit
Laryngoscope and blades
Suction catheters
Yankauer suction tip (or as requested); McGill forceps
Face mask, head strap, variety of endotracheal tubes (with obturator), oral and nasal airways, connectors for masks or endotracheal tubes, sterile anesthetic lubricant (for the endotracheal tube and obturator), syringes (to inflate the tube cuff), tongue blades, topic anesthetic for instillation into the larynx (e.g., LTA kit), ordinary and esophageal stethoscopes, etc.
Monitoring devices for blood pressure and pulse, electrocardiogram, oxygen and carbon dioxide monitors, oxygen alarm
Ordinary intravenous (IV) line, central venous and arterial lines and the trays to insert them, and appropriate gauges

Ether screen, IV standards, drape clips, padded
    armboards, etc.
Nasogastric tubes, etc. (as requested)

Special notes

Induction is facilitated by a quiet atmosphere.
Circulator stands at the head of the table particularly during endotracheal intubation, to assist in patient care measures such as manipulating the trachea (thereby enabling the anesthetist to better visualize the glottis) and injecting premeasured intravenous drugs.
Suction should be ready at all times.

Chapter 6

CONDUCTION ANESTHESIA

SPINAL, EPIDURAL, CAUDAL

Definition

Central nerve blocks performed by injecting anesthetic solutions intrathecally (into the subarachnoid space), into the epidural space, or into the caudal canal.

Discussion

These anesthetics are employed for procedures on the lower abdomen and lower extremities. The composition and concentration of the anesthetic solution will determine the duration of the block. The position of the patient immediately following the injection of the anesthetic solution influences the level and distribution of the block.

Preparation of the patient

Position of the patient is determined by type of block being administered, procedure being performed, condition of the patient, and the preference of the anesthetist. Position may be sitting, lateral, or prone.

Sitting: With back arched and feet supported on a stool (spinal or epidural)

Lateral: With knees, hips, back, and neck flexed (spinal or epidural)

Prone: Flexed at the waist (caudal or hypobaric spinal)

Following the injection of the agent (after an interval determined by anesthetist) the patient is placed in the selected operative position.

For prolonged procedures or for postoperative analgesia, continuous epidural or caudal anesthesia is established by inserting a catheter into the appropriate space at the time of the initial needle placement. Increments of anesthetic solution may then be administered.

Skin preparation and draping

Usually performed by the anesthetist. These materials may be included in the prepackaged disposable tray.

Equipment

Stool (for patient's feet, sitting position)
Sitting stool (for anesthetist)

Supplies

Appropriate sterile disposable tray (spinal, epidural, caudal)
Additional agents, needles, catheters, etc. (as requested)

Special notes

Circulator may be requested to set up intravenous line.

Circulator is usually requested to assist in maintaining the patient's position during administration of the block.

Adhesive tape secures intravenous line and anesthetic catheter.

Do not dispose of the tray items until the anesthetist has the appropriate information needed for the anesthetic record.

The patient, although often sedated, may be alert enough to hear; therefore, discussion of the diagnosis, other medical information, and idle conversation should be limited accordingly.

Patient privacy should always be maintained.

REGIONAL, LOCAL, TOPICAL

Definition

Application of an anesthetic agent that may be either injected around a peripheral nerve trunk, adjacent to or directly into the surgical site, or applied directly to the surface to be treated.

Discussion

Regional nerve block (e.g., brachial plexus block, ankle block) is achieved by depositing an agent immediately adjacent to a larger peripheral nerve(s). This anesthetic is used primarily for surgery upon the extremities. Intercostal nerve block or field block is used in limited abdominal surgery (e.g., gastrostomy, inguinal herniorrhaphy).

Local anesthesia refers to the injection of anesthetic agent into or adjacent to the site of surgery so that smaller nerves are directly anesthetized.

In *topical anesthesia* the anesthetic agent is absorbed through the tissue (usually mucous membrane) to anesthetize the area immediately beneath (e.g., ophthalmic, gingival) or to anesthetize a larger nerve trunk that lies close to the surface (e.g., glossopharyngeal nerve block).

These modalities may be used in combination or conjunction with general anesthesia or heavy sedation. Hyaluronidase (Wydase) may be added to the injectable agent to promote more rapid spread and more rapid resolution of the local edema related to the injection. Epinephrine (Adrenalin) added to the anesthetic solution will prolong its effect.

Preparation of the patient

The patient is positioned to expose the site of the proposed injection or application. In local or topical anesthesia this site is often identical to the site of the surgery, whereas in regional anesthesia the site may be remote from that of surgery.

Skin preparation

Regional: Performed by the anesthetist or surgeon; when the block is established the surgical site is prepared in the usual fashion.

Local: Skin preparation for the injection and the surgery is usually the same.

Topical: Usually none required.

Supplies

Skin preparation tray (regional or local)
Needles and syringes (regional or local)
Medicine cup (for anesthetic agent)
Sponges
Anesthetic agent(s)

Special notes

Circulator may be responsible for insertion of an intravenous line.

Determine type of anesthesia and required supplies prior to bringing patient into the operating room.

Be aware of special needs (e.g., use of two tourniquets, or double-cuff tourniquet) or retrograde intravenous block.

The patient, although often sedated, may be alert enough to hear; therefore, discussion of the diagnosis, other medical information, and idle conversation should be limited accordingly.

Observe measures to maintain patient's privacy.

Part III

SURGICAL PROCEDURES

Operative procedures as in all medical treatments are performed to provide correction of a problem, yet rendering as little harm to the patient as possible. With few exceptions, the paramount need is for exposure or ability to visualize the operative field while preserving the patient's capacity to heal.

An appropriately placed, carefully performed incision provides the exposure necessary for the execution of a safe and rapid definitive surgical procedure. If possible, an incision is made to avoid entry into an area of scar tissue (from a previous surgery) or local disease process in order to prevent injury to an adherent underlying structure (e.g., vessel or intestine). By employing traction and countertraction, the surgeon protects uninvolved structures.

A protocol has been developed in the performance of skin (and certain mucosal) incisions. A first scalpel (or "skin" knife) is used and then discarded for a second scalpel (or "deep" knife). Underlying tissues are serially incised and distracted by the use of toothed forceps, retractors, clamps, sponges, etc., until the surgical site is exposed. In each anatomic site different instruments may be employed, but this general principle is applicable. In specialized procedures utilizing endoscopes, the operating microscope, electrosurgical equipment, lasers, a plasma scalpel, ultrasound modalities, etc. the technique is altered accordingly.

In procedures when potential contamination is inherent (e.g., intestinal surgery) the wound is protected throughout. Upon closure of the incision the sterile operating team regowns and regloves, the field is redraped, and the instruments, electrosurgical pencil, etc. are replaced.

Chapter 7

NECK SURGERY

THYROIDECTOMY

Definition

Removal of all or a portion of the thyroid gland.

Discussion

The thyroid is a highly vascular gland composed of two lobes connected by a narrow bridge (isthmus). It is located on the anterior aspect of the trachea adjacent to the second, third, and fourth rings. Thyroid lobectomy is performed for the treatment of some thyroid nodules and carcinomas. Total thyroidectomy is indicated for certain carcinomas and to relieve tracheal or esophageal compression. Infrequently, a portion of the gland may be substernal necessitating a more extensive procedure.

Procedure

The incision is made above the sternal notch. The platysma muscle is incised and retracted. The strap muscles are separated or divided. Blunt and sharp dissection are employed until the thyroid is exposed. Care is taken to avoid injury to the recurrent and superior laryngeal nerves and the parathyroid gland. The gland is mobilized. All or a portion of the gland is removed. Hemostasis is obtained. The wound may be irrigated and a drain may be inserted. Incision is closed in layers by interrupted stitches.

Preparation of the patient

The patient is supine with a rolled sheet or small sandbag placed between the scapulae (extending the neck). A padded footboard is placed on the table. Table is positioned in reverse Trendelenberg. Arms may be extended on armboards. Apply electrosurgical dispersive pad.

Skin preparation

Begin at the anterior neck extending upward to just below the infra-auricular border and lower lip, and downward to 2.5 to 5 cm (1 to 2 inches) above the nipples; continue down to the table at the neck, around the shoulders, and at the sides.

Draping

Folded towels, a sterile adhesive plastic drape (optional), and a sheet with a small fenestration

Equipment

Electrosurgical unit
Suction
Footboard extension (padded) for table

Instrumentation

Thyroid tray
Limited procedure tray
Spring retractor
Right-angle clamps with fine points (2)
Lahey clamps (extra available)

Supplies

Basin set
Blades (2) No. 10, (1) No. 15
Needle magnet or counter
Suction tubing
Electrosurgical pencil
Dissectors (e.g., peanut)
Small drain (e.g., ¼" Penrose)
Fine suture (e.g., 4-0 silk to mark line of incision) or
    marking pen
Bulb syringe

Special notes

A fine silk suture may be pressed against the neck to mark the line for incision.

Usually straight Crile or mosquito clamps are used. Have extra clamps on hand, for the surgeon may prefer to clamp and cut many times before ligating.

The dressing is secured by a "thyroid collar" (e.g., Queen Anne's dressing). After the wound is dressed in the usual manner, a collar is made with a towel folded in thirds lengthwise. The towel is wrapped around the neck and the ends of the collar are crossed and secured by adhesive tape.

The scrub person should keep the back table sterile until the patient is extubated, breathing satisfactorily, and taken from the room (i.e., prepared for tracheostomy if airway becomes compromised).

In many institutions a tracheostomy tray accompanies the patient to the recovery room, and later to the patient's room until any consideration of airway obstruction secondary to edema or hematoma has passed.

PARATHYROIDECTOMY

Definition

Removal of one or more of the four parathyroid glands located behind the thyroid gland.

Discussion

Parathyroidectomy is performed to excise adenomas, carcinomas, and hyperplasia; only normal or atrophic glands are left intact. Removal of all parathyroid tissue results in tetany and death.

Procedure

See approach for Thyroidectomy, p. 43. Thyroid gland is mobilized. Parathyroid glands are identified and resected as indicated. Some parathyroid tissue (amount is controversial) is left intact. Hemostasis is achieved, the wound may be irrigated, and a drain may be inserted. The incision is closed in layers by interrupted stitches.

Preparation of the patient, Skin preparation, Draping, Equipment, Instrumentation, and Supplies

See Thyroidectomy, p. 43.

Special notes

As for thyroidectomy, a fine silk suture may be pressed against the neck to mark the line for the incision. A marking pen may be used instead.

Have ready several pathology slips and biopsy containers for the many specimens.

A special "thyroid collar" (Queen Anne's dressing) may be applied after the wound is dressed in the usual manner. A collar is made with a towel folded in thirds lengthwise. The towel is wrapped around the neck and the ends of the towel are crossed and secured by adhesive tape.

The scrub person should keep the back table sterile until the patient is extubated, breathing satisfactorily, and taken from the room (i.e., prepared for tracheostomy if airway becomes compromised).

THYROGLOSSAL DUCT CYSTECTOMY

Definition

Excision of a cyst and duct in the midline of the neck including a portion of the hyoid bone.

Discussion

The duct is an embryologic remnant extending from the foramen caecum at the base of the tongue through the hyoid bone to the thyroid gland. When a ductal sinus or cyst is present it is usually found inferior to the hyoid bone.

Procedure

An incision is made between the hyoid bone and thyroid cartilage. The platysma muscle is incised and retracted. Strap muscles are separated and divided. Sharp and blunt dissection are employed to mobilize the cyst and duct. A central portion of the hyoid bone is removed to prevent recurrence, and the cephalad portion of the duct is ligated. The specimen is excised. The wound is closed with interrupted stitches. A drain may be employed.

Preparation of the patient

The patient is supine with a folded sheet (adult), towel (child), or small sandbag placed between the scapulae to extend the neck; the shoulders are lowered (to give better exposure). Arms may be extended on armboards. Additional measures such as padded restraints on extremities may be needed for the pediatric patient. Apply electrosurgical dispersive pad.

Skin preparation, Draping, and Equipment

See Thyroidectomy, p. 43.

Instrumentation

Limited procedure tray
Minor orthopedic procedures tray
Right-angle clamps with fine points (2)

Supplies

Basin set
Blades, adults (2) No. 10, (1) No. 15; children (2) No.
   15
Suction tubing
Needle magnet or counter
Electrosurgical pencil
Dissectors (e.g., peanut)
Drain (e.g., ¼" Penrose)

Special notes

Bone cutters, rongeurs, and periosteal elevator
from Minor orthopedic procedures tray may be
needed to remove a portion of the hyoid bone.

Infrequently, the tract of the duct may be identified by injecting the duct with a solution of methylene blue.

Chapter 8

BREAST PROCEDURES

BREAST BIOPSY

Definition

Removal of tissue to determine the nature of a breast lesion.

Discussion

Frozen section can be performed on the specimen immediately, if indicated.

Procedure

The incision is generally made over the lesion. For central lesions, a circumareolar incision may be employed. The lesion is grasped and dissected free. The specimen may be sent for frozen section. After hemostasis is obtained, a drain may be inserted. Subcuticular tissue is approximated. Skin is closed with fine subcuticular suture or fine interrupted skin stitches. A safety pin or stitch secures the drain.

Preparation of the patient

The patient is supine with arm on the affected side extended on an armboard; the other arm may be tucked in at the patient's side. Apply electrosurgical dispersive pad.

If local anesthesia is employed, see circulator responsibilities, p. 28.

Skin preparation

Use a *gentle* circular motion beginning at the lesion extending from neckline to lower ribs, including a wide margin beyond the midline and under the arm down to the table on the affected side. For lesions in the upper outer quadrant, include the axilla.

Draping

Folded towels and sheet with a small fenestration

Equipment

Electrosurgical unit

Instrumentation

Basic/Minor procedures tray

Supplies

Basin set
Blades (2) No. 15
Electrosurgical pencil
Needle magnet or counter
Small drain (e.g., ¼" Penrose)
Safety pin

Special notes

Circulator must confirm with patient the side of the lesion.

Exercise all precautions in handling excised tissue to avoid misidentification of biopsies when multiple specimens are taken.

Circulator is responsible for specimen being sent to laboratory immediately for frozen section. Do *not* put specimen in formalin.

Notify pathologist if the patient is awake.

MASTECTOMY

Definition

Removal of the breast.

Partial Mastectomy. Excision of a breast tumor with appropriate tumor-free margins.

Subcutaneous Mastectomy. Removal of all breast tissue; overlying skin and nipple are left intact.

Simple Mastectomy. Removal of entire breast only.

Radical Mastectomy:

Modified Radical Mastectomy. Removal of breast and axillary lymph nodes; most frequently performed radical procedure.

Classic Radical Mastectomy. Includes the removal of the entire breast, pectoralis muscles, axillary lymph nodes, fat, fascia, and adjacent tissues. A skin graft may be necessary for skin closure. Less frequently employed, unless there is an invasion of deeper structures.

Extended Radical Mastectomy. En bloc removal of the breast, axillary contents, pectoralis muscles, and internal mammary lymph nodes. Resection of the ribs and sternum may also be included. A skin graft may be required for closure of the wound; rarely performed today.

Discussion

Partial mastectomy followed by radiation treatments is now more widely employed.

A subcutaneous mastectomy is recommended for patients with small, centrally located, noninvasive lesions including chronic cystic mastitis, gynecomastia, and for patients with a strong family history of breast cancer who require prophylactic mastectomy.

A simple mastectomy is usually reserved for patients with no lymph node involvement or for elderly or poor-risk patients who cannot tolerate a more extensive procedure.

Radical mastectomy is performed on patients with malignant lesions in which axillary fat and lymphatic tissues are excised and pectoral muscles may be removed to more widely encompass any potential tumor.

Procedure

In *partial mastectomy* the incision is usually made over the lesion. The skin is elevated and the breast mass is excised. Hemostasis is obtained. The wound may be irrigated. A drain may be inserted. Skin is closed with interrupted stitches. A safety pin or skin stitch secures the drain.

In *subcutaneous mastectomy* the incision is generally made in the inframammary fold. If the breast is small (or in male patients with gynecomastia) a circumareolar incision may be employed. The skin is elevated and all subcutaneous and connective tissues are removed with the nipple and the skin left intact. Hemostasis is obtained. The wound may be irrigated. A drain may be inserted. A prosthesis may be inserted at this time. The skin is closed.

In *modified radical mastectomy* usually a transverse or longitudinal incision is used. Skin flaps are developed and often pectoralis fascia is dissected free from underlying structures. The axillary contents are dissected free from vascular and nervous structures and are removed. Care is taken to avoid injury to the nerve supply to various muscles. After hemostasis is achieved, the skin flaps are approximated over drains or suction catheters (e.g., Hemovac). A skin graft may be required for skin closure.

In *classic radical mastectomy* additional structures including the pectoralis major and minor muscles and the intervening lymphatic and fatty tissues are excised.

Preparation of the patient

The patient is supine with arms extended on armboards; a folded sheet is under the shoulder on the affected side. Apply electrosurgical dispersive pad.

Skin preparation

Using a *gentle* circular motion begin at the lesion extending up to the neckline, and down to the umbilicus with a wide margin beyond the midline. Prepare around the shoulder, under the arm, including the axilla and arm, and down to the table on the affected side. Apply electrosurgical dispersive pad.

Draping

The patient's arm on the affected side is held up in a tube (or impervious) stockinette as a drape sheet is placed under the axilla. The field around the breast is draped with folded towels. The arm is brought through the fenestration of a laparotomy sheet.

Equipment

Electrosurgical unit
Suction

Instrumentation

Major procedures tray
Additional curved Crile clamps and large towel
    clips
Hemoclip appliers (small, medium, large)
Rake retractors (4 or 6 prong)

Supplies

Basin set
Blades, several No. 10
Electrosurgical pencil
Suction tubing
Needle magnet or counter
Tube (or impervious) stockinette
Hemoclips (small, medium, large)
Electrosurgical pencil holder, optional
Dermatome (for skin graft), e.g., Brown, and necessary supplies including:
    mineral oil, saline, tongue blades, and petrolatum impregnated gauze
Drainage unit (e.g., Hemovac)
Pressure dressing

Special notes

Circulator must confirm with patient the side of the lesion.

If mastectomy is to follow a breast biopsy, the patient is reprepared, and redraped, the team is regowned and gloved, and the instruments are changed.

Prepare gently to avoid potential of dislodging tumor cells.

Circulator will hold out the prepared arm to receive the double (or impervious) stockinette; the arm is then held by scrubbed personnel.

Check coagulation and cutting settings on the electrosurgical unit. Often a great deal of the dissection is performed with the cautery. Keep the electrosurgical pencil tip clean as necessary. The use of two electrosurgical pencils may be indicated so that a clean tip will always be available. Avoid a burn injury to the patient by protecting the electrosurgical pencil not in use by keeping it in a holder.

Several knife blade changes may be required because of the fibrous nature of the tissues incised; notify surgeon when a blade is new.

If skin graft is necessary, one thigh must be prepared and draped along with the main operative site.

Irrigation is usually water, not saline, to lessen the survival of tumor cells.

Estrogen and progesterone assays may be requested on the specimen.

Chapter 9

ABDOMINAL EXTRAINTESTINAL SURGERY

ABDOMINAL LAPAROTOMY

Definition

An opening made through the abdominal wall into the peritoneal cavity for the purpose of exploration, diagnosis, and treatment.

Procedure

The skin is incised with the "skin" knife. Subcutaneous tissue is incised with the "deep" knife or electrosurgical unit. Blood vessels may be clamped or cauterized. Fascia is incised and the underlying muscles are retracted or transsected. The surgeon grasps the peritoneum and incises it with the "deep" knife. A scissors (usually a Metzenbaum, infrequently a curved Mayo) is used to complete the peritoneal incision. The abdomen is explored. Wound edges are retracted accordingly by Deaver and/or Richardson retractors or by a self-retaining retractor (e.g., Balfour). The surgery is performed. The wound and/or peritoneal cavity may be irrigated and the irrigation fluid removed by suction. Drains may be employed, often through stab wound incisions. The peritoneum is usually closed with a continuous suture. Two toothed forceps or several Pean or Kocher clamps may be used to grasp the peritoneum to assist in its exposure. The abdomen is closed in layers, or less often, in a single layer. The skin is approximated using Adson tissue forceps and suture material or skin staples. For infected cases, skin and subcutaneous tissues may be left open and drained.

Preparation of the patient

The patient is supine; arms may be extended on armboards. Check with the surgeon regarding insertion of a urinary catheter (e.g., Foley). Apply electrosurgical dispersive pad.

Skin preparation

Determine site of incision; begin cleansing at this point. Include area from nipples to midthighs, and down to the table at the sides. For women, vaginal preparation may be indicated.

Draping

Four folded towels and a laparotomy sheet

Equipment

Suction
Electrosurgical unit

Instrumentation

Major procedures tray
Self-retaining retractor (e.g., Balfour)
Hemoclip appliers, variety (available)

Supplies

Basin set
Blades (2) No. 10, (1) No. 15
Needle magnet or counter
Suction tubing
Electrosurgical pencil
Hemoclips, variety (available)

Special notes

Once the abdomen is entered, the only free sponges used are laparotomy pads (lap pads). Some surgeons request that rings be attached to the lap pads. All x-ray-detectable 4″ × 4″ sponges must be mounted on a sponge forceps (frequently referred to as a spongestick).

Many surgeons prefer to use lap sponges lightly moistened by warm saline after the peritoneal cavity has been entered.

ABDOMINAL HERNIORRHAPHY

Definition

Repair of a musculofascial defect, through which various organs or tissues may present.

Types

Inguinal (Direct, Indirect) and Femoral. The musculofascial defect is in the groin, the herniated tissues presenting through the posterior inguinal wall medial to the deep inferior epigastric vessels (direct); or through the deep inguinal ring and inguinal canal, emerging at the superficial inguinal ring (indirect); or through the femoral canal (femoral).

Umbilical. Within the umbilicus (or about the umbilicus: paraumbilical); most often seen in children or obese adults.

Epigastric. Defect in the abdominal wall between the xiphoid process and the umbilicus through which fat protrudes.

Incisional (Ventral). A defect within the scar of a surgical incision (abdominal).

Discussion

Hernias are either reducible or irreducible, that is, incarcerated. The contents of an incarcerated hernia may become strangulated, compromising the viability of trapped tissues necessitating their resection in addition to the herniorrhaphy.

Procedures

Several techniques are employed for each of these hernia types. Usually an incision is made over the site of the defect. Blunt and sharp dissection are employed to expose the hernia sac and surrounding musculofascial defect. With incisional hernias, the peritoneal cavity may be entered. The hernia sac may be allowed to retract, be sutured over (imbricated), or excised. The musculofascial defect may be closed employing a wide variety of techniques and suture materials, and occasionally a mesh prosthesis. The subcutaneous tissue and skin are approximated.

Preparation of the patient

The patient is supine with the arm on the affected side extended on armboard. Apply electrosurgical dispersive pad. If local anesthesia is employed, see circulator responsibilities, p. 31.

Skin Preparation

Inguinal and Femoral. Begin at the incision extending from umbilicus to midthigh (including a wide margin beyond the midline), and down to the table on the sides; external genitalia are prepared last.

Umbilical. Begin at the incision extending from the nipples to upper thighs, and down to the table at the sides.

Epigastric. Begin at the incision extending from the clavicles to the upper thighs, and down to the table at the sides.

Incisional. Begin at the site of the previous incision; prepare widely enough to allow for extension of the incision.

Draping

Folded towels and a fenestrated sheet

Equipment

Electrosurgical unit

Instrumentation

Basic/Minor procedures tray
Self-retaining retractor (e.g., Adson), optional

Supplies

Basin set
Blades (2) No. 10, (1) No. 15
Needle magnet or counter
Penrose drain (small, for retraction), optional
Dissectors (e.g., peanut)
Electrosurgical pencil
Skin closure strips, optional

Special notes

The small Penrose drain (used to isolate the spermatic cord) is moistened in saline and passed on a Pean clamp.

Synthetic mesh such as Mersilene or Marlex is often used to repair recurrent hernias or large ventral defects.

CHOLECYSTECTOMY

Definition

Removal of the gallbladder.

Discussion

This procedure may be performed to treat chronic or acute cholecystitis, with or without cholelithiasis, to remove a malignancy, or to remove polyps.

Related procedures include:

Cholecystotomy. The establishment of an opening into the gallbladder to allow drainage of the organ and removal of stones. A tube (e.g., Foley, Pezzer, or Malecot) is then placed in the gallbladder to establish external drainage (cholecystostomy). This is performed when the patient cannot tolerate cholecystectomy.

Choledochoscopy. The insertion of a choledochoscope into the common bile duct in order to directly visualize stones and facilitate their extraction.

Choledochotomy. The opening of the common bile duct to remove stones. It is performed to relieve choledocholithiasis or otherwise drain an obstructed common bile duct. Drainage is usually established by placing a T-tube in the duct (choledochostomy).

Procedure

The incision is right subcostal, right paramedian, or midline. The gallbladder is grasped (generally with a Pean clamp). The cystic duct, cystic artery, and the common bile duct are exposed. The cystic artery is clamped (using two right-angle clamps) and ligated with a suture passed on a long instrument or by Hemoclips, as is the cystic duct. The gallbladder is mobilized by incising overlying peritoneum and removed. The underlying liver bed may be reperitonealized. A drain, usually a 1-inch Penrose, is inserted. The drain exits a stab wound or less often the incision. The wound is closed in layers. A safety pin or skin stitch secures the drain. The skin is closed by interrupted stitches or skin staples.

Cholangiogram. Performed prior to the ligation of the cystic duct. A catheter is passed through the stump of the cystic duct into the common bile duct. A suture or special cystic duct clamp secures the catheter. Prior to taking x-ray films, all extraneous metal clamps, retractors, etc. are removed from the field. The catheter is tested with saline for leakage and then radiopaque dye is injected. X-ray films are taken. The catheter is removed and the cystic duct is ligated.

Choledochoscopy. The common bile duct is exposed and traction sutures are placed through it. A longitudinal incision is made in the duct and a variety of stone-removing forceps, scoops, and irrigation and balloon catheters may be employed to explore for and extract stones either proximally (hepatic bile ducts) or distally (bile duct). A choledochoscope may also be employed. Further cholangiograms may then be taken. The duct is usually closed over a T-tube drain.

Preparation of the patient

The patient is supine; both arms may be extended on armboards. Some surgeons position the patient with a roll under the right upper flank, which facilitates interpretation of the cholangiogram, "separating" the biliary tree from the spine. A preliminary x-ray film may be taken to ensure correct placement of the cassette. Apply electrosurgical dispersive pad.

Skin preparation

Begin at the incision, either right subcostal (most frequently used), right paramedian, or midline; extending from the axilla to just above the pubic symphysis, and down to the table at the sides.

Draping

Folded towels and a laparotomy sheet

Equipment

Roll (for positioning)
Suction

Electrosurgical unit
X-ray cassette

Instrumentation

Major procedures tray
Long Metzenbaum scissors
Hemoclip appliers (various sizes and lengths)
Biliary tract tray (for common duct exploration)

Supplies

Basin set
Blades (1) No. 10, (1) No. 15
Hemoclips (various sizes)
Electrosurgical pencil
Needle magnet or counter
Drain (e.g., 1″ Penrose)
Dissectors (e.g., peanut)
Culture tubes (aerobic and anaerobic)

For Cholangiogram:
Catheter (surgeon's preference) and radio-
   paque dye (e.g., Hypaque or Renografin
   60)
Small basins (2) for saline and dye
Biliary tract tray
Syringes (2) 30 ml

For Choledochoscopy:
Choledochoscope
Normal saline 1000 ml
Flexible tubing (e.g., cystoscopy tubing)
Polyethylene tubing (surgeon's preference)
Arterial line pressure bag

Special notes

Correct positioning of the patient is imperative
to assure accurate visualization of the biliary tract.
   Test drains for patency.
   Drains are anchored with a skin stitch.

Instruments coming into contact with bile are isolated in a basin.

Syringes filled with saline or radiopaque dye must be labeled to avoid confusion and ensure successful x-ray exposures.

A "scout" film is taken before surgery begins.

Observe x-ray precautions, see p. 20.

Protective goggles may be worn for choledochoscopy.

DRAINAGE OF PANCREATIC CYST (PSEUDOCYST)

Definition

Internal drainage of a pseudocyst is performed by anastomosing the cyst wall to an adjacent hollow viscus (stomach, duodenum, jejunum), or less frequently, by external drainage or marsupialization.

Discussion

A pseudocyst of the pancreas is so named because this "cyst" does not have an epithelial lining as does a true cyst. These cysts develop secondary to pancreatic trauma or acute pancreatitis in which pancreatic fluid and/or blood has been encased in adhesions that later form the cyst wall. As the cyst often contains pancreatic enzymes, internal drainage is preferable to external drainage to avoid external fistula and excoriation of skin.

Procedure

A vertical or transverse incision is made. The cyst is indentified and anastomosed to an adjacent viscus. An incision is made into the anterior wall of the hollow viscus (e.g., stomach), to gain access to the posterior wall to which the anastomosis is made. Prior to suturing the cyst, the contents are aspirated to facilitate the anastomosis and to avoid spillage of pancreatic fluid into the operative field. If biliary tract disease is responsible for the pancreatitis, a concomitant biliary tract procedure is performed (e.g., cholecystectomy and/or common bile duct exploration). The abdomen is closed in layers. A drain may be used.

Preparation of the patient

The patient is supine; arms may be extended on armboards. Apply electrosurgical dispersive pad.

Skin preparation

Begin at the incision (vertical or transverse) extending from nipples to upper thighs, and down to the table at the sides.

Draping

Folded towels and a laparotomy or transverse sheet
(depending on incision)

Equipment

Electrosurgical unit
Suction

Instrumentation

Major procedures tray
Biliary tract tray
Hemoclip appliers (various sizes and lengths)

Supplies

Basin set
Electrosurgical pencil
Suction tubing
Blades (2) No. 10, (1) No. 15
Needle magnet or counter

Retention type catheter (e.g., Pezzer)
Hemoclips (small, medium, large)
Umbilical tapes
Dissectors (e.g., peanut)

Special notes

The trocar (on the Biliary tract tray) attached to suction tubing may be used to aspirate the cyst.

PANCREATICODUODENECTOMY (WHIPPLE PROCEDURE)

Definition

Removal of the head of the pancreas, the entire duodenum, the very proximal portion of the jejunum, the distal third of the stomach, and the distal half of the common bile duct, with the reestablishment of continuity of the biliary, pancreatic, and gastrointestinal tract.

Discussion

This procedure is usually performed for regional malignancy or benign, obstructive, chronic pancreatitis.

Procedure

Approach is through a transverse, midline, or paramedian incision. The operability of the findings is assessed. The distal stomach, extrahepatic biliary tract, the head of the pancreas, and the entire duodenum are mobilized. The distal stomach, the distal common bile duct, and the neck of the pancreas are resected. A total pancreatectomy, splenectomy, cholecystectomy, and vagotomy may be included. If tumor has invaded the base of the mesocolon, portal vein, aorta, vena cava, or superior mesenteric vessels, this procedure is abandoned and a lesser procedure, usually a bypass (of the biliary tree and/or stomach) will be performed. The proximal end of the jejunum is anastomosed to the distal pancreas. The common bile duct is anastomosed to the jejunum in end-to-side fashion. The distal stomach is anastomosed to the jejunum also in end-to-side fashion. Stapling devices may be used in mobilizing and transsecting multiple blood vessels and in the transsection of the stomach and the gastrojejunal anastomosis. Various plastic stents may be placed in the biliary or pancreatic anastomoses. The wound is drained. The abdomen is closed in layers.

Preparation of the patient

The patient is supine; arms may be extended on armboards. Apply electrosurgical dispersive pad.

Skin preparation

Begin at the incision (transverse, midline, or paramedian) extending from nipples to upper thighs, and down to the table at the sides.

Draping

Folded towels and a laparotomy or transverse sheet (depending on incision)

Equipment

Electrosurgical unit
Suction

Instrumentation

Major procedures tray
Biliary tract tray
Gastrointestinal procedures tray
Long instruments tray (available)
Harrington retractors
Hemoclip appliers (various sizes and lengths)
Automatic stapling device, optional

Supplies

Basin set
Electrosurgical pencil
Suction tubing
Blades (2) No. 10, (1) No. 15
Hemoclips, variety sizes
Dissectors (e.g., peanut)
Needle magnet or counter
Staples, optional
Drains, for retraction: e.g., 1" Penrose; for drainage:
    e.g., Jackson-Pratt, Hemovac
Umbilical tapes

Special notes

Verify with blood bank that number of units of blood ordered are ready and available.

Weigh sponges.

Keep accurate record of amount of irrigation used.

Scrub person may receive specimen in a basin.

Keep all soiled instruments isolated in a basin.

PANCREATECTOMY

Definition

Removal of the entire pancreas.

Discussion

Partial pancreatectomy usually refers to the removal of the tail portion of the pancreas. The extent of the procedure performed depends on the site and nature of the lesion. Indications for pancreatectomy include ductal obstruction, pancreatic stones, pancreatic cysts, trauma, benign or malignant tumors, and endocrine tumors. If total pancreatectomy is performed for benign disease or a malignancy restricted to a very distal portion of the pancreas, a small portion at the head of the pancreas may remain and be attached to the duodenum along with the common bile duct.

Procedure

A transverse, midline, or right paramedian incision is made. The abdomen is explored. If total pancreatectomy is to be performed, see Pancreaticoduodenectomy, p. 66. If only the distal portion of the pancreas is removed, the pancreas is mobilized by dissecting it from numerous vascular attachments, transsecting the gland at the appropriate point, and the proximal portion of the pancreas remaining is oversewn. The operative site is usually drained. The wound is closed in layers.

Preparation of the patient, Skin preparation, Draping, Equipment, Instrumentation, Supplies, and Special notes

See Pancreaticoduodenectomy (Whipple Procedure), p. 66.

DRAINAGE OF ABSCESS(ES) IN THE REGION OF THE LIVER

Definition

Evacuation of purulent material within a confined space in or about the liver.

Discussion

The location of the abscess is determined by sonogram, CT scan, or other x-ray study. A radiologist may aspirate and drain the abscess percutaneously. If percutaneous drainage is inadequate, open surgical drainage is performed. The abscesses are classified as left and right subdiaphragmatic, or subhepatic, and intrahepatic. Multiple abscesses may be present.

Procedure

An incision is made posteriorly along the 12th rib extraperitoneally, or anteriorly, either extraperitoneally or transperitoneally. The abscess is identified and cultures are taken. The abscess is evacuated and may be irrigated with an antibiotic solution. Drains are placed. The wound is closed in layers.

Preparation of the patient

The patient is supine; arms may be extended on armboards for an upper midline or subcostal approach. For a posterolateral approach the patient is in the lateral position with the right side uppermost. The left arm is extended on an armboard; the right arm is supported by a Mayo stand padded with a pillow (or a double armboard may be used). The left leg is extended and the right leg is flexed with a pillow between the legs and padding around the feet and ankles. Position is secured by wide adhesive tape from the shoulders, hips, and legs to the table. Apply electrosurgical dispersive pad.

Skin preparation

For a *subcostal approach* begin at the incision extending from axilla to just above the pubic symphysis, and down to the table at the sides.

For a *posterolateral approach* begin at the incision (eighth interspace) extending from the shoulder to the iliac crest and down to the table anteriorly and posteriorly.

Draping

Folded towels and a laparotomy or transverse sheet (depending on incision)

Equipment

Electrosurgical unit
Suction

Instrumentation

Major procedures tray
Long instruments tray
Biliary tract tray (available)
Harrington retractor

Supplies

Basin set
Electrosurgical pencil
Suction tubing
Blades (2) No. 10, (1) No. 15
Needle magnet or counter
Drainage materials
Culture tubes (aerobic and anaerobic)
Antibiotic irrigation, optional

Special notes

Determine position of the patient.

All instruments that come in contact with the abscess are isolated in a basin.

"Clean" closure of the abdomen requires regowning, regloving, redraping, and a Basic/Minor procedures tray.

Protect skin under adhesive tape with tincture of benzoin.

HEPATIC RESECTION

Definition

Refers to a small wedge biopsy, local excision of tumors, or a major lobectomy.

Discussion

Indications for hepatic resection include trauma, cysts, or tumors, benign (e.g., hemangioma) and malignant (e.g., primary or secondary, i.e., metastatic). A preoperative CT scan or angiogram delineates the pathology.

Procedure

The incision is determined by the section of the liver to be resected. Feasibility of resection is determined. If a thoracoabdominal incision is employed, the abdominal portion is incised first. The thoracic portion of the incision is made incising the diaphragm. Hepatic artery, portal vein, and major biliary ducts are controlled by vascular forceps or vessel loops. The liver parenchyma is divided, pausing to ligate major vascular and biliary channels. Careful technique is necessary when approaching the posterior surface where the hepatic veins enter the inferior vena cava. If bleeding is excessive the vena cava may be controlled by the insertion of balloon catheters intracavally. After hemostasis is obtained and the bile ducts are ligated, the exposed parenchyma may be covered by greater omentum or absorbable hemostatic agents. The area is drained. The abdomen is closed in layers.

Preparation of the patient

For partial left lobe excision a subcostal approach is employed; the patient is supine with arms extended on armboards. For major resection the approach is thoracoabdominal; the patient is in a modified (45°) lateral position with right side uppermost. The left arm is extended on an armboard; the right arm is supported by a Mayo stand padded with a pillow (or a double armboard may be used). The left leg is extended and the right leg is flexed with a pillow between the legs and padding around the feet and ankles. The position is secured by wide adhesive tape from the shoulders, hips, and legs to the table. Apply electrosurgical dispersive pad.

Skin preparation

For a subcostal approach begin at the incision extending from the axilla to just above the pubic symphysis, and down to the table at the sides. For a posterolateral approach begin at the incision (eighth interspace) extending from the shoulder to the iliac crest, and down to the table anteriorly and posteriorly.

Draping

Folded towels and a transverse or laparotomy sheet

Equipment

Electrosurgical unit
Suctions (2)
Hypothermia mattress (available)
Manometer (for measuring portal pressure)
Cell Saver, optional

Instrumentation

Major procedures tray
Long instruments tray
Gastrointestinal procedures tray
Biliary tract tray (available)
Thoracotomy tray (for thoracoabdominal approach)
Hemoclip appliers (various sizes and lengths)

Supplies

Basin set
Blades (3) No. 10
Electrosurgical pencil
Suction tubing
Hemoclips, various sizes
Dissectors (e.g., peanut)
Needle magnet or counter
Hemostatic agents (e.g., Helistat, Hemopad, Thrombostat, Avitene, cryoprecipitate)
Vessel loops, optional

For Thoracoabdominal Approach Add:
Chest tubes (e.g., Argyle)

Intrapleural sealed drainage unit (e.g., Pleurevac)
Y-connector
Bulb syringe

Special notes

Inquire if hypothermia mattress is necessary.

Confirm with blood bank that the number of units ordered are ready and available.

Special liver sutures are available.

Cavitron or plasma scalpel may be employed.

Weigh sponges.

Keep accurate record of the amount of irrigation used.

Protect skin under adhesive tape with tincture of benzoin.

SPLENECTOMY

Definition

Removal of the spleen.

Discussion

Most common indication for splenectomy is accidental injury; other indications include hematologic disorders, congenital anemia (splenic anemia), neutropenia, tumors, cysts, or splenomegaly, as in portal hypertension. Splenectomy may also be indicated as the result of trauma during surgery, as in gastrectomy or mobilization of the splenic flexure of the colon; an attempt is made to preserve the traumatized spleen with suture techniques and hemostatic agents. Splenectomy is avoided whenever possible to avoid the necessity for indefinite protection against pneumococcal pneumonia. Accessory spleens may be present in perisplenic tissues; rarely they are found in more removed sites.

Procedure

A midline or left subcostal incision is made. The spleen is identified and the splenic hilum is isolated, taking care not to injure the tail of the pancreas. The splenic vessels (may be multiple) are divided and ligated. The enlarged spleen may be adherent to surrounding structures including the parietal peritoneum and diaphragm. The spleen is removed. The wound may be irrigated. Hemostasis is achieved and the wound is closed in layers. If optimal hemostasis cannot be achieved or there is a question of pancreatic injury, a closed suction unit may be employed.

Preparation of the patient

The patient is supine; arms may be extended on armboards for an abdominal approach. Rarely, a thoracoabdominal approach is indicated for massive splenomegaly.

Skin preparation

Begin at the incision extending from the axilla to just above the pubic symphysis, and down to the table at the sides.

Draping

Folded towels and a laparotomy or transverse sheet
(depending on incision)

Equipment

Electrosurgical unit
Suction
Cell Saver, optional

Instrumentation

Major procedures tray
Biliary tract tray

Gastrointestinal procedures tray
Long instruments tray (available)
Harrington retractors
Hemoclip appliers (various sizes and lengths)
Automatic stapling device, optional

Supplies

Basin set
Electrosurgical pencil
Suction tubing
Blades (2) No. 10, (1) No. 15
Hemoclips, various sizes
Dissectors (e.g., peanut)
Hemostatic agents (e.g., Thrombostat, Avitene, Helistat)
Needle magnet or counter
Drains, for retraction: e.g., 1″ Penrose for drainage: e.g., Jackson-Pratt or Hemovac
Umbilical tapes
Staples, optional

Special notes

Verify with blood bank that the number of units of blood ordered are ready and available.

Weigh sponges.

Keep accurate record of amount of irrigation used.

Scrub person may receive specimen in a basin.

Chapter 10

GASTROINTESTINAL SURGERY

ESOPHAGOSCOPY

Definition

Endoscopic visualization of the esophagus.

Discussion

Esophagoscopy is performed to diagnose malignancies, esophagitis, hiatal hernia, strictures, and varices; to remove tissues or secretions for study; for direct therapeutic manipulations such as removal of a foreign body, injection or coagulation of varices, or insertion of a plastic prosthesis to relieve strictures. Flexible fiberoptic esophagoscopy is most often performed in the gastrointestinal (GI) laboratory.

n applies topical anesthesia (usually
ead of the table is lowered. The pa-
ld by an assistant and it is raised or
ndoscopist directs until the esopha-

goscope is passed (the neck will be extended). The entire esophagus including the esophagogastric junction and proximal stomach may be examined. Manipulations for diagnosis and treatment are performed. The scope is removed.

Preparation of the patient

The patient is supine with shoulders even with or a little over the break at the head of the table to permit lowering of the head. Anesthesia is usually topical with sedation and/or analgesia administered intravenously by the anesthetist. See Bronchoscopy, p. 203 for topical anesthesia tray.

Draping

Patient may be covered with a drape sheet. A drape sheet covers the back table.

Skin preparation

None.

Equipment

Fiberoptic light source
Suction

Instrumentation

Fiberoptic esophagoscope, suction, biopsy forceps, sponge carriers, grasping forceps, dilators, and bougies
Fiberoptic light cord

Supplies

Small basin (with saline and syringe)
Lubricating jelly
Bronchoscopy sponges (on carrier)
Aspirating tubes (e.g., Lukens)
Specimen containers

Needle, e.g., 25 gauge (to remove biopsy)
Suction tubing
Topical anesthetics (as for Bronchoscopy, p. 203)

Special notes

Check with surgeon regarding topical anesthesia.

Gloves are worn.

Protective goggles should be worn.

Pass forceps in the closed position and guide them into the scope as requested.

Remove specimens from forceps with a needle to avoid damaging cells.

Hold aspirating tubes upright and pinch off suction tubing as necessary to prevent aspiration of specimen.

Careful labeling and handling of specimens is essential. (Have several labels and requisitions ready.)

GASTROSCOPY

Definition

Endoscopic visualization of the stomach and proximal duodenum.

Discussion

Gastroscopy is performed for diagnosis, aspiration of gastric contents, removal of a foreign body, or tissue biopsy. Flexible fiberoptic gastroscopy is usually performed in the gastrointestinal (GI) laboratory or at the patient's bedside. For percutaneous gastrostomy, which is aided by the passage of a fiberoptic gastroscope, see Gastrostomy, p. 86.

Preparation of the patient, Skin preparation, and Draping

See Esophagoscopy, p. 77.

Equipment

Electrosurgical unit
Fiberoptic light source
Suction

Instrumentation

Rigid fiberoptic gastroscope, suction-electrocoagu-
    lator and cord, biopsy forceps, grasping forceps,
    cautery
Fiberoptic light cord

Supplies

Small basin (with saline and syringe)
Lubricating jelly
Needle, e.g., 25 gauge (for specimen removal)
Specimen containers
Aspirating tubes
Suction tubing
Topical anesthetics (as for Bronchoscopy, see p. 203)

Special Notes

See Esophagoscopy, p. 77.

COLONOSCOPY

Definition

Endoscopic visualization of the large intestine from
rectum to cecum (and occasionally the very terminal ileum).

Discussion

Total colonoscopy is usually performed in the gastrointestinal (GI) laboratory or the radiology department. Exceptions to this include colonoscopy performed during open laparotomy or certain pediatric

examinations when general anesthesia is required. Colonoscopy limited to the distal colon may be performed in the operating room by inserting only a portion of the colonoscope or by employing a flexible fiberoptic sigmoidoscope. See Sigmoidoscopy, below, for Procedure, Preparation of the patient, Skin preparation, Draping, Equipment, Instrumentation, and Supplies.

SIGMOIDOSCOPY

Definition

Endoscopic visualization of the anal canal, rectum, and sigmoid colon.

Discussion

The procedure is performed for diagnosis, excision of polyps, biopsy of lesions, etc. Sigmoidoscopy is performed in the operating room under sedation or anesthesia when the patient is unable to tolerate the procedure because of pain and tenderness, or for biopsy, polypectomy, etc. when these procedures are too risky outside the operating room environment.

Procedure

Rigid Sigmoidoscopy. The anus is digitally lubricated and examined. Anoscopy may be performed. The sigmoidoscope is inserted and advanced under direct visualization until obstructed by an unyielding angulation of the lumen or to the full length of the scope. Definitive inspection of the mucous membrane is done as the scope is withdrawn. Air may be insufflated to distend the lumen for better visualization. A variety of instruments may be used via the scope, for example, biopsy forceps, suction-electrocoagulator, snare, clip applicator, etc. Scopes are usually 18 to 19 mm in diameter; larger diameters to 30 mm may be employed when anesthesia is given.

Flexible Sigmoidoscopy. Digital examination and anoscopy are performed. The tip of the scope is inserted and under direct visualization the scope is advanced by various torquing and advancement motions to the length of the scope (30 or 65 cm) or until resistance, patient discomfort, or inability to see the lumen ahead is reached. Definitive examination is done on withdrawal. Various accessory instruments (e.g., electrosurgical biopsy forceps, snare, cytology brush, irrigating tube) may be employed.

Preparation of the patient

Positions for rigid sigmoidoscopy include jackknife, modified lateral/Sims', or lithotomy. The modified lateral/Sims' position is generally preferred for flexible sigmoidoscopy, although the jackknife position may be employed. Apply electrosurgical dispersive pad.

Jackknife. The table is flexed and the patient is prone with arms extended on armboards angled toward the head of the table with the hands pronated, a pillow is placed in front of the legs, and a roll is placed at the ankles. Buttocks are distracted by 3-inch or 4-inch adhesive tapes anchored to the underside of the table (pull tapes toward patient's head before anchoring them for maximal exposure) when surgery (e.g., hemorrhoidectomy) is performed. When general anesthesia is employed, chest rolls are required.

Lithotomy. The patient's legs are placed in stirrups and the buttocks are elevated by a folded towel. Buttocks may be distracted by 3-inch or 4-inch adhesive tapes anchored to the stirrups.

Modified Lateral/Sims'. The patient lies on the left side with left arm extended on an armboard and the right arm flexed over it on a pillow (or a double armboard may be used). The back is angled so that the anal area extends just over the table's edge. The left leg is straight and the right leg is flexed, or both legs may be flexed with a pillow between the knees; additional padding is required at the feet and ankles. Buttocks are distracted by a 3-inch or 4-inch adhesive tape on the right buttock (uppermost) anchored to the underside of the table.

Skin preparation

None.

Draping

Patient may be covered with a drape sheet. A drape sheet covers the back table.

Equipment

Stirrups or pillow and rolls for positioning
Double armboard, optional

Rigid:
Fiberoptic light source
Suction
Electrosurgical unit

Flexible:
Fiberoptic light source with a combined air insufflation and irrigation capacities
Suction (connects directly to the channel of the scope)
Electrosurgical unit

Rigid:
Sigmoidoscopy tray, suction-electrocoagulator and cord, biopsy forceps, snare, clip applicators, grasping forceps

Flexible:

Flexible sigmoidoscope, electrosurgical biopsy forceps, suction, endoscopy snare, polyp grasper, irrigating tube, cytology brush

Supplies

Gloves
Lubricant
Suction tubing
Long cotton swabs

Special notes

Protect skin under adhesive tape with tincture of benzoin.

Adequate padding is required for female breasts and male genitalia.

Gloves are worn.

Protective goggles should be worn.

Lubricate scope.

Clean scope immediately following use.

Rigid:

Assist surgeon by guiding suction, forceps, etc. into scope, and remove biopsy tissue as necessary.

Flexible:

Be prepared to help stabilize scope. Assist surgeon by passing biopsy forceps, endoscopic snare, polyp grasper, etc. as necessary.

The surgeon may direct the scrub person to open and close the endoscopy snare and biopsy forceps.

VAGOTOMY AND PYLOROPLASTY

Definition

Vagotomy. The transection of the vagus nerves (or peripheral divisions) performed at the level of the distal esophagus, or at the gastric cardia, to reduce gastric secretion in patients with peptic ulcers.

Pyloroplasty. The enlargement of the gastric outlet, which will enhance emptying of the stomach.

Discussion

Vagotomy may be truncal or selective. In truncal vagotomy the main trunks of the vagus nerve are interrupted, including branches to the stomach and other abdominal viscera. Selective vagotomy (of which there are several modifications) is performed about the gastric cardia, so that primarily gastric vagal nerves are interrupted. Pyloroplasty is performed in conjunction with vagotomy to enhance gastric emptying, which is otherwise delayed when vagus nerves have been transsected.

Procedure

The upper abdomen is exposed through a midline, paramedian, or high transverse incision. Physical findings are assessed and either truncal or selective vagotomy is performed. Hemoclips are applied to the severed nerve trunks. Small sections of vagus nerve are sent to the pathology laboratory to confirm that neural tissue was actually divided. Pyloroplasty is then performed. The most commonly performed procedure is the Heineke-Mikulicz, in which the pyloroduodenal junction is incised longitudinally and closed transversely. In patients with severe bleeding a gastrotomy or duodenotomy may be necessary to identify and control the bleeding site.

Preparation of the patient

The patient is supine; arms may be extended on armboards. Apply electrosurgical dispersive pad.

Skin preparation

Begin at the midline extending from the axilla to the pubic symphysis, and down to the table at the sides.

Draping

Folded towels and a laparotomy or transverse sheet

Equipment

Electrosurgical unit
Suction

Instrumentation

Major procedures tray
Long instruments tray
Gastrointestinal procedures tray
Blunt nerve hook (e.g., Smithwick)
Hemoclip appliers (various sizes and lengths, especially long)

Supplies

Basin set
Blades (3) No. 10, (1) No. 15
Needle magnet or counter
Suction tubing
Electrosurgical pencil
Penrose drains (2) long, 1" (for traction on esophagus)
Hemoclips, assorted sizes

Special notes

Left and right vagus nerve specimens must be kept separate and labeled accurately.

GASTROSTOMY

Definition

Establishment of an artificial opening into the stomach exiting onto the skin of the abdominal wall.

Discussion

A gastrostomy, either temporary or permanent, is used to drain the stomach or allow for liquid feedings for patients with esophageal stricture or tumor. A catheter (e.g., Foley) maintains the patency of the gastrostomy tract. Recently, *percutaneous gastrostomy*, a nonoperative method, has been employed. A flexible fiberoptic gastroscope is passed into the stomach, which is distended with air. The lighted tip of the scope is impacted on the gastric wall. A second operator passes a catheter through a percutaneous stab wound aiming at the transilluminated gastroscope tip. Gastrostomy is often performed as an adjunct to a more extensive procedure. In a debilitated patient gastrostomy may be performed under local anesthesia.

Procedure

A gastrostomy (feeding) as an isolated procedure is performed through a limited transverse left upper abdominal incision. The peritoneal cavity is entered, the gastric wall is identified, and concentric pursestring sutures are placed. A small incision is made into the stomach (within the innermost pursestring suture) through which a catheter is passed. The pursestring sutures are secured. The catheter can exit through the incision or preferably a separate stab wound. The gastric wall is sutured at a few points to the peritoneal surface of the stab wound. The abdomen is closed in layers.

Preparation of the patient

The patient is supine; arms may be extended on armboards. Apply electrosurgical dispersive pad.

Skin preparation

Begin at the incision (usually transverse left upper abdominal) extending from nipples to upper thighs, and down to the table at the sides.

Draping

Folded towels and a transverse sheet

Equipment

Suction
Electrosurgical unit

Instrumentation

Major procedures tray
Hemoclip appliers

Supplies

Basin set
Blades (2) No. 10, (1) No. 15
Needle magnet or counter
Gastrostomy catheter (e.g., Foley, Pezzer)
Electrosurgical pencil
Suction tubing
Hemoclips, assorted
Catheter plug

Special notes

Have suction ready as soon as the incision into
the stomach is made.

GASTRECTOMY

Definition

Removal of the stomach and reestablishment of the
continuity of the gastrointestinal tract.

Discussion

Subtotal (partial) gastrectomy refers to the excision
of a portion of the stomach performed primarily for
peptic ulcer disease or tumor of the distal stomach.

A vagotomy (see p. 84) may be included. Gastrointestinal continuity is reestablished by anastomosing of the gastric remnant to the proximal duodenum (Billroth I) or to the proximal jejunum (Billroth II, or a modification of it).When treating malignancies, the greater omentum, lymph nodes, and adjacent organs (e.g., spleen) are removed.

Total gastrectomy is often performed because of malignancy or uncontrollable bleeding. Continuity of the gastrointestinal tract is established by anastomosing the distal esophagus to the proximal jejunum, usually with the creation of a pouch or reservoir. (The duodenum or an isolated segment of colon can also replace the resected stomach.) The lymph nodes, adjacent organs, and greater omentum are removed when treating malignancies.

Procedure

The incision may be upper midline or bilateral subcostal. For total gastrectomy a thoracoabdominal incision may be necessary. The pathology is identified and its operability assessed. The stomach is mobilized by clamping and dividing the vascular attachments. The greater omentum, and sometimes the spleen, are resected in continuity with the stomach en bloc when malignancy is present. According to the extent of the resection and the type of anastomosis to be fashioned, the duodenum or jejunum is mobilized and anastomosed to the gastric remnant (or distal esophagus) anterior or posterior to the transverse colon. A retrocolic anastomosis requires an incision to be made in a relatively avascular portion of the transverse mesocolon. Anastomosis is facilitated by the use of automatic stapling devices, or a wide variety of sutures and suturing techniques may be employed. A side-to-side jejunal pouch may be required when total gastrectomy is performed. A drain (e.g., Jackson-Pratt or Hemovac) is inserted. If pleural space has been entered, an intrapleural sealed drainage unit (e.g., Pleurevac) is necessary. The wound is closed in layers. Drains are anchored.

Preparation of the patient

For an upper midline or bilateral subcostal approach the patient is supine. For a thoracoabdominal approach the patient is in a modified (45°) lateral/Sims' position with the left side uppermost. The right arm is on an armboard; the left arm is supported by a Mayo stand padded with a pillow (or a double armboard may be used). The right leg is extended and the left leg is flexed with a pillow between the legs, and padding around the feet and ankles. A pillow folded longitudinally may be necessary to support the back. The position is secured by wide adhesive tape from the shoulders, hips, and legs to the table. Apply electrosurgical dispersive pad.

Skin preparation

For an upper midline or bilateral subcostal approach begin at the incision extending from the axilla to just above the pubic symphysis, and down to the table at the sides. For a thoracoabdominal approach begin at the incision extending from the shoulder to the iliac crest, and down to the table anteriorly and posteriorly.

Draping

Folded towels and a transverse or laparotomy sheet

Equipment

Suction
Electrosurgical unit
Pillows, pads for positioning (for thoracoabdominal approach)

Instrumentation

Major procedures tray
Long instruments tray
Gastrointestinal procedures tray

Hemoclip appliers (various sizes and lengths)
Long blunt nerve hooks (2), e.g., Smithwick
Automatic stapling devices, optional
Large self-retaining retractor (e.g., Balfour)

Supplies

Blades (2) No. 10, (1) No. 15
Basin set
Needle magnet or counter
Suction tubing
Electrosurgical pencil
Hemoclips, variety
Staples, optional

For Thoracoabdominal Approach add:

Chest tubes (e.g., Argyle)
Intrapleural sealed drainage unit (e.g., Pleurevac)
Y-connector
Bulb syringe

Special Notes

Check that blood has been ordered and is available.

Weigh sponges.

Keep accurate record of irrigation fluid used.

Have rubber-shod clamps ready (prevents tissue damage to bowel).

Keep all soiled instruments isolated in a basin.

Have long, free ties ready.

Frozen section may be requested.

Surgeon may request a "clean" closure of the abdomen; this requires regowning, regloving, redraping, and a Basic/Minor procedures tray.

SMALL BOWEL RESECTION

Definition

Excision of a segment of the small intestine to remove an obstruction, a gangrenous portion of bowel, a perforation, or source of a hemorrhage, etc.; the remaining small bowel is anastomosed to a segment of more distal small bowel or colon.

Discussion

Small bowel resection is infrequently performed as an isolated procedure, as for inflammatory bowel disease, rare primary tumors, and mesenteric infarctions. More often, the small bowel is resected in the course of other procedures because of adhesive obstructive bowel disease, tumors of adjacent organs, and inflammatory processes such as diverticulitis or tubo-ovarian abscess.

Procedure

As An Isolated Procedure. An incision is made so that the entire small bowel is accessible, especially if the patient has had previous surgery and there are adhesions. The mesentery is divided ligating vascular structures; the affected segment is excised, and continuity of the bowel is restored by suturing the ends of the remaining small bowel together. An automatic stapling device may be employed or one or two layered anastomoses may be performed. The abdomen is closed in layers.

As Part of Another Procedure. Similar steps are taken leaving the resected segment attached to the adherent organ also to be resected (e.g., colon, ovary).

Preparation of the patient

The patient is supine; arms may be extended on armboards. Apply electrosurgical dispersive pad.

Skin preparation

Begin at the incision (often right paramedian) extending from nipples to upper thighs, and down to the table at the sides.

Draping

Folded towels and a laparotomy sheet

Equipment

Suction
Electrosurgical unit

Instrumentation

Major procedures tray
Long instruments tray
Gastrointestinal procedures tray
Hemoclip appliers (variety)
Self-retaining retractor (e.g., Balfour)
Automatic stapling devices, optional

Supplies

Basin set
Blades (2) No. 10, (1) No. 15
Hemoclips, assorted sizes
Electrosurgical pencil
Needle magnet or counter
Staples, optional

CUTANEOUS ILEOSTOMY

Definition

Formation of temporary or permanent opening of
the ileum, which is brought out onto the abdomen as
a stoma.

Discussion

Cutaneous ileostomy is performed to divert the fecal
stream in resection of the colon and rectum (permanent end ileostomy); to protect a distal anastomosis,
for example, ileo-anal (temporary loop ileostomy);

or to relieve inflammatory bowel disease of the colon with or without distal resection. A continent ileostomy (Koch pouch) consists of a stoma in continuity with a pouch of folded and sutured ileum that serves as a reservoir. The patient catheterizes the stoma to empty the pouch.

Procedure

The abdomen is entered, usually through a right paramedian or midline incision. A disc of skin and subcutaneous fat is excised at the ileostomy site; the anterior rectus sheath is incised and a small fragment removed. The incision is deepened into the peritoneum. The ileum is cleared of its mesentery for several centimeters, divided, and the proximal end is passed through the stoma site onto the abdominal wall. The distal end of the ileum is sutured or stapled closed. The proximal end is everted on itself and sutured circumferentially.The mesentery of the terminal ileum is sutured to the parietal peritoneum to prevent internal hernia. Alternatively, a loop ileostomy may be performed. The abdomen is closed. An ileostomy appliance is placed over the stoma.

Preparation of the patient

The patient is supine; arms may be extended on armboards. Apply electrosurgical dispersive pad.

Skin preparation

Begin at midline extending from above nipples to the upper thighs, and down to the table on the sides.

Draping

Folded towels and a laparotomy sheet

Equipment

Suction
Electrosurgical unit

Instrumentation

Major procedures tray
Long instruments tray
Gastrointestinal procedures tray
Hemoclip appliers (various sizes and lengths)
Automatic stapling device, optional

Supplies

Basin set
Blades (3) No. 10, (1) No. 15
Needle magnet or counter
Electrosurgical pencil
Suction tubing
Hemoclips, various sizes
Marking pen, optional
Staples, optional
Ileostomy appliance (e.g., Karaya Seal)

APPENDECTOMY

Definition

Excision of the appendix, usually performed to remove the acutely inflamed organ.

Discussion

An incidental appendectomy may be performed in
conjunction with other abdominal surgery.

Procedure

An incision is made in the right lower abdomen
either transversely oblique (McBurney) or vertically
for primary appendectomy. The appendix is identified and its vascular supply ligated. The appendix is
ligated, that is, the stump tied off with absorbable suture. The appendix is removed and the stump may
be inverted in the cecum, cauterized with chemicals
or electrocoagulation, or simply left alone after liga-

tion. Another technique is to devascularize the appendix and invert the entire appendix into the cecum. The wound is closed in layers except when an abscess has occurred with acute appendicitis. A drain may be placed into the abscess cavity exiting through the incision or a stab wound. Antibiotic irrigation may be used.

Preparation of the patient

The patient is supine; arms may be extended on armboards. Apply electrosurgical dispersive pad.

Skin preparation

Begin in lower right quadrant (McBurney incision is most frequently used) extending from nipples to upper thighs, and down to the table at the sides.

Draping

Folded towels and a laparotomy sheet

Equipment

Electrosurgical unit

Instrumentation

Basic/Minor procedures tray

Supplies

Basin set
Blades (3) No. 10
Needle magnet or counter
Electrosurgical pencil
Culture tube (aerobic and anaerobic)
Drain (e.g., Penrose, ¼", optional)
Antibiotic irrigation, optional

Special notes

Instruments used for amputation of the appendix are to be isolated in a basin.

There may be no skin closure of the wound if the appendix has ruptured.

COLOSTOMY

Definition

Formation of a permanent or temporary opening into the colon brought out onto the abdominal wall as a stoma.

Discussion

A colostomy is intended to be permanent or temporary. A *temporary colostomy* is performed to divert the fecal stream from the distal colon, which may be obstructed by tumor or inflammation, or requires being "put at rest" because of an anastomosis or a pouch procedure. A temporary colostomy may be created in the transverse colon or the sigmoid colon. The proximal and distal portions of the colon remain connected (loop colostomy) or separated (double barrel colostomy). In a Hartmann procedure a sigmoid colostomy is formed and the distal end of the colon is either brought out as a mucous fistula or closed and returned intraperitoneally.

A *permanent colostomy* is performed to treat malignancies of the colon; other indications include irrevocable rectal stricture, irrevocable anal incontinence, and inflammatory bowel disease. A permanent colostomy can be fashioned similar to a temporary colostomy, but most often is an end colostomy.

Procedure

The incision depends on the segment of the colon to be used, unless performed in conjunction with another procedure. The segment of colon is mobilized. The colon can be brought out through the main incision or through an adjacent site from which a disc of skin and subcutaneous tissue has been excised. The underlying rectus fascia, muscle, and peritoneal layers are incised to accommodate the colon. The appropriate segment of the colon is excised between clamps (atraumatic clamps may be used on the retained portions of bowel) or an automatic stapling device may be employed. An "end" segment or loop of colon is brought through the stoma site and (usually) sutured to the peristomal skin. In a loop colostomy a rod or bridge may be placed under the colon to avoid retraction. The wounds are closed and a colostomy pouch is applied over the stoma.

Preparation of the patient

The patient is supine; arms may be extended on armboards. Apply electrosurgical dispersive pad.

Skin preparation

Begin at the incision (check with surgeon) extending from nipples to upper thighs, and down to table at the sides.

Draping

Folded towels and a laparotomy or transverse sheet (depending on incision)

Equipment

Electrosurgical unit
Suction

Instrumentation

Major procedures tray
Long instruments tray

Gastrointestinal procedures tray
Self-retaining retractor (e.g., Balfour), optional

Supplies

Basin set
Blades (2) No. 10
Suction tubing
Electrosurgical pencil
Penrose drain, 1″ (retraction on colon)
Glass rod and tubing with colostomy pouch (e.g.,
    Karaya Seal or plastic bridge) and loop colos-
    tomy set (e.g., Hollister)

Special Notes

Instruments used on the bowel are isolated in a
basin.

Specimen may be received in a basin.

"Clean" closure of the abdomen requires regowning, regloving, redraping, and Basic/Minor
procedures tray.

CLOSURE OF COLOSTOMY

Definition

Reestablishment of colonic continuity and the repair
of the abdominal wall.

Discussion

This procedure can be simple or involved, particularly the anastomosis between a sigmoid end colostomy and the proximal rectal remnant.

Procedure

For an *end colostomy* an incision circumscribes
the stoma, which is dissected free of abdominal wall
structures. An appropriate incision is made to en-

able intra-abdominal dissection permitting anastomosis at the site of the distal colon. The distal segment is mobilized and anastomosed to the proximal end; an end-to-end automatic stapling device can facilitate the procedure. The wound is closed; subcutaneous tissue and the skin of the stoma site can be left open to avoid infection.

For a *loop or double barrel colostomy* an elliptical incision is made around the stoma(s). The colonic loop is dissected free of scar tissue and skin and the anastomosis is performed. The proximal and distal segments may need to be resected in order to perform anastomosis on well-vascularized bowel of satisfactory diameters. The abdomen is closed, often leaving the subcutaneous tissue and skin packed open to prevent wound infection.

Preparation of the patient

The patient is supine; arms may be extended on armboards. Apply electrosurgical dispersive pad.

Skin preparation

Cover colostomy stoma with a sponge soaked in preparation solution. Begin just beyond the perimeter of the stoma extending from nipples to midthighs, and down to the table at the sides. Cleanse the area immediately around the stoma and the stoma itself last. Discard each sponge after cleansing the stoma.

Draping

Folded towels and a laparotomy or transverse sheet

Equipment

Electrosurgical unit
Suction

Instrumentation

Major procedures tray
Long instruments tray

Gastrointestinal procedures tray
Automatic stapling device, optional
Self-retaining retractor (e.g., Balfour), optional

Supplies

Basin set
Blades (3) No. 10, (1) No. 15
Needle magnet or counter
Suction tubing
Electrosurgical pencil
Staples, optional
Packing (e.g., Adaptic dressing, 4″ × 4″ sponges, optional)

Special notes

Instruments used on the bowel are isolated in a basin.

"Clean" closure of the abdomen requires regowning, regloving, redraping, and Basic/Minor procedures tray.

RIGHT HEMICOLECTOMY

Definition

Resection of the right half of the colon (a portion of the transverse colon, the ascending colon, and the cecum) and a segment of the terminal ileum and their mesenteries; an anastomosis is performed between the ileum and the transverse colon (ileocolostomy).

Discussion

Indications for right hemicolectomy are tumors, bleeding, inflammation, or trauma; obstruction is less often encountered than in the left half of the colon.

Procedure

A right paramedian, midline, or oblique right midabdominal incision is made. The distal small bowel and the midtransverse colon are identified, and their vascular attachments ligated and divided. The appropriate segment of colon is excised between clamps (atraumatic clamps may be used on the portions of the retained bowel) or an automatic stapling device may be employed. The terminal ileum and midtransverse colon are anastomosed by various suture techniques or staples. Care is taken to avoid injury to structures including the right ureter, duodenum, inferior vena cava, and common bile duct. The incision is closed in layers.

Preparation of the patient

The patient is supine; arms may be extended on armboards. Check with the surgeon regarding insertion of a Foley catheter before beginning to prepare the patient. Apply electrosurgical dispersive pad.

Skin preparation

Begin at the incision (right paramedian, midline, or oblique right midabdominal) extending from nipples to upper thighs, and down to the table at the sides.

Draping

Folded towels and a laparotomy sheet

Equipment

Electrosurgical unit
Suction

Instrumentation

Major procedures tray
Long instruments tray
Gastrointestinal procedures tray
Hemoclip appliers (various sizes and lengths)
Automatic stapling devices, optional

Harrington retractor
Self-retaining retractor (e.g., Balfour)

Supplies

Basin set
Blades (3) No. 10, (1) No. 15
Electrosurgical pencil
Suction tubing
Needle magnet or counter
Hemoclips (various sizes)
Staples, optional

Special notes

Scrub person may receive specimen in a basin.
Instruments used on the colon are isolated in a basin.
"Clean" closure of the abdomen requires regowning, regloving, redraping, and a Basic/Minor procedures tray.

TRANSVERSE COLECTOMY

Definition

Resection of a segment of the transverse colon with an end-to-end anastomosis to reestablish continuity of the colon.

Discussion

Transverse colectomy is usually performed as treatment for a malignancy or a stricture caused by inflammatory bowel disease.

Procedure

A vertical or transverse incision may be used. The transverse colon and hepatic and splenic flexures are mobilized by dividing vascular mesenteric attachments and supporting connective tissues. The appropriate segment of colon is excised between clamps (atraumatic clamps may be used on the portions of the retained bowel) or an automatic stapling device may be employed. An anastomosis is fashioned between the proximal and distal colon, and the mesenteric defect is closed; sufficient mobility must be achieved to enable the anastomosis to be tension free. Injury to the stomach, pancreas, spleen, and superior mesenteric vessels is avoided. The wound is closed in layers.

Preparation of the Patient

The patient is supine; arms may be extended on armboards. Check with surgeon regarding insertion of a Foley catheter before beginning preparation. Apply electrosurgical dispersive pad.

Skin Preparation

Begin at the incision (midline or transverse) extending from nipples to upper thighs, and down to the table at the sides.

Draping

Folded towels and a transverse or laparotomy sheet (depending on incision)

Equipment

Electrosurgical unit
Suction

Instrumentation

Major procedures tray
Gastrointestinal procedures tray
Automatic stapling device, optional
Hemoclip appliers (various sizes)
Harrington retractor
Self-retaining retractor (e.g., Balfour)

Supplies

Basin set
Blades (3) No. 10
Suction tubing
Electrosurgical pencil
Hemoclips (various sizes)
Needle magnet or counter
Staples, optional

Special notes

Instruments used on the colon are isolated in a basin.

Specimen can be received in a basin.

Ends of the bowel may be covered with lap pads or surgical gloves and tied with umbilical tape to prevent contamination of the abdomen.

"Clean" closure of the abdomen requires re-gowning, regloving, redraping, and a Basic/Minor procedures tray.

ANTERIOR RESECTION OF THE SIGMOID COLON AND RECTUM

Definition

Involves the excision of the sigmoid colon and when applicable the rectosigmoid and the proximal two thirds of the rectum with the anastomosis of the distal descending or proximal sigmoid colon to the remaining segment of the rectosigmoid or rectum.

Discussion

This procedure is performed for benign (e.g., diverticulitis) or malignant conditions.

Procedure

A vertical or transverse incision can be used. The lower descending, sigmoid, and rectosigmoid colon (and proximal rectum) are mobilized by dividing mesenteric vascular attachments. In procedures for malignancy, greater portions of the mesentery are excised to include additional lymph-node-bearing tissue. The ureters are identified and protected. The appropriate segment of colon is excised, and the bowel is anastomosed with sutures or staples. Tension is avoided on the anastomosis by mobilizing more proximal colon as necessary. The abdomen is closed in layers.

Preparation of the patient

The patient is supine; arms may be extended on armboards. Check with surgeon regarding insertion of a Foley catheter before beginning preparation. Apply electrosurgical dispersive pad.

Skin preparation

Begin at the incision (vertical or transverse) extending from nipples to upper thighs, and down to the table at the sides.

Draping, Equipment, Instrumentation, and Supplies

See Right Hemicolectomy, p. 101.

ABDOMINOPERINEAL RESECTION OF THE RECTUM

Definition

Excision of the rectum, usually including a portion of the sigmoid colon, through an abdominal (anterior) and a perineal approach.

Discussion

This procedure is performed most often for the treatment of rectal malignancy, but also for inflammatory bowel disease, irreversible sphincter injuries, etc. Abdominoperineal resection of the rectum may be combined with resection of the proximal colon as well.

Procedure

A vertical or transverse abdominal incision is made. The extent and level of the pathology is determined. The portion of the colon to be removed is mobilized by dividing the mesenteric vascular attachments to the bowel, carrying the dissection to the rectum. The ureters and other adjacent organs are identified and otherwise avoided unless they are to be removed. The colon is transsected proximally. The distal portion (the transsected end of which is protected from spillage by use of lap pads, clamps, and/or a rubber glove secured by umbilical tapes) is dissected into the depths of the pelvis transsecting the lateral rectal stalks (middle hemorrhoidal vessels) to the level of the coccyx. Perirectal connective and adipose tissue are removed with malignancies. In benign disease the dissection stays close to the bowel wall. A stoma site is fashioned by excising a disc of skin and tunneling into the peritoneum through the rectus muscle. The end of the proximal portion of the colon (or ileum) is passed through the tunnel without tension and assuring good vascularity, and is sutured to the peristomal skin. The abdomen may then be closed or if simultaneous perineal dissection is performed, the "abdominal" surgeon remains to assist from above. As the perineal portion is completed, the surgeon above closes the abdomen. The colostomy is sutured. The "perineal" surgeon closes the anus with a heavy gauge pursestring suture. An elliptical sagittal incision is made into the perianal and perirectal tissues and deepened, incising the levator muscles; the pelvis is entered and the previously dissected distal colon and proximal rectum are passed into the perineal wound. The rectum is excised avoiding the urethra and prostate or vagina. Hemostasis is achieved. The perineal wound is closed in layers over one or more drains. A colostomy pouch is placed over the stoma.

Preparation of the patient

The patient is usually in modified lithotomy/Sims' position with the sacrum elevated on folded towels or a sandbag, or the procedure is begun with the patient supine and later moved to lithotomy or modified lateral/Sims' position. Check with the surgeon regarding insertion of Foley catheter before beginning the preparation. Apply electrosurgical dispersive pad.

Skin preparation

Modified lithotomy: Begin at the incision (midline, left paramedian, or transverse) extending from the nipples to lower thighs, and down to the table at the sides. Prepare genitalia (add a vaginal preparation for females), extending to the table at the perineal area; prepare anus last and discard each sponge.

Supine: Begin at the pubic symphysis extending downward over the labia. Cleanse each inner thigh working toward the perineum. Prepare vagina, then perineum, and anus last (discarding each sponge).

Modified lateral/Sims': Begin at suprapubic area extending from the iliac crest to midthighs, and down to the table anteriorly and posteriorly. Prepare genitalia and anus last.

Draping

Modified lithotomy: Drape sheet (under buttocks), leggings, folded towels (abdomen), and a laparotomy or transverse sheet (a hole will be cut for perineal exposure)

Supine: Folded towels and a laparotomy or transverse sheet

Modified lateral/Sims': Folded towels and a laparotomy or transverse sheet

Lithotomy: Same as modified lithotomy

Equipment

Electrosurgical unit
Suction
Stirrups (depending on position)

Instrumentation

Major procedures tray
Long instruments tray
Gastrointestinal procedures tray
Basic/Minor procedures tray for perineal approach
(when both abdominal and perineal approach
are performed)
Hemoclip appliers (various sizes and lengths)
Large retractors (e.g., Harrington, Israel, Balfour)

Supplies

Basin set
Blades (4) No. 10, (1) No. 15
Needle magnet or counter (2 for simultaneous approach, 3 for "clean" set up)
Electrosurgical pencils (2 for simultaneous approach, 3 for "clean" set up)
Pouch for electrosurgical pencils
Suction tubing
Hemoclips, assorted sizes
Extra glove and umbilical tape (for proximal end of
a specimen before it is passed through the perineal wound)
Vessel loop or umbilical tape (retraction)
Marking pen (stoma site), optional
Colostomy pouch (e.g., Karaya Seal)
Drainage supplies (e.g., Penrose, Hemovac, Foley
catheter)

Special notes

For modified lithotomy position the abdominal
and perineal approaches are performed by two
teams simultaneously (a second scrub nurse is necessary). For a two-stage procedure the patient is

prepared and draped for the second stage after the abdomen is closed.

Isolate all instruments used on the colon in a basin.

The scrub person may receive specimen in a basin.

Since there are two separate surgical fields additional care must be exercised to avoid confusion when counting sponges, needles and sharps, and instruments.

"Clean" closure of the abdomen requires regowning, regloving, redraping, and a Basic/Minor procedures tray.

Using a pouch prevents inadvertent activation of a second electrosurgical pencil not in use.

HEMORRHOIDECTOMY

Definition

Excision of distended veins, anal skin, anoderm (externally), and mucous membrane (internally).

Discussion

Hemorrhoidectomy refers to the removal of enlarged veins and/or hemorrhoidal tissues, which are often associated with local anal problems such as fissures (anal ulcer) and fistula. Anesthesia may be regional, local, or general (or a combination). Following the induction of anesthesia proctosigmoidoscopy is performed.

Procedure

The proximal portions of the hemorrhoidal complex are suture-ligated and the hemorrhoid is excised by scalpel, cautery, or laser. Less often cryosurgery is employed (usually reserved for limited outpatient procedures). If the anus is stenotic the distal internal sphincter may be incised. A mucous membrane flap and/or skin flaps may be employed to cover denuded areas. Care is taken not to excise too much skin, anoderm, or mucous membrane and to avoid injury to the sphincter mechanism.

Preparation of the patient

See Sigmoidoscopy, p. 81.

Skin preparation

Preparation is minimal. Begin inside tape margins discarding each sponge after wiping the anus.

Draping

Jackknife: Folded towels and a laparotomy sheet
Lithotomy: Drape sheet under buttocks, leggings, folded towels, drape sheet over abdomen
Modified lateral/Sims': Folded towels and a laparotomy sheet

Equipment

Stirrups or pillow and roll for positioning
Electrosurgical unit

Instrumentation

Rectal procedures tray
Rectal retractors, including Sims', Hill-Ferguson, and Sawyer; curettes

Supplies

Blades (1) No. 10, (1) No. 15
Needle magnet or counter
Small basin
Hemostatic agent (e.g., Surgicel, Gelfoam)
Suction tubing
Electrosurgical pencil
Lubricant

Pressure dressing (e.g., petrolatum impregnated gauze, 4″ × 4″ sponges)

Special notes

Protect skin under adhesive tape with tincture of benzoin.

Be prepared for sigmoidoscopy prior to procedure.

Lubricate retractors.

Carbon dioxide laser may be used. See Appendix, p. 570 for safety precautions.

PILONIDAL CYSTECTOMY AND SINUSECTOMY

Definition

Refers to the removal of a cystic mass containing hair, skin, tissue debris, etc., most often located in the sacrococcygeal area.

Discussion

Pilonidal cysts are most frequently found in the sacrococcygeal region, but can occur about the perineum, hands, etc. When acutely or chronically infected, surgical treatment is indicated. These cysts may be very extensive with multiple and deep sidetracts.

Procedure

An incision is made about the cyst or into the cyst directly. Necrotic tissue, hair, tissue debris, etc. are curetted and/or excised. The cyst wall is sometimes excised. The wound can be packed open, partially closed, or completely closed by means of tissue flaps.

Preparation of the patient

The patient is in jackknife position (the table is flexed) with arms extended on armboards angled toward the head of the table and the hands pronated, a pillow in front of the legs, and a roll at the ankles. Buttocks are distracted by 3-inch or 4-inch adhesive tapes anchored to the underside of the table (pull tapes toward patient's head before anchoring for maximal exposure).

Skin preparation

Begin at the sacrum extending from the iliac crests to the upper thighs. Cleanse anus last discarding each sponge afterward.

Draping

Folded towels and a laparotomy sheet

Equipment

Pillow and roll for positioning
Electrosurgical unit
Suction

Instrumentation

Rectal procedures tray
Extra probes (available)
Curettes

Supplies

Small basin
Blades (1) No. 10, (2) No. 15
Suction tubing
Electrosurgical pencil
Needle magnet or counter
Methylene blue with needle and syringe, optional
Pressure dressing

Special notes

Protect skin under adhesive tape with tincture of benzoin.

THIERSCH PROCEDURE

Definition

Placement of a circumanal device to restrict complete rectal prolapse (procidentia).

Discussion

Prosthetic materials include various sutures, fascia, Mersilene tape, folded Marlex mesh, vascular prostheses, etc. The Thiersch procedure often ultimately fails when the prosthetic material extrudes with ensuing local infection. The procedure may be repeated after the infection subsides.

Procedure

Two incisions, 1 cm each, are made diametrically opposite around the anus. A large curved hemostat is passed deep in the perianal tissues external to the sphincter (avoiding the vagina), encircling the sphincter, and exiting the opposite incision. The prosthetic material is passed through the tunnel created by the clamp. This maneuver is repeated for the other hemicircumference (prosthesis completely encircles anal canal). The prosthetic ends are sutured (or stapled) after an appropriate degree of constriction is determined. The sutured segment is replaced deep in the wound. Wounds may be irrigated with an antibiotic solution. The wounds are closed.

Preparation of the patient

The procedure may be performed under regional, local, or general anesthesia. The patient may be in the jackknife, lithotomy, or modified lateral/Sims' position (see Sigmoidoscopy, p. 81). A sigmoidoscopy may be performed prior to the procedure.

Skin preparation

Preparation is minimal. Begin inside tape margins discarding each sponge after wiping the anus.

Draping

Jackknife: Folded towels and a laparotomy sheet
Lithotomy: Drape sheet under buttocks, leggings, towels, drape sheet over abdomen
Modified lateral/Sims': Folded towels and a laparotomy sheet

Equipment

Electrosurgical unit
Suction
Pillow and roll or stirrups (for positioning)

Instrumentation

Rectal procedures tray
Rectal retractors, including Sims', Hill-Ferguson, and Sawyer
Ligature carrier, optional

Supplies

Blades (1) No. 10, (2) No. 15
Needle magnet or counter
Small basin
Suction tubing
Electrosurgical pencil
Lubricant
Prosthesis
Antibiotic irrigation and bulb syringe (optional)

Special notes

Protect skin under tape with tincture of benzoin.
Be prepared for sigmoidoscopy prior to procedure.
Lubricate retractors.
Check with surgeon regarding prosthesis material.

RIPSTEIN PROCEDURE (PRESACRAL RECTOPEXY)

Definition

An anterior (abdominal) approach to correct complete rectal prolapse (procidentia) by mobilizing the rectum within the abdomen (and pelvis) and fixing it to the presacral fascia and periosteum by an encircling band of material such as a Teflon, Marlex, or Mersilene mesh.

Discussion

If the sigmoid colon is extremely redundant a portion of it may be resected.

Procedure

A vertical or transverse incision is used. The rectum is dissected from its supporting tissue attachment. A mesh of Marlex (or Mersilene, Teflon, etc.) is sutured (or stapled) to the presacral periosteum taking care to avoid the local venous plexus. The mesh is placed around the bowel to anchor it to the sacrum without restricting the rectum too tightly. A resection proximally may be performed. The abdomen is closed in layers.

Preparation of the patient

The patient is supine; arms may be extended on armboards. Check with surgeon regarding insertion of a Foley catheter. Apply electrosurgical dispersive pad.

Skin preparation

Begin at the incision (vertical or transverse) extending from nipples to upper thighs, and down to the table at the sides.

Draping

Folded towels and a laparotomy or transverse sheet

Equipment

Electrosurgical unit
Suction

Instrumentation

Major procedures tray
Long instruments tray
Gastrointestinal procedures tray (available)
Harrington retractor
Self-retaining retractor (e.g., Balfour)
Hemoclip appliers (assorted sizes and lengths)
Stapler (fascia)

Supplies

Basin set
Electrosurgical pencil
Blades (3) No. 10
Suction tubing
Needle magnet or counter
Hemoclips (variety)
Mesh or banding materials
Staples, optional

Special notes

Check with surgeon regarding prosthetic material to be used.

Chapter 11

GYNECOLOGIC AND OBSTETRIC SURGERY

DILATATION OF THE CERVIX AND CURETTAGE OF THE UTERUS (D & C)

Definition

The gradual enlargement of the cervical canal and removal (by scraping) of endocervical or endometrial tissue for histologic study.

Discussion

The procedure is usually performed to diagnose cervical or uterine malignancy, control dysfunctional uterine bleeding, complete incomplete abortion, aid in evaluating infertility, and relieve dysmenorrhea. Fractional curettage differentiates between endocervical and endometrial lesions.

Procedure

A weighted speculum is placed in the vaginal vault. The cervix is grasped with a tenaculum. A sound is passed through the cervical canal into the uterine cavity to determine its depth and angulation. The cervix is dilated with graduated dilators. The uterine cavity may be explored with stone forceps. The uterine cavity is curetted. Curettings are removed with stone forceps and collected on Telfa placed in the posterior fornix. A small serrated curette is used to scrape the uterine walls again; or when D & C is performed to remove placental tissue, a large, blunt curet and ovum forceps are used.

If fractional D & C is performed, endocervical curettings are obtained *before* the uterus is sounded to avoid bringing endometrial cells into the cervical os.

Preparation of the patient

Following the administration of regional or general anesthesia, the patient is positioned in lithotomy. Arms may be extended on armboards.

Skin preparation

Begin at the pubic symphysis and extend downward over the labia. Cleanse each inner thigh. The vaginal vault and cervix are cleansed using sponge sticks (three). The perineum and anus are cleansed with remaining sponges. Discard each sponge after wiping the anus. The patient's bladder is usually drained with a straight catheter.

Draping

Drape sheet under the buttocks, leggings, and drape sheet over the abdomen

Equipment

Stirrups

Instrumentation

Dilatation and currettage (D & C) tray

Supplies

Telfa (for specimen)
Perineal pad
T-binder

Special notes

Stirrups are well padded to avoid nerve damage.

Lift both legs at the same time when putting the patient in stirrups to prevent postoperative lumbosacral strain.

Raise and lower legs slowly to prevent disturbances caused by rapid alterations in venous return.

Instruments are set up on back table for surgeon; usually a scrub person is not required.

CONIZATION OF THE UTERINE CERVIX

Definition

The excision of tissue around the cervical os.

Discussion

This procedure is performed to diagnose and/or treat conditions such as cervicitis, epithelial dysplasia, and carcinoma in situ. "Cold" conization refers to scalpel and scissors dissection. "Hot" conization refers to tissue removal by use of electrocautery.

Procedure

A weighted speculum is placed in the vaginal vault. The outer portion of the cervix is grasped with a tenaculum. Dilatation and Curettage (see p. 118) is performed. The cervix may be stained with Schiller's or Lugol's solution. Sutures are placed at the 3 o'clock and 9 o'clock positions. The cervix may be injected circumferentially with a phenylephrine

Neo-Synephrine) solution. The uterine canal is carefully sounded. An incision is made circumferentially around the cervical os using the knife or cautery. Alternatively, a cervical cyst may be electrodesiccated with a needle electrode. Bleeding may be controlled with sutures and/or ball electrode desiccation or a hemostatic agent.

Preparation of the patient

Following the administration of regional or general anesthesia, the patient is positioned in lithotomy. Arms may be extended on armboards. Apply electrosurgical dispersive pad.

Skin preparation

Preparation may be omitted (check with surgeon); see Dilatation and Curettage, p. 118 for vaginal preparation.

Draping

Drape sheet under the buttocks, leggings, and drape sheet over the abdomen

Equipment

Stirrups
Electrosurgical unit

Instrumentation

Dilatation and curettage (D & C) tray
Cervical cone tray

Supplies

Telfa (for specimen)
Electrosurgical pencil (with blade, needle, and/or ball tip)
Blade No. 11

Small basin(s)
Schiller's or Lugol's solution, optional
Long cotton-tipped applicators, optional
Neo-Synephrine 1:20,000 (reduces bleeding) with
    needle and syringe, optional
Hemostatic agent (e.g., Surgicel, Thrombostat)
Perineal pad
T-binder

Special notes

See Dilatation and Curettage, p. 118.

THERAPEUTIC ABORTION BY SUCTION CURETTAGE

Definition

The vacuum aspiration of uterine contents usually performed to terminate early pregnancy.

Discussion

Procedure is also performed for missed and incomplete abortions.

Procedure

This procedure is similar to dilatation and curettage until the cervix is dilated. An appropriate suction curette is inserted through the dilated cervix into the uterine cavity. The controlled suction apparatus is activated. The curette is rotated 360° with a back-and-forth motion while traction is maintained on the cervix. The endometrial cavity is curetted with a sharp curette and a brief suction curettage is repeated.

Preparation of the patient, Skin preparation, and Draping

See Dilatation and Curettage, p. 118.

Equipment

Stirrups
Controlled suction apparatus (e.g., Berkely Vacu-
    rette Machine)

Instrumentation

Dilatation and curettage (D & C) tray
Disposable vacuum curettes (assorted sizes, curved
and straight)
Aspiration tubing

Supplies

Lubricant
Perineal pad
T-binder

Special notes

See Dilatation and Curettage, p. 118.
Evacuation is done using all available vacuum
(in Berkely unit, better than 73 cm of mercury is recommended).
Surgeon connects suction tip to the aspiration
tubing. Circulator or scrub person attaches tubing to
controlled suction unit and activates it on surgeon's
request.
A gauze tissue bag is used inside the collection
bottle to collect specimen. Send gauze tissue bag
and contents to pathology laboratory.

MARSUPIALIZATION OF BARTHOLIN'S
DUCT CYST

Definition

The incision and drainage of a vulvovaginal cyst
and the suturing of the cyst wall to the edges of the
incision.

Discussion

The cyst wall is composed primarily of the duct of the gland; by not excising the cyst the secretory function of the gland may be preserved.

Procedure

A vertical incision is made in the vaginal mucosa over the center of the cyst (outside the hymenal ring). The cyst is incised and drained. The lining of the cyst is everted and sutured to the vaginal mucosa with interrupted stitches. If cystectomy is necessary, the cyst is mobilized using sharp and blunt dissection. The intact cyst is excised. The mucosa is approximated; a drain may be inserted.

Preparation of the patient

Following the administration of local, regional, or general anesthesia, the patient is positioned in lithotomy. Arms may be extended on armboards. Apply electrosurgical dispersive pad.

Skin preparation

See Dilatation and Curettage, p. 118. Patient's bladder may be catheterized with a straight catheter; check with surgeon.

Draping

Patient is draped with a sheet under the buttocks, leggings, and a fenestrated sheet. The surgeon and the assistant may be seated. A drape sheet is fastened beneath the fenestration; the sheet lies across the surgeon's lap and an instrument lap tray is placed on the surgeon's lap. Some surgeons prefer to stand, eliminating the need for the extra drape sheet and lap tray.

Equipment

Stirrups
Electrosurgical unit

Instrumentation

Cervical cone tray

Supplies

Culture tubes (2) (aerobic and anaerobic cultures)
    and swabs
Smear slides (2)
Disposable syringe and long 15- or 18-gauge nee-
    dle, optional
Lap tray, optional
Electrosurgical pencil
Drain (e.g., Penrose ¼"), optional
Perineal pad
T-binder

Special notes

Stirrups are well padded to avoid nerve
damage.
Lift both legs at the same time when putting the
patient in stirrups to prevent postoperative lumbosacral strain.
Raise and lower legs slowly to prevent circulatory disturbances caused by rapid alterations in venous return.

CULDOSCOPY

Definition

Culdoscopy is the introduction of an endoscope
through the posterior vaginal wall that provides visualization of the pelvic structures.

Discussion

Once frequently employed as a diagnostic tool, culdoscopy has largely been replaced by laparoscopy, in which positioning of the patient is easier and better visualization of the pelvis is achieved. See Laparoscopy, p. 131 for Procedure, Preparation of the patient, Instrumentation, and Supplies.

VAGINAL HYSTERECTOMY

Definition

Removal of the uterus through a vaginal approach.

Discussion

Indications for this procedure include diseases of the uterus restricted to benign conditions in which the uterus is not greatly enlarged, and conditions in which poor pelvic muscular support is present necessitating anterior and posterior colporrhaphy.

Procedure

A weighted vaginal speculum is placed in the vaginal vault. The cervix is grasped with a tenaculum. Dilatation and curettage may be performed. A phenylephrine (Neo-Synephrine) solution may be injected into the vaginal incision sites. An incision is made anterior to the cervix in the vaginal wall. The bladder is reflected from the cervix using sharp, then blunt dissection, exposing the peritoneum of the anterior cul-de-sac, which is then incised posteriorly. The uterosacral ligaments are ligated and divided. The uterus is placed on traction. The cardinal ligaments and uterine arteries are ligated and divided, and the uterus is delivered. If the ovaries are to be preserved, the ovarian vessels are preserved and the remaining structures in the broad ligament are ligated and divided. After the specimen is removed the incisions into the cul-de-sac and vaginal apex are repaired. The uterosacral and round ligament stumps may be sutured to the angles of the vaginal vault closure. An anterior and/or posterior colporrhaphy may be performed (see p. 129). The vagina may be packed.

Preparation of the patient

Following the administration of regional or general anesthesia, the patient is positioned in lithotomy. Arms may be extended on armboards. Apply electrosurgical dispersive pad.

Skin preparation

Begin at the pubic symphysis and extend downward over the labia. Cleanse each inner thigh. The vaginal vault and cervix are then cleansed using sponge sticks (three). The perineum and anus are cleansed with the remaining sponges. Discard each sponge after wiping the anus. The bladder may be drained with a straight catheter.

Draping

The patient is draped with a sheet under the buttocks, leggings, and a fenestrated sheet. Usually the surgeon and the assistant are seated. A drape sheet is fastened beneath the fenestration; the sheet lies across the surgeon's lap and an instrument lap tray is placed on the surgeon's lap. Some surgeons prefer to stand, eliminating the need for the extra drape sheet and lap tray.

Equipment

Electrosurgical unit
Suction
Stirrups

Instrumentation

Vaginal hysterectomy tray

Supplies

Blades (2) No. 10
Needle magnet or counter
Basin set
Lap tray, optional
Neo-Synephrine 1:20,000, with local syringe and
    needle, optional
Suction tubing
Electrosurgical pencil
Foley catheter drainage unit
Gauze packing (e.g., 1"), optional
Vaginal cream
Perineal pad
T-binder

Special notes

In addition to the operative permit a sterilization
permit may be required.

Stirrups are well padded to avoid nerve
damage.

Lift both legs at the same time when putting the
patient in stirrups to prevent postoperative lumbosacral strain.

Raise and lower legs slowly to prevent circulatory disturbances caused by rapid alterations in venous return.

Instruments for the lap tray often include a
weighted speculum, a tenaculum, retractors, curved
Mayo scissors, and hysterectomy clamps (e.g.,
Heaney, curved Kocher).

ANTERIOR AND/OR POSTERIOR
COLPORRHAPHY

Definition

Repair and reinforcement of musculofascial support of the bladder and the urethra (anteriorly) and distal rectum (posteriorly), preventing protrusion of the structures through the vaginal wall.

Discussion

Cystocele (or cystourethrocele) presents with symptoms of nuisance protrusion anteriorly into the vagina with urinary retention and/or stress incontinence. *Rectocele* presents posteriorly and may be associated with difficulties in defecation. These conditions may present simultaneously or independently to varying degrees. An associated *enterocele* (herniation through the rectouterine pouch) may also occur. This latter entity can also present with uterine prolapse or in patients in whom hysterectomy has been performed. Multiparity is the most common cause for these entities. Repair may be performed to correct any of these conditions alone, in combination, or to complement a vaginal hysterectomy.

Procedure

The cervix (if present) is grasped with a tenaculum. For *anterior colporrhaphy* the anterior vaginal mucosa is incised in the midline. The incision is deepened into the musculofascial wall reflecting the bladder anteriorly, mobilizing the urethra, and exposing the urethrovesical junction. Plication sutures are placed in the musculofascial tissues to restore the urethrovesical angle and support of the bladder. Care is taken not to overtighten the repair. Excess of the previously stretched vaginal mucosa is excised and the mucosal incision is approximated.

For *posterior colporrhaphy* an incision is made at the mucocutaneous junction reflecting the attenuated vaginal mucosa proximally to expose the rectocele. Perirectal fascia is separated from the mucosa and plicated. The levator muscles are approximated at the midline to an appropriate degree of tension. The excess vaginal mucosa is excised and the mucosal incision is closed. A vaginal pack may be placed.

Preparation of the patient

Following the administration of regional or general anesthesia, the patient is positioned in lithotomy. The arms may be extended on armboards. Apply electrosurgical dispersive pad.

Skin preparation

Begin at the pubic symphysis and extend downward over the labia. Cleanse each inner thigh. The vaginal vault and cervix are then cleansed using spongesticks (three). The perineum and anus are cleansed with the remaining sponges. Discard each sponge after wiping the anus. The patient is catheterized with an indwelling or straight catheter.

Draping, Equipment, Instrumentation, and Supplies

See Vaginal Hysterectomy, p. 126.

Special notes

Stirrups are well padded to avoid nerve damage.

Lift both legs at the same time to prevent postoperative lumbosacral strain.

Raise and lower legs slowly to prevent circulatory disturbances caused by rapid alterations in venous return.

Instruments for the lap tray often include a

weighted speculum, a tenaculum, retractors, curved Mayo scissors, and Allis clamps.

LAPAROSCOPY

Definition

The introduction of an endoscope through the anterior abdominal wall following the establishment of a pneumoperitoneum.

Discussion

Laparoscopy permits visualization of the pelvic structures without open laparotomy. It is used to identify causes of infertility, pelvic mass, ectopic pregnancy, etc.; it may also be employed for elective sterilization.

Procedure

The vagina is retracted and the anterior lip of the cervix is grasped with a tenaculum. A self-retaining cannula is inserted in the cervix. Two towel clips are placed on the inferior rim of the umbilicus and a 2-mm incision is made. Traction is placed on the towel clips and a Verres needle is inserted through the incision into the peritoneal cavity. Proper placement of the needle is ascertained. Polyethylene tubing connected to the insufflation device is connected to the Verres needle. Pneumoperitoneum is established with approximately 2 liters of gas (carbon dioxide or nitrous oxide). The needle is withdrawn and the incision is enlarged to 1 cm. Towel clips provide traction as the trocar and sleeve (angled toward the pelvis) are inserted. The trocar is withdrawn from the sleeve and the proper location of the sleeve is ascertained. The carbon dioxide tubing is attached to the sleeve to keep the abdomen inflated.

The laparoscope is inserted and the light source connected. The abdomen is examined. If a procedure such as tubal ligation is performed, a second (lower) incision may be made, which allows for the insertion of accessory instruments through the initial incision, or a single-puncture laparoscope may be used. At the completion of the procedure the gas is permitted to escape through the sleeve. Incisions are closed with a subcuticular stitch or skin closure strips.

Preparation of the patient

Following the administration of local, regional or general anesthesia, the patient is placed in modified lithotomy (45°) position. Arms may be extended on armboards. The table is positioned in Trendelenburg; for extreme Trendelenburg, shoulder braces are required. Apply electrosurgical dispersive pad.

Skin preparation

Begin at the umbilicus extending from nipples to pubic symphysis, and down to the table at the sides. Follow this by a vaginal preparation beginning at pubic symphysis and extending down over the labia. Cleanse each inner thigh. Prepare vaginal vault and cervix using spongesticks (three). Perineum and anus are prepared last, discarding each sponge after wiping the anus. Catheterize patient with a straight catheter.

Draping

Drape sheet under the buttocks, leggings, and a special laparoscopy sheet or other fenestrated sheet.

Equipment

Insufflation device (e.g., Eder CO_2 and N_2O, Wolf CO_2)
Fiberoptic light source
Electrosurgical unit

Suction
Shoulder braces, optional

Instrumentation

Laparoscopy tray
Uterine retractor, tenaculum, and uterine manipulator
For chromotubation (infertility detection): Intrauter-
ine cannula (e.g., Cohen)

Supplies

Suction tubing (for uterine manipulator)
Blade No. 15 or No. 11
Skin closure strips, optional
For infertility add: plastic tubing, syringe containing
dye, e.g., methylene blue

Special notes

Lift both legs at the same time when putting the
patient in stirrups to prevent postoperative lumbosacral strain.

Raise and lower legs slowly to prevent circulatory disturbances caused by rapid alterations in venous return.

Laparoscope lens warmer may be used. Antifogging solution may be applied to lens before use
and wiped off to prevent fogging (e.g., Ultrastop,
pHisoHex).

Regarding insufflation device: check amount of
gas in tanks before starting, tighten all connections,
and prefill unit with carbon dioxide.

TOTAL ABDOMINAL HYSTERECTOMY

Definition

Removal of the entire uterus through an abdominal
incision.

Discussion

Some indications for total abdominal hysterectomy are endometriosis, adnexal disease, postmenopausal bleeding, dysfunctional uterine bleeding, and benign and malignant tumors.

Procedure

A Pfannenstiel, vertical, midline, or paramedian incision is employed. The peritoneal cavity is entered and a self-retaining retractor is placed. The patient is placed in Trendelenburg position and the intestines are protected with warm moist (saline) laparotomy pads. The round ligaments of the uterus are ligated, divided, sutured, and tagged with a hemostat. After identifying the ureters, the broad ligaments are incised, and the bladder is reflected from the anterior aspect of the cervix. The infundibulopelvic ligaments are ligated and divided. If the ovaries are to be preserved the ovarian ligament is ligated and divided adjacent to the uterus (avoiding the ureters). The uterosacral ligaments are ligated and divided. The cardinal ligaments are likewise divided. The vagina is incised circumferentially and the uterine specimen removed. A "free" sponge (soaked in preparation solution) may be placed in the vagina prior to closure. After hemostasis is secured the vaginal cuff is closed; a drain may be used. The stumps of the uterosacral and round ligaments are sutured to the angles of the vaginal closure. The pelvic peritoneum is approximated and the wound is closed. The free sponge is removed.

Preparation of the patient

The patient is supine; arms may be extended on armboards. Apply electrosurgical dispersive pad.

Skin preparation

A vaginal and an abdominal preparation (separate trays) are required. Put the patient's legs in a froglike position and prepare as for Dilatation and Curettage, p. 118. Insert a Foley catheter and connect it to continuous drainage. Return the patient's legs to their original position and replace the safety belt. For abdominal preparation begin at the incision (usually Pfannenstiel) extending from nipples to midthighs, and down to the table at the sides.

Draping

Folded towels and a transverse or laparotomy sheet

Equipment

Suction
Electrosurgical unit

Instrumentation

Major procedures tray
Abdominal hysterectomy tray
Self-retaining retractor (e.g., Balfour or O'Connor-O'Sullivan)

Supplies

Blades (3) No. 10
Basin set
Needle magnet or counter
Suction tubing
Electrosurgical pencil
Foley catheter drainage unit
Perineal pad

Special notes

Sterilization permit may be required in addition to the routine surgical permit.

Have spongesticks available throughout procedure.

Instruments that come in contact with the cervix or vagina are isolated in a basin.

Specimen may be received in a basin.

Counts are taken three times (at closure of vaginal cuff, peritoneum, and skin).

If a "free" sponge has been placed in the vagina prior to closure, it is included in the sponge count and *must* be removed from the vagina at the termination of the procedure before the patient leaves the room.

SALPINGO-OOPHORECTOMY

Definition

The removal of a fallopian tube and corresponding ovary.

Discussion

Salpingo-oophorectomy is performed for a variety of nonmalignant diseases that include acute and chronic infections, cysts, tumors, and hemorrhage (tubal pregnancy). Malignancy of a tube or ovary will usually necessitate hysterectomy with excision of the opposite adnexae.

Procedure

A low midline, paramedian, or Pfannenstiel incision is employed. The peritoneal cavity is entered and a self-retaining retractor is placed. The patient is placed in Trendelenburg position. The intestines are protected by laparotomy pads. If adhesions are present the affected tube and ovary are isolated from surrounding organs. The infundibulopelvic ligament is ligated and divided, as is the broad ligament attachment of the tube and ovary. The tube and ovary are excised. The site of an adnexal excision may be reperitonealized. The wound is closed in layers.

Preparation of the patient

The patient is supine; arms may be extended on armboards. Apply electrosurgical dispersive pad.

Skin preparation, Draping, and Equipment

See Total Abdominal Hysterectomy, p. 133.

Instrumentation

Major procedures tray
Self-retaining retractor (e.g., Balfour, or O'Connor-O'Sullivan)
Somer's clamp

Supplies

Blades (2) No. 10, (1) No. 15
Basin set
Needle magnet or counter
Suction tubing
Electrosurgical pencil

Special notes

For bilateral salpingo-oophorectomy, a sterilization permit in addition to the routine surgical permit may be required.

Have spongesticks available throughout the procedure.

TUBAL STERILIZATION

Definition

The interruption of the fallopian tubes resulting in sterilization.

Discussion

Puerperal sterilization is best performed 24 to 36 hours after vaginal delivery, although it is performed at other times, that is, during Cesarean section or as an elective surgery. Approaches include minilaparotomy, laparoscopy, and posterior colpotomy. For details of the laparoscopic approach, see Laparoscopy, p. 131.

Procedure

Minilaparotomy. A small incision is made suprapubically. An opening is made into the peritoneal cavity. Each tube is grasped with a Babcock forceps and the tubal procedure performed (excision of, cauterization of, or application of a clip on a section of tube). The peritoneum is approximated. The wound is closed in layers.

Posterior Colpotomy. A weighted speculum is placed in the vagina. The cervix is retracted anteriorly with a tenaculum. A transverse incision is made into the vaginal mucosa posterior to the cervix and extended through the peritoneum to enter the cul-de-sac. Each tube is grasped with a Babcock forceps and the tubal procedure performed. The colpotomy site is closed with through-and-through sutures including the vaginal mucosa and peritoneum.

Preparation of the patient

Minilaparotomy. Patient is supine; arms may be extended on armboards.

Posterior Colpotomy. Patient is in lithotomy; arms may be extended on armboards.

Patient may be catheterized with a straight catheter; check with surgeon. Apply electrosurgical dispersive pad.

Skin preparation

Minilaparotomy. Begin at the incision (check with surgeon) extending from nipples to midthighs.

Posterior colpotomy. Begin at pubic symphysis and extend downward over the labia. Cleanse each inner thigh. Use spongesticks (three) to cleanse vaginal vault and cervix. The perineum and anus are cleansed with remaining sponges; discard each sponge after cleansing the anus.

Draping

Minilaparotomy: Folded towels and laparotomy sheet

Posterior colpotomy: Drape sheet under buttocks, leggings, and drape sheet over the abdomen

Equipment

Minilaparotomy: Electrosurgical unit

Posterior colpotomy: Suction, electrosurgical unit

Instrumentation

Minilaparotomy:

Basic/Minor procedures tray
Hemoclip appliers (small, medium)

Posterior Colpotomy:

Cervical cone tray
Babcock forceps (long)
Weighted speculum
Hemoclip appliers, long (small, medium)

Supplies

Minilaparotomy:

Blades (2) No. 15
Basin set
Needle magnet or counter
Electrosurgical pencil
Hemoclips (small, medium)

Posterior Colpotomy:

Blade No. 10
Suction tubing
Needle magnet or counter
Basin set
Electrosurgical pencil
Hemoclips (medium)

Special notes

Put specimens in separate containers labeled right and left tube segment.

TUBOPLASTY OF THE FALLOPIAN TUBES

Definition

The reestablishment of patency to the fallopian tubes.

Discussion

Tuboplasty is usually performed when the patient seeks a reversal of a sterilization procedure. Success depends on the amount of tubal destruction.

Procedure

Usually a Pfannenstiel incision is employed. The peritoneal cavity is entered and a self-retaining retractor is placed. Tubal patency may be demonstrated by the injection of methylene blue through a cervical cannula. Tuboplasty is performed according to the site obstruction, for example, cornual resection with reimplantation, tubal resection with anastomosis, and fimbrioplasty. The operating microscope is often used. A laser beam may be directed through the microscope to open adhesions of the fimbria and to lyse lesions within the tubes; for laser precautions, see Appendix, p. 570. The abdomen is closed in layers. The cervical cannula is removed.

Preparation of the patient

Following the induction of anesthesia, a catheter or cannula is inserted in the cervix for subsequent instillation of dye. If this step is to be included, the patient must initially be placed in lithotomy position.

After the catheter (connected to extension tubing and a syringe filled with dye) is secured, the patient is returned to the supine position. The safety belt is replaced. Care is taken not to dislodge the catheter. Apply electrosurgical dispersive pad.

Skin preparation

If the catheter will be inserted into the cervix, a vaginal preparation is required in addition to the abdominal preparation; see Dilatation and Curettage, p. 118. For abdominal preparation, begin at the incision (usually Pfannenstiel) extending from nipples to midthighs, and down to the table at the sides.

Draping

Folded towels, transverse or laparotomy sheet and microscope cover

Equipment

Stirrups
Suction
Electrosurgical unit
Microscope

Instruments

Dilatation and curettage (D & C) tray
Major procedures tray (includes probe)
Micro instruments (e.g., smooth and toothed forceps, tying forceps, Castroviejo needle holder, scissors)
Beaver knife handle
Mosquito hemostats (6 curved, 2 straight)
Frazier suction tips (assorted)

Supplies

Basin set

Blades (2) No. 10, (1) No. 15, (1) No. 11
Beaver blade
Needle magnet
Electrosurgical pencil (blade and needle tips)
Suction tubing
Pediatric Foley or special cannula, extension tubing,
    syringe eyedropper
Dye (e.g., methylene blue)
Perineal pad

Special notes

Stirrups are well padded to avoid nerve
damage.
Lift both legs at the same time when putting the
patient in stirrups to prevent postoperative lumbosacral strain.
See Appendix, p. 570 for laser precautions.
Raise and lower legs slowly to prevent disturbances caused by rapid alterations in venous return.
While the patient is in lithotomy position, an extension tubing is connected to the catheter or cannula. A syringe filled with dye solution is attached to
the catheter. During the abdominal phase of the
procedure, the circulator may be requested to inject
the dye.

PELVIC EXENTERATION

Definition

The en bloc removal of the rectum, distal sigmoid
colon, the urinary bladder and the distal ureters, internal genitalia, pelvic lymph nodes, pelvic peritoneum, a portion of the levator muscles, and the
creation of an ileal or colonic loop urinary diversion;
the hypogastric vessels are no longer removed.

Discussion

The primary indication for this procedure is radio-
resistant or recurrent cervical carcinoma. Total pel-

vic exenteration implies the excision of the internal genitalia, rectum, and bladder necessitating a permanent colostomy and a urinary diversion. If malignancy has spread beyond the pelvis or there are significant medical risks, this procedure is abandoned. The rectum may be spared and anterior exenteration is performed. Posterior exenteration is usually not performed for gynecologic malignancy, but may be done for rectal malignancy. The morbidity and mortality for this procedure is significant.

Procedure

A generous midline incision is employed. The abdomen is explored. Frozen section may be done. The order of the procedure varies with the operator. The urinary diversion (see Ileal Conduit, p. 188) may be done first or later in the procedure. Pelvic lymphadenectomy is done removing the fatty tissues about the iliac vessels, extending into the obturator fossa. The ligamentous attachment of the uterus and adnexae are separated from the pelvic wall and the rectum is mobilized from its posterior and lateral attachments (see Abdominoperineal Resection, p. 106). The bladder and urethra are mobilized and excised (see Cystectomy, p. 171). From the perineal approach (often by a second team) the anus and distal rectum are excised (see Abdominoperineal Resection, p. 106). The distal vagina may be preserved or reconstructed later on. The specimen is removed en bloc. A colostomy is created and the pelvic floor closed. The abdomen is closed in layers. Appropriate stomal pouches are applied.

Preparation of the patient

A nasogastric tube, urinary catheter, and rectal tube may be inserted before surgery. Antiembolic stockings may be requested. Central venous pressure monitoring is established. Following the administration of general anesthesia, the patient is placed in a modified lithotomy position with the legs tilted forward. Folded towels may be used to elevate the buttocks. The legs and feet are padded with towels or foam pads to avoid injury at pressure points. Table may be positioned in Trendelenburg. Apply electrosurgical dispersive pad.

Skin preparation

Begin at the midline extending from nipples to knees, and down to the table at the sides. Prepare perineum and genitalia next; a vaginal preparation is required for women. Cleanse the anus last, discarding each sponge after use.

Draping

The patient is draped with a sheet under the buttocks and leggings. The abdomen is draped with folded towels and individual drape sheets or a laparotomy sheet. If a laparotomy sheet is used it will be cut to expose the patient's perineum (for an elliptical incision below the anus).

Equipment

Electrosurgical unit
Suctions (2)
Stirrups
Scales (to weigh sponges)

Instrumentation

Major procedures tray
Long instruments tray
Vascular procedures tray
Kidney tray
Gastrointestinal procedures tray
Abdominal hysterectomy tray (female)
Abdominal prostatectomy tray (male)
Self-restraining retractors (e.g., Balfour, O'Connor-O'Sullivan)
Hemoclip appliers (all sizes and lengths)

Supplies

Blades (4) No. 10, (1) No. 15, (1) No. 11, (1) No. 12
Basin set
Needle magnet or counter
Suction tubing
Electrosurgical pencils (2)
Pouches (2) for electrosurgical pencils
Dissectors (e.g., peanut)
Penrose drains, umbilical tapes, and vascular loops
    (for retraction)
Hemoclips (all sizes)
Graduate
Asepto syringe
Robinson catheters, various sizes (available)
Pouches for colostomy and urostomy (e.g., Karaya
    Seal)
T-binder

Special notes

Confirm with laboratory that blood is available
as ordered.
Weigh sponges.
Keep accurate record of amount of irrigation
used.
Be prepared for many frozen sections.
Keep all soiled instruments isolated in a basin.
"Clean" closure of the abdomen requires re-
gowning, regloving, redraping, and a Basic/Minor
procedures tray.
Check specimen for instruments and sponges.

SHIRODKAR PROCEDURE

Definition

The placement of an encircling tape ligature at the
level of the internal os to maintain the integrity of the
cervical canal.

Discussion

This procedure is performed to correct the incompetent cervix during mid or later pregnancy to prevent spontaneous abortion. Incompetency is related to previous laceration or congenital weakness. The procedure is best performed before the cervix actually dilates.

Procedure

A transverse incision is made in the vaginal mucosa at its junction with the anterior aspect of the cervix. The bladder is reflected away. A similar incision is made posteriorly. A tape ligature is passed on a ligature carrier to encircle the cervix with both ends exiting in the anterior incision. The tape is tightened and sutured. The posterior portion of the tape loop may be sutured to the vaginal mucosa. The mucosal wounds are closed. Thus, a tape ligature encircles the cervix (cerclage). An alternate procedure, McDonald, may be employed, in which a suture of Mersilene (No. 4) is placed in a pursestring fashion around the four quadrants of the cervix and tied to effect competency.

Preparation of the patient

Following the administration of regional or general anesthesia, the patient is placed in lithotomy position. Arms may be extended on armboards. Apply electrosurgical dispersive pad.

Skin preparation

Extreme care must be taken to do the vaginal preparation *very gently*. Begin at the pubic symphysis and extend down over the labia. Cleanse each inner thigh. Gently cleanse vaginal vault and cervix with spongesticks (three). The perineum and anus are cleansed with the remaining sponges. Discard each sponge after wiping the anus.

Draping

Drape sheet under the buttocks, leggings, and a
    drape sheet over the abdomen

Equipment

Stirrups
Electrosurgical unit, optional

Instrumentation

Dilatation and curettage (D & C) tray
Cervical cone tray
Short Heaney retractors
Ligature carrier

Supplies

Tape ligature (e.g., 5-mm Mersilene tape)
Perineal pad
T-binder

Special notes

See Dilatation and Curettage, p. 118.

CESAREAN SECTION

Definition

Delivery of the fetus through incisions in the abdominal wall and the uterus.

Discussion

There are numerous indications for this means of delivery, including mechanical (cephalopelvic) disproportion, fetal distress, malrotation, and placenta previa. Previous cesarean section is no longer regarded as an absolute indication for this procedure.

Procedure

A low transverse or vertical incision consistent with the estimated size of the fetus is made. The rectus muscles are separated and the peritoneum incised. The bladder is reflected from the lower uterine segment and the uterus incised. The amniotic sac is entered and fluid aspirated. The fetal head is delivered using manual pressure or by obstetric forceps and counterpressure on the fundus. The newborn's airway is aspirated gently and the delivery completed. Oxytocin is usually administered intravenously. The umbilical cord is clamped and cut. The baby is transferred to the neonatal team. Hemostasis is secured and the placenta delivered. The uterine incision is closed in a single or a double layer. The previously incised peritoneum of the lower uterine segment is sutured to its anatomic position. Tubal ligation may be performed. The wound is closed in layers.

Preparation of the patient

The patient is supine; arms may be extended on armboards. Insert a Foley catheter and connect it to continuous drainage.

Skin preparation

Begin at the incision (infraumbilical vertical or low transverse) extending from nipples to midthighs, and down to the table at the sides. DO NOT prepare the vagina.

Draping

The patient is draped with folded towels and a laparotomy (or transverse) sheet. An additional sheet is needed to cover a second back table for the infant.

Equipment

Suction
Electrosurgical unit
Heat lamps and bassinet with a warmer
Identification bands (3)
Ink pad (for footprint, single use), optional

Instrumentation

Cesarean section tray
Delivery forceps
Cord clamp

Supplies

Basin set
Electrosurgical pencil
Suction tubing
Blades (2) No. 10
Bulb syringe (to aspirate infant's nose and mouth)
Test tubes, 2 (for cord blood)
Drain (e.g., Penrose) optional

Special notes

Have oxytocin, usually 20 units, ready for anesthetist to administer intravenously. This will help the uterus to contract, minimize blood loss, and aid in expulsion of the placenta.

Once the uterus is opened, immediate suctioning is necessary.

Following delivery of the infant, the cord is clamped and cut and the infant is given to the pediatrician.

Records pertaining to the birth are completed according to hospital policy.

Two newborn identification bands are put on the infant, and one newborn identification band is put on the mother (in addition to her own armband), before either mother or infant leaves the delivery room.

Cord blood is sent to the laboratory in two test tubes.

As soon as the head is delivered, the scrub person hands the bulb syringe to the surgeon to aspirate amniotic fluid from the infant's nose and mouth. The bulb syringe is passed off the table with the infant.

For prophylaxis of gonococcal or Chlamydial ophthalmia neonatorum, erythromycin 0.5% ointment, tetracycline 1% ointment, or silver nitrate 1% solution (single-use tubes or ampules) is instilled into each conjunctival sac.

Counts are taken prior to the closure of the uterus, the peritoneum, and the skin.

Chapter 12

GENITOURINARY SURGERY

HYPOSPADIAS REPAIR

Definition

Refers to the correction of a condition in which the anterior urethra terminates at some point on the ventral surface of the penis proximal to its normal position.

Discussion

This condition is a relatively common congenital anomaly. Hypospadias can be noted distally (glandular), midpenile, penoscrotal, and perineal. The ventral aspect of the penis is often shortened causing a downward curvature (chordee). When very distal, the deformity is minimal and may not require correction; proximal locations necessitate surgery to avoid difficulty in urination and coitus. Continence is usually not affected because the urinary sphincters are not involved. Circumcision should not be performed on infants with hypospadias to preserve skin useful in correcting the deformity. Correction may be delayed until full penile growth occurs.

Procedure

The chordee is repaired by lysing the fibrous tissue on the ventral aspect of the penis. The absent portion of the urethra is reconstructed out of the foreskin. In circumcised patients other tissues, for example, a segment of vein, ureter, or skin from a non-hair-bearing area such as the inner aspect of the arm, may be used. An incision is made on the ventral aspect of the penis. The reconstructed urethra, splinted from within by a catheter, is placed in a tunnel over which the remaining foreskin is grafted. Numerous procedures can be used according to the severity of the defect; some require a second stage to restore urethral continuity.

Preparation of the patient

The patient is supine with the legs apart; arms may be extended on armboards. The safety strap is replaced above the patient's knees. Children are maintained in a froglike position; care must be taken to adequately secure the child (see Pediatric General Information, p. 467) while preventing trauma to skin and pressure points. Apply electrosurgical dispersive pad (pediatric size for children).

Skin preparation

Begin cleansing the ventral surface of the penis extending from umbilicus to lower thighs, and down to the table at the sides. Cleanse rectum last (discarding sponges afterward).

Draping

Cuffed towel under the scrotum, folded towels around pubic area, and a laparotomy sheet (adults) or pediatric laparotomy sheet (children)

Equipment

Electrosurgical unit

Instrumentation

Adults:
Basic/Minor procedures tray
Urethral sounds

Infants and Children:
Pediatric minor procedures tray
Lacrimal duct probes

Supplies

Blades (2) No. 15
Needle magnet or counter
Basin set
Catheter (e.g., Foley)
Electrosurgical pencil

EPISPADIAS REPAIR

Definition

Correction of a congenital absence of the upper wall of the urethra proximal to the glans; urethra opens on the dorsal aspect of the penis.

Discussion

This deformity most often occurs at the abdomino-penile junction and can be associated with deformities of the bladder and urinary sphincter. Circumcision should not be performed on infants with epispadias to preserve skin useful in correcting the deformity. Repair is necessary to effect continence and ability to copulate.

Procedure

If a lesser deformity exists distally, the tissues are mobilized, sutured over the defect, and the meatus opened at the tip of the glans. For more proximal defects the urethra is corrected in similar fashion to that employed for hypospadias (see p. 151). A suprapubic incision is made to expose the prostatic urethra. Redundant tissue of the prostatic urethra is excised. Catgut sutures approximate the prostatic urethra and vesical neck over a probe or catheter recreating the continence mechanism. A suprapubic cystostomy is placed to provide temporary urinary diversion. The wound is closed.

Preparation of the patient, Skin preparation, Draping, Equipment, and Instrumentation

See Hypospadias Repair, p. 151.

Supplies

Blades (2) No. 15
Needle magnet or counter
Basin set
Electrosurgical pencil
Catheters, urethral: e.g., Foley
    suprapubic cystostomy: e.g., Pezzer, Malecot

CIRCUMCISION

Definition

The excision of the foreskin.

Discussion

Circumcision may be performed as a prophylactic health measure, to correct phimosis (constriction of the foreskin), to treat recurrent balanitis (inflammation of the glans penis), or as a religious rite.

Procedure

If phimosis is present a dorsal slit is made. Adhesions are lysed. A circumferential incision is made at the reflection of the foreskin which is then excised. Hemostasis is achieved and the wound approximated using absorbable suture.

Preparation of the patient, Skin preparation, Draping, and Equipment

See Hypospadias Repair, p. 151.

Instrumentation

Adults:
Limited procedure tray
Probe and grooved director

Infants and Children:
Pediatric minor procedures tray
Circumcision clamp (e.g., Gomco, Plastibell)

Supplies

Blades (2) No. 15
Electrosurgical pencil
Needle magnet or counter
Basin set
Catheter, e.g., Foley (adult)

Special notes

Consider the special needs of the Jewish patient for ritual circumcision.

PENILE IMPLANT

Definition

Insertion of a prosthesis in the penis for the treatment of impotence.

Discussion

Although the procedure permits the patient to engage in sexual intercourse, it does not treat the underlying cause. Many varieties of prostheses are available including semirigid, flexible, and dynamic (inflatable prosthesis with reservoir).

Procedure

A Foley catheter is usually inserted. If a single-rod prosthesis is used a dorsal incision is made proximal to the glans, and a tunnel is made between the corpora cavernosa. Hemostasis is achieved. Using a double-rod prosthesis requires incisions being made into a corpora cavernosa; the tunnel is dilated with a clamp and Hegar dilators. The prosthesis is inserted. When using a dynamic (inflatable) prosthesis the tunica albuginea incision is made toward the base of the penis or in the low suprapubic region. The corpora cavernosa are dilated and the prosthesis cylinders are placed. The reservoir is placed in the prevesical space and the pump is placed in the scrotum by means of subcutaneous tunnels also made through the initial incision. The wounds are closed.

Preparation of the patient

The patient is supine with legs separated; arms may be extended on armboards. Replace safety strap above the knees. Apply electrosurgical dispersive pad.

Skin preparation

Begin on the dorsum of the penis extending from umbilicus to the lower thighs, and down to the table at the sides.

Draping

Cuffed towel under the scrotum, folded towels around pubic region, and a laparotomy sheet

Equipment

Electrosurgical unit

Instrumentation

Basic/Minor procedures tray
Ruler and/or caliper
Andrews suction tip 9½"
Hegar dilators
Senn retractors (2) blunt
Metzenbaum scissors, long, 9"

Supplies

Blades (1) No. 10, (2) No. 15
Basin set
Needle magnet or counter
Electrosurgical pencil (needle tip)
Foley catheter
Dissectors (e.g., peanut)
Antibiotic solution and bulb syringe, optional
Prostheses and necessary equipment (e.g., syringes,
    needles, connectors)

Special notes

Check with the surgeon regarding the size and
type of implant.

The prosthesis should be sterilized and handled
in strict accordance with manufacturer's recommen-
dations; extra precautions must be observed to
avoid contamination of the prosthesis with lint, glove
powder, etc. to minimize foreign body reaction.

Prepackaged sterile prostheses should not be
opened until the surgeon confirms the size.

MARSHALL-MARCHETTI-KRANTZ PROCEDURE

Definition

Suspension of the bladder neck and proximal urethra to the symphysis pubis.

Discussion

This procedure is performed to correct urinary stress incontinence caused by weakness of the support of the bladder neck and proximal urethra. If there are other causes of incontinence, for example, neurologic problems, this surgery is not appropriate. Elevation of the bladder neck restores continence.

Procedure

A Pfannenstiel incision is used. After displacing the muscles, a self-retaining retractor is employed. The prevesical space of Retzius is entered. The bladder is identified and reflected from the vagina. The urethra is exposed. Sutures are placed in the paraurethral tissues, suspending them to the periosteum at the symphysis pubis. At intervals, counterpressure is applied by a gloved hand vaginally. The space of Retzius may be drained. The wound is closed in layers.

Preparation of the patient

The patient is in modified lithotomy position; arms may be extended on armboards. Apply electrosurgical dispersive pad.

Skin preparation

Begin at the incision (Pfannenstiel) extending from nipples to lower thighs, and down to the table at the sides. Follow this by a vaginal preparation beginning at the pubic symphysis and extending down over the labia. Cleanse each inner thigh. Prepare vaginal vault and cervix using spongesticks (three). The perineum and anus are prepared last, discarding each sponge after wiping the anus. A Foley catheter is inserted and connected to straight drainage.

Draping

Drape sheet under the buttocks, leggings, folded towels and a transverse sheet (abdomen)

Equipment

Stirrups
Electrosurgical unit
Suction

Instrumentation

Major procedures tray
Self-retaining retractor (e.g., Balfour)
Hemoclip appliers (assorted sizes and lengths)
Heaney needle holders

Supplies

Basin set
Blades (2) No. 10, (1) No. 15
Electrosurgical pencil
Suction tubing
Hemoclips (assorted)
Drain (e.g., Penrose or Jackson-Pratt)

Special notes

Stirrups are well padded to avoid nerve damage.

Lift both legs at the same time when putting the patient in stirrups to prevent postoperative lumbosacral strain.

Raise and lower legs slowly to prevent disturbances caused by rapid alterations in venous return.

Extra gloves are needed for the assistant who applies vaginal counterpressure.

HYDROCELECTOMY

Definition

Excision of a portion of the tunica vaginalis testis with evacuation of fluid contained therein.

Discussion

A hydrocele is an accumulation of serous fluid around the testis within the tunica vaginalis resulting from trauma or infection, or occurring spontaneously. In children indirect inguinal hernia may accompany the hydrocele.

Procedure

An inguinal or scrotal approach may be employed. In the inguinal approach the testis and spermatic cord are delivered into the inguinal wound. The hydrocele fluid is aspirated through a small incision or with a needle and syringe. Excessive sac wall is excised or may be wrapped around and sutured behind the epididymis. Hemostasis is achieved. If a hernia is present, it is repaired (see Inguinal Herniorrhaphy, p. 58, adult; p. 481, pediatric). The incision is closed.

Preparation of the patient

The patient is supine with legs apart; arms may be extended on armboards. Apply electrosurgical dispersive pad.

Skin preparation

Scrotal approach: Begin at the scrotum extending from the umbilicus to lower thighs, and down to the table at the sides.

Inguinal approach: Begin at the inguinal area on the affected side extending from the umbilicus to lower thighs, and down to the table at the sides.

Draping

Cuffed towel under the scrotum, folded towels around the pubic area, and a laparotomy sheet

Equipment

Electrosurgical unit

Instrumentation

Basic/Minor procedures tray (adult)
Pediatric minor procedures tray (child)

Supplies

Basin set
Blades (1) No. 10, (2) No. 15 (adult); (2) No. 15
    (child)
Needle magnet or counter
Penrose drain, small (retraction)
Syringe (30 ml) and needle (20 gauge)
Scrotal suspensory support (adults)

VASECTOMY

Definition

Excision of a segment of the vas deferens with ligation of the distal and proximal ends.

Discssion

The procedure is done bilaterally for the purpose of
male contraception or to prevent orchitis prior to
prostatectomy. Occasionally the vas may be multiple or absent on either side.

Procedure

The vas is palpated through the scrotum before
the anesthetic is administered. A scrotal incision is
made, the vas is seized, and it is freed of surrounding
tissue. A segment of vas is excised and the ends ligated. The severed ends may be cauterized or
crushed with a clamp prior to ligation. The severed
ends may be allowed to retract or may be buried
within the scrotal connective tissue and sutured in
place. The wound is closed. The procedure is
repeated on the other side.

Preparation of the patient

The patient is supine with legs apart; arms may be extended on armboards (or one arm may be tucked in at the side). The safety strap is fastened above the patient's knees. Apply electrosurgical dispersive pad.

Skin preparation

Begin at the scrotum extending from above the pubic symphysis to the lower thighs. Prepare perianal area last, discarding each sponge after wiping over the anus.

Draping

Folded towels and a laparotomy sheet

Equipment

Electrosurgical unit

Instrumentation

Vasectomy tray

Supplies

Electrosurgical pencil
Blade (1) No. 15
Scrotal support
Small basin

Special notes

Local anesthesia is frequently employed.

An ice pack may be applied to the scrotum immediately postoperatively.

In addition to the surgical permit a sterilization permit may be required.

VASOVASOSTOMY

Definition

Anastomosis of the severed ends of the vas deferens.

Discussion

The procedure is performed to reestablish continuity of the vas deferens in the previously vasectomized patient to restore fertility.

Procedure

A scrotal incision exposes the vas deferens above and below the site of the previous ligation. The scar tissue is excised from both ends of the vas. Under magnification sutures are placed in the mucosal lining of the lumen. The muscularis is approximated separately. The wound is closed.

Preparation of the patient, Skin preparation, and Draping

See Vasectomy, p. 161.

Equipment

Electrosurgical unit
Loupes or microscope

Instrumentation

Basic/Minor procedures tray
Vasovasostomy microscopic instruments, e.g., 1 tissue forceps, 2 curved smooth forceps, 1 curved tying forceps, 1 Castroviejo needle holder, 1 vas holder

Supplies

Basin set
Blades (1) No. 15, (1) No. 11

Electrosurgical pencil with needle tip
Scrotal support

Special notes

Check with the surgeon regarding use of loupes or microscope.
Have ice pack ready (optional).

CUTANEOUS VASOSTOMY

Definition

Establishment of an opening of the vas onto the scrotal skin.

Discussion

Cutaneous vasostomy is performed to drain an infected epididymis or testis, in which an incised loop of vas is sutured to the scrotal skin. Vasography may be done by injection of contrast media into the severed end(s). The wound or wounds usually close spontaneously after the precipitating episode subsides.

Procedure

An incision is made over the vas, which is seized and freed of surrounding tissue. The vas is divided and the severed ends are sutured to the scrotal skin.

Preparation of the patient, Skin preparation, Draping, Equipment, Instrumentation, and Supplies

See Vasectomy, p. 161.

SPERMATOCELECTOMY

Definition

Excision of a cystic swelling of the spermatic ductal system, usually at the epididymis.

Discussion

This condition is a benign cystic swelling of the sperm-conveying ductal system, usually of the epididymis. If fertility is a consideration and the excision of the cyst interrupts the duct, a side-to-side anastomosis of the epididymis and vas (epididymovasostomy) is performed to maintain continuity of the system.

Procedure

A scrotal incision is made and the pathology assessed. The cystic mass is excised. If an obvious interruption of the ductal system is created, anastomosis is performed using fine absorbable sutures with the aid of loupes or a microscope. The anastomosis may be tested for patency using a blunt needle (e.g., 20 gauge), syringe, and methylene blue dye. The incision is closed.

Preparation of the patient, Skin preparation, Draping, Equipment, Instrumentation, and Supplies

See Vasovasostomy, p. 163.

ORCHIECTOMY

Definition

Removal of one or both testicles.

Discussion

The procedure is performed for endocrine control of prostatic carcinoma, primary tumors of the testes, severe testicular trauma, or irreversible vascular compromise after testicular torsion.

Procedure

For benign disease or endocrine control the incision can be made transcrotally or inguinally. The testis is identified, the spermatic cord ligated, and the testis removed. The procedure is repeated bilaterally as indicated. For primary testicular malignancy, high ligation of the spermatic cord is done. Radical lymphadenectomy may be performed through an abdominal incision; lymph-node-bearing fatty tissues from the level of the renal vessels, and about the aorta, to the level of the transsection of the spermatic cord are removed. A testicular prosthesis may be placed at the time of orchiectomy, at a later date, or not at all.

Preparation of the patient, Skin preparation, Draping, Equipment, Instrumentation, and Supplies

See Hydrocelectomy, p. 159.

Special notes

In addition to the surgical permit, a sterilization form may be required.

CYSTOSCOPY

Definition

Endoscopic examination of the interior of the urethra, the bladder, and ureteral orifices.

Discussion

Cystoscopy is indicated for diagnosis of urinary tract symptoms (e.g., hematuria, pyuria), to catheterize the ureters, to obtain a biopsy specimen, to treat lesions, and for follow-up examination of an operative or endoscopic procedure.

Procedure

A well-lubricated cystoscope is inserted in the urethra; the urethra may be dilated initially with a sound. In the presence of a stricture the urethra is dilated with filiform sounds. The urethra is inspected as the cystoscope is advanced into the bladder. The obturator is removed and a urine specimen is obtained. The bladder is filled with irrigation fluid and under direct visualization the bladder, ureteral orifices, bladder neck, and urethra are examined. A panendoscope, a resectoscope, or a ureteral catheterizing endoscope may be required.

Preparation of the patient

The patient is usually on the cystoscopy table in the lithotomy position. Regional, general, or topical anesthesia may be employed. If a procedure in addition to cystoscopy is performed, apply electrosurgical dispersive pad.

Skin preparation

Women: See Dilatation and Curettage, p. 118.
Men: Cleanse entire pubic area including scrotum and perineum.

Draping

Leggings and a fenestrated sheet

Equipment

Extra IV standard pole for hanging irrigation fluid

Fiberoptic light source
Electrosurgical unit (available)

Instrumentation

Cystoscope (telescope, obturator, and sheath)
Fiberoptic light cord
Stopcock
Hemostat
Urethral sounds
Syringe (30 ml)
Medicine glass, syringe (10 ml), penile clamp (for topical anesthetic instillation)
Graduated pitcher (to measure residual urine)

Supplies

Topical anesthetic (e.g., lidocaine (Anestacon))
Lubricant
Irrigation solution (e.g., 2000 or 3000 ml distilled water)
Disposable cystoscopic irrigation tubing
Catheters (as requested)
Test tubes (for specimen collections)

Special notes

Well-padded knee supports avoid pressure on neurovascular structures in the popliteal space.

The scrub person prepares the instrument table; a scrub person is usually not required during the procedure.

If a procedure in addition to cystoscopy is performed the irrigation solution should be nonelectrolytic and isotonic (e.g., glycine, sorbitol).

Particular care must be taken to position patients with hip problems carefully.

Care is taken not to damage lensed telescopes and fiberoptic light cords.

For bladder fulguration a resectoscope is needed; for lithopaxy add a lithotrite and corresponding scope; for ureteral catheterization add catheterizing telescope and ureteral catheters.

Replace irrigation solution as necessary.

Instruments may be disinfected with a 2% aqueous glutaraldehyde solution (e.g., Cidex; rinse them very well).

CYSTOSTOMY

Definition

An opening is made into the bladder.

Discussion

Cystostomy is performed for purposes of urinary diversion to relieve obstruction and to "protect" the site of a more distal surgical procedure, such as a vesicourethral anastomosis. This procedure may be done independently or as an adjunct to another procedure. The procedure may be performed as a suprapubic laparotomy or percutaneously with the bladder distended.

Procedure

A low vertical or transverse incision is used. The bladder may be distended by a urethral catheter (if a catheter can be inserted). The dome of the bladder is incised and a Pezzer or Malecot catheter is inserted and secured with absorbable sutures to obtain a watertight closure. The catheter exits the main incision, or preferably a stab wound, and is secured to the skin with a stitch. The wound is closed; drainage is optional. Tube cystostomy may complement other open bladder procedures (e.g., lithotomy). A urethral catheter may be placed until the cystostomy tract matures to minimize leakage.

Preparation of the patient

The patient is supine; arms may be extended on armboards. Trendelenburg position may be requested. A suprapubic puncture approach is frequently performed under local anesthesia. Check with the surgeon regarding insertion of Foley catheter and instillation of irrigation or antiseptic fluids.

Skin preparation

Males: Begin at the suprapubic region extending from 7.5 cm (3 inches) above the umbilicus to the lower thighs, and down to the table at the sides; the genitalia are included.

Females: Begin with the vaginal preparation (see Dilatation and Curettage, p. 118) after placing patient's legs in a froglike position. Return patient's legs to supine position. Replace safety strap above knees. Proceed with abdominal preparation beginning at the suprapubic region.

Draping

Folded towels and a laparotomy sheet

Equipment

Electrosurgical unit
Suction

Instrumentation

Suprapubic Laparotomy:
Major procedures tray
Long instruments tray
Urethral sounds
Catheter stylet
Trocar (available)
Hemoclip appliers (assorted sizes and lengths)

Percutaneous Approach:
Limited procedure tray
Catheter stylet, and trocar

Supplies

Basin set
Blades (2) No. 10, (1) No. 15, (1) No. 11

Needle magnet or counter
Electrosurgical pencil
Suction tubing
Foley catheter and sealed drainage unit
Irrigation solution and syringe (e.g., 30 ml with cone
    tip)
Hemoclips (small, medium, large)
Catheter for cystostomy (e.g., Pezzer, Malecot)

Special notes

Irrigating solutions should be sterile, isotonic, and at body temperature.

The circulator may be requested to unclamp the urethral catheter when the bladder is incised.

CYSTECTOMY

Definition

Removal of the urinary bladder.

Discussion

A partial cystectomy may be performed when the lesion is localized. Total radical cystectomy is performed depending on infiltration of the lesion, evidence of metastases, and the ability of the patient to tolerate the procedure. Prior to cystectomy a urinary diversion procedure, for example, bilateral ureterosigmoidostomy, ureteroileostomy (ileal-loop) or cutaneous ureterostomy, must be performed.

This procedure is performed most often for malignancy primary to the bladder or in adjacent organs. Other indications include neurologic disorders, radiation injury, congenital defects, intractable infection, and severe trauma. When malignant disease is present the depth of infiltration, presence of metastases, and general condition of the patient will dictate the extent of the procedure. Superficial bladder lesions are treated transcystoscopically by various modalities, with radiation therapy, or by partial cystectomy. Total radical cystectomy is performed when an infiltrating lesion is restricted to the bladder and there are no distant metastases. In conjunction with cystectomy a urinary diversion procedure is performed, either a cutaneous ureterostomy or, preferably, an ileal conduit (ureteroileostomy) or a colonic conduit (ureterocolostomy). Pelvic lymphadenectomy may be performed as well.

Procedure

A midline or low transverse incision is made, the operative field explored, and the extent of the pathology assessed. The bladder is dissected from its vascular supply. The prostate and seminal vesicles are included in the specimen. The distal ureters, urethra, and vasa are divided and ligated. In the female, hysterectomy (see Total Abdominal Hysterectomy, p. 153) including the proximal vagina, urethra, and distal ureters are included in the specimen. Urinary diversion (see Ileal Conduit, p. 188) is then performed or it may have been performed prior to cystectomy. A closed-system wound drain may be employed. The wound is closed in layers.

Preparation of the patient

Males: The patient is supine; arms may be extended on armboards for a suprapubic approach.
Females: The patient is placed in lithotomy position (while the urethra and bladder are mobilized), and then the patient is moved into supine position for a suprapubic approach for the cystectomy.
Apply electrosurgical dispersive pad.

Skin preparation

Suprapubic: Begin at the suprapubic area extending from nipples to lower thighs, and down to the table at the sides.

Vaginal: Begin at the pubic symphysis and extend downward over the labia. Cleanse each inner thigh. The vaginal vault is cleansed using spongesticks (three). The perineum and anus are cleansed with remaining sponges; discard each sponge after wiping the anus.

Draping

Suprapubic approach: Folded towels and a transverse sheet
Vaginal approach: Drape sheet under the buttocks, leggings, and a laparotomy sheet

Equipment

Electrosurgical unit
Suction

Instrumentation

Suprapubic Approach:
Major procedures tray
Long instruments tray
Kidney procedures tray
Gastrointestinal procedures tray
Abdominal hysterectomy tray (available)
Self-retaining retractor (e.g., Balfour, O'Connor-O'Sullivan)
Hemoclip appliers (assorted sizes and lengths)

Vaginal Approach:
Basic/Minor procedures tray
Dilatation and curettage (D & C) tray

Supplies

Suprapubic Approach:
Basin set
Blades (2) No. 10, (1) No. 15, (1) No. 11, (1) No. 12
Needle magnet or counter

Suction tubing
Electrosurgical pencil
Dissectors (e.g., peanut)
Hemoclips (assorted sizes)
Urostomy or ileostomy pouch
Drain (e.g., Hemovac, Jackson-Pratt, Penrose)

Vaginal Approach:
Basin set
Blades (1) No. 10, (1) No. 15, (1) No. 11, (1) No. 12
Needle magnet or counter
Suction tubing
Electrosurgical pencil

Special notes

Verify with blood bank that blood ordered is available.

An automatic stapling device may be used to perform the intestinal anastomosis; it may also be used in the construction of the ileal or colonic conduit.

TRANSURETHRAL RESECTION OF THE PROSTATE (TURP) AND/OR LESIONS OF THE BLADDER OR BLADDER NECK (TURB)

Definition

Transurethral resection is the piecemeal removal of prostatic tissue and/or lesions of the bladder or bladder neck transcystoscopically.

Discussion

The procedure is particularly desirable when the patient is a poor surgical risk, thereby eliminating the need for open prostatectomy. If carcinoma is present, following histologic studies of the resected specimen, open prostatectomy may be indicated in the good-risk patient.

Procedure

The urethra may be dilated. Cystoscopy is performed to assess the hypertrophy and inspect the bladder. The resectoscope complete with sheath and obturator is passed. The irrigation tubing, fiberoptic light cord, and cautery cable are connected. The obturator is removed and the operating element with the foroblique telescope and cutting loop is inserted through the sheath. The bladder is continuously irrigated. The urethra and bladder trigone are reexamined. Electrodissection is employed to remove pieces of prostatic hypertrophied tissue. At intervals the fragments of tissue and blood clots are washed out of the bladder; the Ellik evacuator and Toomey syringe may be employed. Total removal of all fragments of tissue is desired. When resection is complete the bladder and prostatic fossa are examined for residual unattached fragments of tissue. Adequate hemostasis is ensured and the resectoscope sheath is removed. A Foley catheter (with 30-ml bag) is inserted into the bladder, filled with 5 to 10 ml of fluid, and then drawn into the prostatic fossa where an additional 12 to 25 ml of fluid is introduced to provide additional hemostasis.

Preparation of the patient

The patient is in lithotomy position on the cystoscopy table. Regional or general anesthesia may be employed. Apply electrosurgical dispersive pad.

Skin preparation

Cleanse entire pubic area including scrotum and perineum.

Equipment

Electrosurgical unit
Fiberoptic light source
IV standard for irrigation fluid

Instrumentation

Resectoscope (complete with sheath, obturator), cutting loops, operating element, foroblique telescope, rotating contact, rubber tips, electro-surgical cord
Fiberoptic light cord
Evacuator (e.g., Ellik) and basin of glycine solution
Urethral dilators
Hemostat
Strainer or screen
Various collection devices
Stopcock
Toomey syringe
Syringe, 30 ml

Supplies

Lubricant
Isotonic (nonhemolytic) irrigant (e.g., sorbitol or glycine)
Disposable irrigation system
Foley catheter with 30-ml balloon and drainage unit

Special notes

See Cystoscopy, p. 166.

OPEN PROSTATECTOMY

Definition

Excision of the prostate gland via surgical incision.

Discussion

Prostatectomy is usually performed to relieve urinary obstruction caused by benign or malignant disease. There are four approaches to prostatectomy.
1. *Transurethral prostatectomy* is performed most often; see Transurethral Resection of the Prostate, p. 174.

2. *Suprapubic prostatectomy* is performed after incising the bladder which permits correction of associated conditions such as calculi and diverticula. This procedure is not used for malignancy.
3. *Retropubic prostatectomy* avoids entry into the bladder and allows good visualization of the field. Limited malignancies may be treated by this approach.
4. *Perineal prostatectomy* affords excellent visualization and access to the prostate and seminal vesicles and is useful for radical excision of the prostate, which includes the capsule, seminal vesicles, and portions of the vasa. The approach is inadequate to perform iliac node dissection. Perineal prostatectomy may result in impotency, and possible injury to the rectum is increased.

Bilateral vasectomy (see p. 161) is usually performed in conjunction with prostatectomy to avoid retrograde infection.

Procedure

Suprapubic. The bladder is exposed through a transverse or vertical suprapubic incision. The dome of the bladder is incised, and the bladder is aspirated and explored for additional pathology. An incision is made in the bladder posteriorly over the prostate; the prostate is enucleated by finger dissection. Hemostasis is achieved. A transurethral Foley catheter is placed; a suprapubic catheter exits a stab wound incision in the bladder and abdominal wall. A drain may be placed in the prevesical space. The anterior bladder incision and the wound are closed.

Retropubic. A suprapubic incision is made; the prostate and bladder neck are exposed in the prevesical space. The prostate capsule is incised and the gland enucleated by digital dissection. Hemostasis is achieved. A Foley catheter is positioned in the urethra and the capsule is repaired. A drain may be employed. The wound is closed.

Perineal. A tractor is placed in the bladder transurethrally to displace the prostate toward the perineum; a curvilinear incision is made in the perineum. In benign disease the prostate is enucleated from its capsule. For malignancy the entire gland, its capsule, the seminal vesicle, and distal portion of the vasa are excised. Care is taken to avoid injury to the rectum. A urethrovesical anastomosis is performed after a transurethral Foley catheter is placed. The wound is drained and the incision is closed.

Preparation of the patient

Suprapubic and Retropubic: The patient is supine with the legs separated and the arms extended on armboards. Shoulder braces are required when the patient is in Trendelenburg position.

Perineal: The patient is in exaggerated lithotomy position with the knees touching the chest; arms may be extended on armboards. The buttocks are tilted and elevated (e.g., with folded bath towels). Shoulder braces are needed when the patient is in Trendelenburg position.

Apply electrosurgical dispersive pad.

Skin preparation

Suprapubic and Retropubic. Begin at the suprapubic region extending from 7.5 to 10 cm (3 to 4 inches) above the umbilicus, to the lower thighs, and down to the table at the sides. Cleanse perineum and anus last, discarding each sponge after wiping the anus.

Perineal. Begin at the suprapubic region extending from the umbilicus to the lower thighs. Cleanse perineum and anus last, discarding each sponge after wiping the anus.

Draping

Suprapubic: Cuffed towel and a sheet under the scrotum (extending to the foot of the table), folded towels and a laparotomy or transverse sheet (depending on incision)

Retropubic: Folded towels, an impervious sheet from the scrotum to the foot of the table, folded towel over the scrotum and penis (secured by towel clips), and a fenestrated sheet

Perineal: A sheet under the buttocks, leggings, towels around the perineal area, and a fenestrated drape

Equipment

Electrosurgical unit
Suction
Shoulder braces
Stirrups (for perineal approach)

Instrumentation

Major procedures tray
Long instruments tray
Open prostatectomy tray
Prostatic lobe forceps, prostatic enucleator
Boomerang suture passer
Heaney needle holders (2)
Lahey clamps (4)
Otis prostatic urethral sounds
Hemoclip appliers (assorted)

For Suprapubic Add:

Self-retaining abdominal retractor (e.g., Judd-Masson)

For Retropubic Add:

Millin retropubic bladder retractor

For Perineal Add:

Perineal prostatectomy retractors: lateral, anterior, bifurcated, and perineal self-retaining (e.g., Denis-Browne)

Supplies

Basin set
Blades (2) No. 10, (1) No. 15, (1) No. 11, (1) No. 12
Needle magnet or counter
Electrosurgical pencil
Suction tubing
Dissectors (e.g., peanut)
Hemoclips (assorted sizes and lengths)
Irrigation syringe, 30 ml with cone tip
Irrigation solution (e.g., saline)
Lubricant
Hemostatic catheter (e.g., No. 24 Foley with 30-ml
     balloon and drainage bag)
Suprapubic catheter (e.g., Malecot, Pezzer)
Penrose drain, 1"

Special notes

Bladder irrigation fluid should be sterile, isotonic, and at body temperature.

If stirrups are used in positioning, they should be well padded to avoid nerve injury.

NEPHRECTOMY

Definition

Removal of a kidney.

Discussion

This procedure is performed for numerous conditions including hydronephrosis, pyelonephritis, renal atrophy, renal artery stenosis, trauma, and tumors of the kidney and ureter. When the major portion of the ureter is also excised the procedure is termed nephroureterectomy.

Procedure

For benign disease a flank incision is made (with or without rib resection). Gerota's fascia is incised. The kidney and ureter are mobilized. The ureter is divided and the distal end ligated. The vascular pedicle is ligated. For malignant disease a radical nephrectomy is performed. A transperitoneal or anterior retroperitoneal incision is used; for large upper-pole lesions a transthoracic approach may be employed. On the right side the duodenum is protected with moistened laparotomy pads. The vascular pedicle is transsected and lymph-node-bearing tissue is excised. Gerota's fascia is dissected from surrounding tissues. The ureter is divided and the kidney and surrounding fat, adrenal gland, and fascia are removed en bloc. If tumor is present in the renal vein, the vena cava is mobilized and the tumor embolus removed. When the lower ureter is involved in the malignant process ureterectomy is included. When a flank incision is used for the nephrectomy, a secondary lower flank or inguinal incision is used to expose the distal ureter extraperitoneally. The distal ureter is dissected free of surrounding tissues and a small cuff of bladder is excised with the intramural portion of the ureter. The bladder incision is repaired, a suprapubic cystostomy catheter may be placed, and the distal ureter and bladder cuff are delivered into the flank wound and removed with the kidney. The flank incision may be closed with or without drainage. For trauma and some presentations of calculus disease involving only a portion of the kidney, a partial nephrectomy may be performed.

Preparation of the patient

The lateral position is usually the position of choice when the approach is lumbar (flank) or transthoracic; the affected side is up. The patient's waist is over the middle break in the table; the table is flexed. The arm on the unaffected side is extended on an armboard; the arm on the affected side may be supported by a Mayo stand padded with a pillow (or a double armboard may be used). The torso may be stabilized by kidney rests (larger one in front), and/or pillows or sandbags. The leg on the unaffected side is extended and the uppermost leg is flexed with a pillow between the legs; adequate padding is needed around the feet and ankles. The position is secured by wide adhesive tape at the shoulder, thighs, and legs, fastened to the underside of the table.

For the abdominal approach the patient is supine; arms may be extended on armboards. The table is in modified Trendelenburg position. The thorax on the affected side may be elevated for optimal exposure. When nephroureterectomy is performed a flank incision and a secondary lower flank or inguinal incision are employed. The patient is turned from the lateral to the supine position. Particular care is taken to protect the first incision with sponges, towels, and/or drapes. Some surgeons use a single incision extending from beneath the 12th rib to the suprapubic area. The thorax on the affected side may be elevated to achieve adequate exposure.

Skin preparation

Lateral: Begin at the level of the 12th rib extending from the axilla to 2 to 3 inches below the iliac crest, and down to the table anteriorly and posteriorly.

Abdominal: Begin at the incision extending from the axilla to the midthighs, and down to the table at the sides. *Nephroureterectomy* (second incision): carefully prepare from just below the first incision to the midthighs, and down to the table at the sides.

Draping

Nephrectomy: Folded towels and a transverse sheet

Nephroureterectomy: Folded towels, two transverse sheets, and additional drapes to cover the first (flank) incision when two incisions are used; folded towels and a transverse sheet that is cut for a single incision

Equipment

Pillows, kidney rests, etc. (for position support)
Suction
Electrosurgical unit

Instrumentation

Major procedures tray
Long instruments tray
Kidney tray
Thoracotomy tray, Vascular procedures tray, and
    Gastrointestinal procedures tray (available)
Hemoclip appliers (assorted sizes and lengths)

Supplies

Basin set
Blades (2) No. 10, (1) No. 15, (1) No. 11, (1) No. 12
Suction tubing
Needle magnet or counter
Asepto syringe
Hemoclips (assorted sizes)
Dissectors (e.g., peanut)
Penrose drains, long (2) 1" (for retraction and
    drainage)
Wound suction drain, e.g., Jackson-Pratt (available)
Chest tube and a closed chest drainage unit, e.g.,
    Pleurevac (for transthoracic approach)
Suprapubic catheter, (for nephroureterectomy) e.g.,
    Pezzer, Malecot and drainage unit

Special notes

The surgeon may request hypothermia measures (e.g., hypothermia mattress).
Have the patient's x-ray films in room.
Verify with blood bank that blood is available
as ordered.
Protect skin under adhesive tape with tincture of
benzoin.
The scrub person needs to save all perirenal fat
in a small basin of normal saline. The fat may be
used as a bolster to stop bleeding.

When two incisions are employed the patient is repositioned, reprepared, and redraped; an additional instrument tray is unnecessary.

UPPER TRACT UROLITHOTOMY (URETEROLITHOTOMY, PYELOLITHOTOMY, NEPHROLITHOTOMY)

Definition

Removal of calculi from the ureter, renal pelvis, and kidney.

Discussion

Numerous techniques are available in removing calculi from the urinary tract. If lithotriptic procedures (extracorporeal shock wave lithotripsy, ultrasonic, and other nephroscopic and transcystoscopic modalities) are unsuccessful or unavailable, or there are contraindications to these techniques, open surgery is required.

Procedure

Proximal Calculi. A flank incision is made, with rib resection (12th) optional. For stones within the renal parenchyma (nephrolithotomy), temporary interruption of the renal circulation is achieved by occluding the main vessels atraumatically. After the position of the stone is ascertained, the parenchyma incised, and the calculus removed, the kidney is repaired. Fatty tissue may be used to bolster the suture line. Stones in the renal pelvis (pyelolithotomy) or in the proximal ureter (ureterolithotomy) are extracted through incisions overlying the stones. Atraumatic clamps, tapes, or vessel loops occlude the distal ureter to prevent migration of fragments. The collecting system is irrigated and sutured closed.

Distal Calculi. Calculi in the distal ureters are

approached retroperitoneally by inguinal, lower midline abdominal, or transverse oblique incision. The stone is palpated noting that the ureter proximal to it may be dilated. Control of the ureter proximal and distal to the stone is achieved with vessel loops or atraumatic clamps. The ureter is opened and the stone retrieved. Irrigation may be employed and the ureter is closed. Drainage may be employed in any of these approaches. The wound is closed in layers.

Preparation of the patient

The position of the patient is lateral if the stone is in the kidney or proximal ureter; see Nephrectomy, p. 180. The patient is supine for stones in the distal ureter. Apply electrosurgical dispersive pad.

Skin preparation

Lateral approach: See Nephrectomy, p. 180.
Abdominal approach: Begin at the incision extending from axilla to midthighs, and down to the table at the sides.

Draping

Folded towels and a transverse sheet (for lateral or abdominal approach)

Equipment

Kidney rests, pillows, etc. (for position support)
Suction
Electrosurgical unit

Instrumentation

Major procedures tray
Long instruments tray
Kidney tray

Thoracotomy tray, Vascular procedures tray, and
    Gastrointestinal procedures tray (available)
Hemoclip appliers (assorted sizes and lengths)

Supplies

Blades (2) No. 10, (1) No. 15, (1) No. 11, (1) No. 12
Suction tubing
Electrosurgical pencil
Needle magnet or counter
Asepto syringe
Hemoclips (assorted sizes)
Vessel loops and umbilical tapes
Dissectors (e.g., peanut)
Penrose drain, 1″ (retraction)

Special notes

Have the patient's x-ray films in the room.
Have nephroscope and fiberoptic light source
available.
To facilitate calculus extraction, the surgeon
may inject a mixture of calcium chloride, thrombin,
and cryoprecipitate, which forms a "clot" around the
calculus and prevents its migration.

CUTANEOUS URETEROSTOMY

Definition

Establishment of a ureteral stoma on the abdominal
wall.

Discussion

Cutaneous ureterostomy is a form of urinary diversion performed for distal ureteral obstruction caused
by tumor, radiation injury, fibrosis, and intractable
infection. The procedure is usually temporary, later
incorporating the stoma into an ileal-loop conduit or

the anastomosing of the affected ureter to the opposite ureter (ureteroureterostomy).

Procedure

Depending on the level of the obstruction, a flank incision is made. The ureter is exposed and dissected free. The obstruction may or may not be dealt with at this time (depending on the condition of the patient). The ureter, transsected as far distally as possible, exits out a stoma site, and is matured (sutured) to the abdominal skin. A urostomy pouch is placed. The incision is closed.

Preparation of the patient

The patient is supine; arms may be extended on armboards. Apply electrosurgical dispersive pad.

Skin preparation

Begin at the incision extending from nipples to midthighs, and down to the table at the sides.

Draping

Folded towels and a laparotomy sheet

Equipment

Electrosurgical unit
Suction

Instrumentation

Major procedures tray
Long instruments tray
Self-retaining abdominal retractor (e.g., Balfour)
Hemoclip appliers (various sizes and lengths)
Iris scissors and fixation forceps (ureteroureterostomy)

Supplies

Basin set
Blades (2) No. 10, (1) No. 15, (1) No. 11, (1) No. 12
Needle magnet or counter
Suction tubing
Electrosurgical pencil
Dissectors, peanut
Hemoclips (assorted)
Splinting catheter (usually Silastic)
Urostomy pouch

Special notes

For the ureteroureterostomy anastomosis, the ureter is prepared using iris scissors and fixation forceps.

ILEAL CONDUIT

Definition

An isolated segment of ileum into which the ureters are implanted exiting as a urostomy stoma on the abdominal wall.

Discussion

This procedure is performed in conjunction with cystectomy (see p. 171). Creation of an ileal conduit has superseded ureterosigmoidostomy and cutaneous ureterostomy, avoiding the potential of ascending urinary tract infection, diarrhea, skin problems, etc. Most often the ileal segment is brought out as a urostomy stoma, but a continent pouch with a nipple valve may be constructed (Koch). In selected cases when urinary sphincter function remains intact, the ileal segment may be anastomosed as a bladder substitute to the proximal urethra, preserving urinary function. An isolated loop of the sigmoid colon may be used instead of ileum.

Procedure

See Cystectomy, p. 171. The ileal conduit may be constructed prior to or after the bladder is excised. The distal ileum is exposed; a segment (approximately 15 cm) is divided from the ileum, maintaining its mesentery. The continuity of proximal and distal ileum is reestablished. The mesentery is closed over the intervening mesentery of the isolated loop to avoid internal herniation. The proximal end of the isolated loop is closed. The ureters are dissected and anastomosed to the ileal loop. The distal end of the ileal loop is brought out to the stoma site (right lower quadrant of the abdomen). The stoma is sutured to the skin and a urostomy pouch is applied. The abdominal wound is closed. Drainage is optional. Stapling devices may be employed to perform the intestinal anastomoses and closure of the proximal end of the isolated loop.

Preparation of the patient

The patient is supine; arms may be extended on armboards. Apply electrosurgical dispersive pad.

Skin preparation

Begin cleansing at the incision (check with the surgeon). Extend preparation from the nipples to midthighs, and to the table at the sides.

Draping

Folded towels and a laparotomy sheet

Equipment

Electrosurgical unit
Suction

Instrumentation

Major procedures tray

Gastrointestinal procedures tray
Long instruments tray
Self-retaining abdominal retractor (e.g., Balfour)
Hemoclip appliers (assorted sizes and lengths)
Ruler
Automatic stapling device, optional

Supplies

Basin set
Blades (2) No. 10, (1) No. 15, (1) No. 11, (1) No. 12
Needle magnet
Suction tubing
Electrosurgical pencil
Dissectors (e.g., peanut)
Hemoclips
Ureteral stent (e.g., Silastic ureteral catheter)
Urostomy pouch
Staples, optional
Drain (e.g., Penrose), optional

ADRENALECTOMY

Definition

Excision of either or both of the adrenal glands.

Discussion

This procedure is done to excise primary tumors of
the adrenals, benign or malignant (usually unilaterally), or for purposes of modifying an endocrine-
dependent tumor, as in breast or prostatic malignancy. During the entire perioperative period corticosteroid replacement must be administered. Small
fragments of the adrenal cortex may be implanted
in the patient's thigh musculature so that some glandular function is preserved.

Adrenalectomy can be performed employing
an anterior or posterior approach. The posterior approach is less traumatic to the patient, but does not

permit exploration of the abdomen, concomitant oophorectomy when indicated, or other coincidental intra-abdominal procedures. The anterior approach also affords the opportunity to search for ectopic adrenal tissues.

Procedure

Posterior Approach. The patient may be in the lateral position if unilateral adrenalectomy is performed. For bilateral adrenalectomy the patient is prone. An incision is made from the lower ribs (the 12th rib is resected after the muscles are separated) to the posterior iliac crest. The fascia is incised and Gerota's capsule exposed. The adrenal gland is identified and excised taking care not to injure the kidney. The left adrenal vein is divided from the renal vein, and the right adrenal vein is divided from the inferior vena cava. Careful hemostasis of the fragile vasculature is required; clips may be employed. The incision is closed in layers. If the pleura was entered, drainage may be necessary.

Anterior Approach. An upper abdominal longitudinal incision is made. The peritoneal cavity is explored and additional procedures are performed as indicated. The retroperitoneal space is entered on the right after reflecting the duodenum, and on the left through the lesser sac. Precautions are taken to assure that hemostasis is maintained, as noted above. The adrenal gland (one or both) is excised and the wound is closed in layers.

Preparation of the patient

The patient is in the lateral position with the affected side up for unilateral adrenalectomy.

For bilateral adrenalectomy, the abdominal or posterior approach may be employed. For the abdominal approach the patient is supine; arms may be extended on armboards. For the less frequently employed posterior approach, the patient is prone. Following insertion of an intravenous line and endotracheal intubation (while the patient is on the gurney), the patient is carefully rolled over to the prone position onto the table. The arms are extended on armboards angled toward the head of the table with the hands pronated. Chest rolls are placed under the patient from the acromioclavicular joint to the level of the iliac crests to facilitate breathing. Female breasts and male genitalia are protected. A pillow(s) is placed in front of the ankles. Pads may be placed under the elbows and knees. The safety strap is secured across the patient's thighs.

Skin preparation

Lateral position: Begin cleansing at approximately the level of the 12th rib extending from the axilla to 5 to 7.5 cm (2 to 3 inches) below the iliac crest, and down to the table at the sides.

Abdominal approach: Begin cleansing for a right paramedian incision extending from the axilla to midthighs, and down to the table at the sides.

Prone position: Begin cleansing for bilateral curvilinear incisions which begin at the level of the 10th rib and extend to the superior border of the iliac crests. Prepare from the axilla to the upper thighs, and down to the table at the sides.

Draping

Folded towels and a laparotomy sheet (for lateral or abdominal)
Folded towels and a transverse sheet that may be cut to accommodate the incisions (for prone)

Equipment

Pillows, kidney rests, etc. (for positioning)
Electrosurgical unit
Suction

Instrumentation

Major procedures tray
Long instruments tray and Kidney tray

Thoracotomy tray, Vascular procedures tray, and
    Gastrointestinal procedures tray (available)
Hemoclip appliers (assorted sizes and lengths)

Supplies

Basin set
Blades (2) No. 10, (1) No. 15, (1) No. 11, (1) No. 12
Suction tubing
Electrosurgical pencil
Needle magnet or counter
Asepto syringe
Dissectors (e.g., peanut)
Penrose drain, 1" (for retraction)
Hemoclips (assorted), optional

Special notes

Ask the surgeon which approach will be used.

Check with the surgeon and anesthetist regarding need for vasodilating drugs such as phen-
tolamine.

Hormones such as hydrocortisone may be requested.

EXTRACORPOREAL SHOCK WAVE
LITHOTRIPSY (ESWL)

Definition

Disintegration of upper urinary tract calculi by
means of precisely directed shock waves delivered
to the patient immersed in a water bath.

Discussion

The ESWL unit (e.g., Dornier HM3) makes possible
the removal of most upper urinary tract calculi without surgery. Multiple shock waves produced by an
electrode beneath the immersed patient pass from
the water into the body pulverizing the calculus into
sandlike particles that are eliminated in the urine.

The shock waves selectively fragment the stone, which is of a higher density than the surrounding area, thus sparing significant injury to soft tissues and bone, which are more resilient.

A modular lithotripter developed by the manufacturers of the currently employed ESWL system has recently become available. The new lithotripter (Dornier HM4) does not require immersion of the patient. This bath-free unit employs a self-contained water cushion that couples to the patient's body. Patient positioning is achieved by a computer-controlled guidance system that permits focus on the calculus with an even greater degree of accuracy than the existing system. This precision positioning with placement of the x-ray source beneath the treatment table and actuation of the triggering mechanism by the ECG and respiratory motion may decrease the number of shock waves required and reduces radiation exposure to the patient and staff. Sedation of the patient without need for anesthesia is an additional advantage of this newer modification.

Procedure

The patient is safety-strapped onto the "gantry" stretcher, which is then lowered into the immersion tub; the water level should be approximately 5 cm (2 inches) below the overflow outlet. Image intensifiers on either side of the patient are rotated into place. X-ray "window" balloons are inflated to improve the quality of the image (there being less distortion of the beam through air as compared with water). The physician positions the stone on the crosshairs of both monitors by adjusting the gantry. The previously placed waterproofed ECG leads are double-checked noting that the release of the shock waves must appropriately coincide with the cardiac cycle to avoid arrhythmias. The shock waves are then released at the physician's discretion. The patient is repositioned as necessary to maintain the calculus in the crosshairs of the monitors as it is being disintegrated. The voltage is read continuously and altered to change the intensity of the shocks. The total number of shock waves required depends on the size, composition, and location of the calculus, as well as the physique of the patient. Stones begin to fragment after 1200 (sometimes fewer) shocks have been delivered; 2400 shocks is generally considered the maximum dose.

For calculi located in the proximal portion of the ureter (superior to the pelvic brim), the surgeon may attempt to reposition the calculus back into the kidney (renal pelvis) in order to achieve the maximum effect of ESWL. Transcystoscopically under fluoroscopic control, a ureteral catheter is positioned in the ureter immediately distal to the calculus. The ureter is then filled with a lidocaine mixture (e.g., 2% Xylocaine jelly and sterile water 3:1). If the calculus cannot be repositioned into the renal pelvis, the physician may elect to perform ESWL with the stone in the ureter. In that case, two or three additional ureteral catheters may be positioned beside the stone and just distal to the stone to prevent its premature passage while still intact, thereby preventing possibly injury to the ureter. The ESWL procedure is then performed. Alternatively, the physician may try to shatter the calculus using ultrasonic lithotripsy transureteroscopically (see Ultrasonic Lithotripsy, p. 199).

Preparation of the patient

The ESWL procedure may be performed under general or block (spinal, epidural) anesthesia. The patient may be prepared in an anesthesia holding area or the ESWL room. If cystoscopy or ureteroscopy precedes ESWL the patient may be anesthetized in the cystoscopy room. Following the administration of anesthesia the patient is transferred to the gantry stretcher and strapped in for safety and to counter the effects of buoyancy.

Skin preparation

None is required. Following the immersion of the patient in the tub, the circulator wipes his or her

hand along the skin surface area overlying the affected kidney to release air bubbles that could accumulate, thereby reducing the efficiency of the
shock waves.

Draping

None required.

Equipment

If cystoscopy, retrograde pyelography, or ureteroscopy are performed prior to ESWL:
   X-ray cassettes
   Fiberoptic light source for cystoscope
   Extra IV standards for irrigation fluid
Dornier ESWL System components:
   1. Special tub and frame
   2. Localization system
      a. X-ray generator, high-voltage generator,
         control cabinet
      b. Control panel
      c. Two x-ray tube housing assemblies (under
         tub)
      d. Two image intensifiers
      e. Two TV monitors
   3. Shock wave generation unit
      a. Capacitor charging unit
      b. Pulse generator
      c. Shock wave generator
      d. ECG trigger unit
      e. Ellipsoid reflector
      f. Underwater electrode
   4. Patient positioning unit
      Guideway and gantry stretcher
   5. Hydraulic supply system
      a. Suspended telescopic cylinder (vertical)
      b. Two cylinders (horizontal)
      c. Hydraulic supply unit
      d. Accumulator
   6. Water treatment system
   7. Control cabinet

Supplies

When cystoscopy, retrograde pyelography, or ureteroscopy precedes ESWL:

    Specimen bottles, culture tubes
    Ureteral catheters and adaptors (to attach to drainage system)
    Lubricant
    Foley catheters

For ESWL:

    Underwater electrode
    X-ray cassettes

Instrumentation

None required for ESWL.

Cystoscope, ureteroscope, ultrasonic wand (see Ultrasonic Lithotripsy, p. 199) may be requested prior to ESWL procedure.

ESWL Unit Use Procedure
1. Patient data recorded
2. Gantry stretcher adjusted without patient
3. Patient placed and secured on gantry stretcher
4. Gantry stretcher adjusted with patient
5. Patient prepared (reiterate to the patient what will be happening)
6. Gantry stretcher and patient moved into tub
7. Image intensifiers swung into place with balloons inflated
8. X-ray unit adjusted
9. Monitors adjusted
10. ECG triggering unit adjusted
11. Kidney stone located
12. X-ray window ventilated
13. Capacitor charging unit adjusted
14. Shock waves released
15. Shock circuit switched off
16. Image intensifiers moved backward and swung out
17. Patient lifted out of tub

18. Water drained
19. Used electrode removed, new electrode inserted
20. Tub cleaned and disinfected

Special notes

A lithotripter supervisor is essential to the well-run lithotripsy unit. The supervisor is responsible for checking and preparing the lithotripsy equipment and assisting the physician and the anesthetist.

It is absolutely essential for the circulator working with the lithotripsy patient to be thoroughly familiar with the ESWL unit.

The epidural catheter (if used) needs to be protected in the water bath. A partially split $2'' \times 2''$ sponge may be placed at the base of the catheter. The catheter tubing may then be protected by a sterile, plastic adhesive drape which seals it from the water.

Care is required in positioning the patient on the gantry stretcher to avoid undue pressure, particularly on the limbs.

The water temperature of the tub should be maintained at 36°C (97°F). Temperatures below 35°C (95°F) or above 37°C (99°F) should be adjusted.

X-ray balloons ("windows") must be inflated when x-rays are taken and are usually deflated when radiography is completed.

Lead aprons are worn by personnel when x-rays are taken.

The underwater electrode generally needs to be replaced after every 700 to 800 shocks. The plastic sleeve must be removed from the electrode; if the generator is moved forward with plastic sleeve, the mechanism will be damaged.

Towels and blankets are kept in a warmer to dry and cover the patient following emersion from the tub.

Additional charting information is required for the operative procedure report including:

Water temperature

Shock wave voltage
Electrode series
Total number of shock waves delivered
Fluoroscopy time

ULTRASONIC LITHOTRIPSY

Definition

Disintegration of urinary tract calculi located in the ureter by means of ultrasonic waves delivered by a probe inserted transureteroscopically.

Discussion

The ultrasonic lithotripter generates ultrasonic waves that shatter a calculus within the ureter. The pulverized particles are eliminated in the urine. This procedure may be extended to include stones in the renal pelvis which are approached by percutaneous nephrostomy. Extracorporeal shock wave lithotripsy (ESWL) is the preferred method for disintegration of stones in the renal pelvis when applicable.

Procedure

Cystoscopy is performed, and a guidewire is passed into the affected ureter. Under fluoroscopic control a ureteroscope is passed into the ureter over the guidewire. It may be necessary to dilate the ureter using graduated-sized catheters or a dilating pressure balloon catheter. Once the ureter is sufficiently dilated the ureteroscope is passed over the guidewire. The ultrasonic wand is passed through the ureteroscope, and the stone is either shattered or dislodged by ultrasonic waves and removed by suction.

Preparation of the patient, Skin preparation, and Draping

See Cystoscopy, p. 166.

Equipment

Ultrasonic lithotripter unit, foot switch and power cord
Fiberoptic light source for cystoscope
Extra IV standard for irrigation fluid

Instrumentation

Cystoscopy instruments including light cord
Ureteroscope, light cord, alligator forceps
Ultrasonic wand
Bridge adaptor (accommodates ultrasonic wand)

Supplies

Surgical jelly lubricant
Irrigating solution
Suction tubing
Disposable irrigation system
Coated movable core guidewire (e.g., .035″ × 150 cm)
Ureteral catheters and adaptors to connect to drainage
Xylocaine jelly, 2%
Foley catheter and drainage unit
Syringe, 10 ml
Test tubes for specimen collection
Ureteral stent (e.g., double-J stent to avoid obstruction from large calculi)

Special notes

Connect suction to lithotripter wand.
Irrigating solution may be water, normal saline, or lactated Ringer's solution.

ELECTROHYDRAULIC LITHOTRIPSY

Definition

Fragmentation of urinary tract calculi found in the

bladder by means of electrohydraulic shock waves delivered by a probe inserted transcystoscopically.

Discussion

An electrohydraulic lithotripter releases a series of high-voltage sparks that when placed in a 0.15% (or ⅙ normal) saline solution produce a series of sharp, high-amplitude shock waves that crack and fragment the bladder calculi. The fragments may then be eliminated in the urine. These shock waves have no adverse effect on tissue because of tissue flexibility. Only a few surgeons have extended this procedure to include ureteral stones.

Procedure

Cystoscopy is performed. The electrohydraulic lithotripter probe is passed through the cystoscope so that the electrode tip lies 1 to 2 mm from the calculus and 1 to 2 mm from the tip of the cystoscope. The stone is then cracked and fragmented by the hydraulic shock waves.

Preparation of the patient, Skin preparation, and Draping

See Cystoscopy, p. 166.

Equipment

Electrohydraulic lithotripter unit, power cord, foot switch, cable
Fiberoptic light source for cystoscope
Extra IV standard for irrigation fluid

Instrumentation

Cystoscopy instruments including fiberoptic light cord (see Cystoscopy, p. 166)
Extender cable
Disposable probes

Alligator forceps, Wappler forceps, Ellik evacuator,
Toomey syringe (for fragments)

Supplies

Lubricant
Irrigation solution 0.15% (⅙ normal) saline
Disposable irrigation system
Foley catheter and drainage unit

Special notes

Do not reuse electrode.

Sterilize lithotripter extender cable with ethylene oxide gas *only*.

Do not use the electrohydraulic lithotripter on any patient with a pacemaker.

The surgeon may request the irrigating solution to be kept at room temperature.

The irrigating solution of 0.15% (⅙ normal) saline may be prepared in the operating room by adding 500 ml of normal saline to a 3-liter bag of sterile distilled water from which 500 ml have been discarded. Alternatively, 6 ml of concentrated sodium chloride solution (23.4%) can be added to each liter of sterile water.

Chapter 13

THORACIC PROCEDURES

BRONCHOSCOPY

Definition

Endoscopic visualization of the trachea, main bronchi and their openings, and most of the segmental bronchi.

Discussion

This procedure is performed for aspiration of secretions, biopsy, or removal of a foreign object. Rigid and flexible fiberoptic bronchoscopes are used. An advantage of the flexible scope is that more peripheral subdivisions may be inspected, but foreign objects and copious, viscid mucus cannot be removed through its lumen.

Procedure

Rigid. The head is lowered and a well-lubricated scope is inserted into the mouth. The epiglottis is elevated with the tip of the bronchoscope, and the scope is passed into the trachea. The scope is advanced into the bronchi. Bronchoscopy washings, biopsy, etc. may be obtained. A foreign body may be removed. Laser may be employed; see Appendix, p. 572 for precautions. The patient is well suctioned and the scope is removed slowly.

Flexible. Following intubation, the well-lubricated bronchoscope is inserted through the adaptor into the endotracheal tube (secured by the anesthetist) and advanced as necessary. Bronchoscopy washings, biopsy taken with forceps or brush, etc. may be obtained. The patient is well suctioned and the scope is removed slowly.

Preparation of the patient

General anesthesia: The patient is supine; anesthetist moves to the patient's side and the surgeon is at the head of the table. The patient's shoulders are just above the top break in the table so that the head may be lowered.

Topical anesthesia: The patient is usually sitting up at the edge of the table facing the surgeon while the circulator or the scrub person helps support patient from behind. (A footstool is needed).

Skin preparation

None.

Draping

The patient may be covered with a drape sheet. A drape sheet covers the back table. Gloves are worn.

Equipment

Suction
Fiberoptic light source (scope)
Footstool (for patient during topical anesthesia)
Fiberoptic headlight and light source

Topical Anesthesia. Topical anesthetic tray on a Mayo stand. Have available:

Laryngeal mirrors
Lingual spatula
Anesthetic spray
Laryngeal syringe with straight and curved cannulas
Medicine cups (for drugs of preference)
Emesis basin
Luer-lock syringe, 10 ml with 22-gauge needle
Tissues

Instrumentation and supplies

Rigid Bronchoscopy:

Rigid fiberoptic bronchoscope (check size)
Endotracheal adaptor (for anesthetist)
Fiberoptic telescope
Fiberoptic light cords (2)
Suction cannulas
Suction tubing
Specimen collectors (e.g., Lukens tubes)
Sponge carriers (2) (loaded with bronchoscopy sponges)
Biopsy forceps
Grasping forceps
Lubricant
Bronchoscopy sponges
Small basin with sterile saline and syringe (for washings)
Telfa and 25-gauge needle (for removing specimen)
Laser may be employed; see Appendix, p. 572 for precautions

Flexible Bronchoscopy:

Flexible fiberoptic bronchoscope
Endotracheal adaptor (for anesthetist)
Fiberoptic light cord
Biopsy forceps
Brush (and slides and alcohol to collect specimen)

Culture jar for biopsy specimen

Small basin with sterile saline and syringe (for washings)

Suction tubing

Specimen collectors (e.g., Lukens tubes)

Lubricant

Telfa and 25-gauge needle (for removing specimen)

Special notes

Prior to the procedure be certain there is an endotracheal adaptor for the anesthetist.

Antifogging solution may be applied to the lens before use and wiped off to prevent fogging (e.g., Ultrastop, pHisoHex).

Room lights may be turned off and x-ray view boxes turned on.

The patient's upper lip and teeth may be protected with a plastic mouth guard or a damp sponge.

Have a sitting stool for the surgeon.

Hold specimen collector upright and pinch off suction tubing after specimen is obtained or it will be aspirated into the suction unit.

Keep syringe filled with saline ready for washings.

Pass biopsy forceps with tips closed.

Guide forceps and other instruments into the scope as necessary.

Take care not to crush specimens; use a needle only to remove a specimen and place it on Telfa.

Specimens must be dispatched promptly.

MEDIASTINOSCOPY

Definition

Endoscopic visualization of the mediastinum (tracheobroncheal junction, bronchi, aortic arch, and regional lymph nodes).

Discussion

This procedure is performed when a malignancy is suspected. Tissue may be biopsied.

Procedure

A transverse incision is made over the suprasternal notch and extended down to the pretracheal fascia. Hemostasis is achieved. Using blunt dissection the superior mediastinum is entered. The scope is passed. Care is taken to avoid injury to nearby blood vessels. Lymph node tissue may be biopsied. Needle aspiration is employed to identify a nonvascular structure. A specimen may be obtained using biopsy forceps. Hemostasis is achieved. The scope is removed and the wound is closed.

Preparation of the patient

General anesthesia is administered and an endotracheal tube is inserted. The patient is supine with the neck extended by a rolled towel under the shoulders. The anesthetist moves to the patient's side and the surgeon operates at the head of the table. Apply electrosurgical dispersive pad.

Skin preparation

Begin at the suprasternal notch; include the entire neck and shoulders down to the table, extending from chin to nipples.

Draping

Folded towels and a sheet with a small fenestration

Equipment

Electrosurgical unit
Suction
Fiberoptic light source

Instrumentation

Mediastinoscopy tray

Supplies

Basin set
Blade (1) No. 15
Telfa and 22-gauge needle (for specimen removal)

Special notes

Approach is both endoscopic and surgical.

A sponge count is taken before the scope is removed and at closure of the wound.

Remove specimen from biopsy forceps with a needle only to avoid damage to cells.

SEGMENTAL RESECTION OF THE LUNG

Definition

Excision of anatomic subdivisions of the pulmonary lobes; only segments containing diseased tissue are removed (lesion must have a segmental distribution).

Discussion

Indications for this procedure include bronchiectasis, cysts or blebs, benign or metastatic tumors, and tuberculosis.

Procedure

The affected lung is exposed through a posterolateral incision. The diseased segment is identified. The visceral pleura is dissected free from blood vessels and bronchi of the appropriate bronchopulmonary segment. The segmental pulmonary vein and segmental branches of the pulmonary artery are ligated. The segmental bronchus is isolated, doubly clamped, and transsected; suctioning of the area prior to clamping prevents blood and fluid from entering the unaffected lung. The bronchial stump is sutured or stapled. The suture line is tested for air leaks. The pleural space is irrigated. Hemostasis is achieved. A chest tube (one or more) is inserted. The wound is closed in layers. The chest tube is connected to a sealed drainage unit.

Preparation of the patient

The patient is usually in the lateral position with the affected side uppermost. The arm on the unaffected side is positioned on an armboard, and the arm on the affected side is supported by a Mayo stand padded by a pillow (or a double armboard may be used). The torso may be stabilized by kidney rests, and/or pillows or sandbags. The leg on the unaffected side is extended and the leg on the affected side is flexed, with a pillow between the legs and adequate padding around the feet and ankles. The position is secured by wide adhesive tape at the shoulder, hip, and legs anchored to the underside of the table. Slanting the upper section of the table downward encourages drainage to the trachea. Check with the surgeon regarding insertion of a Foley catheter. Apply electrosurgical dispersive pad.

Skin preparation

Begin cleansing for a posterolateral incision extending from the shoulder and arm to the iliac crest, and down to the table anteriorly and posteriorly.

Draping

Folded towels and a transverse sheet (a sterile, adhesive plastic drape and drape sheets may be requested)

Equipment

Electrosurgical unit
Suction

Fiberoptic light source (if headlight is used)
Scale (to weigh sponges)

Instrumentation

Major procedures tray
Thoracotomy tray
Vascular procedures tray
Hemoclip appliers, assorted sizes, long-handled
Long Pean clamps
Stapling devices, optional
Cushing vein retractors

Supplies

Basin set
Suction tubing
Electrosurgical pencils (2)
Needle magnet or counter
Blades (3) No. 10, (1) No. 15
Dissectors (e.g., peanut)
Asepto syringes (2)
Magnetic instrument pad, optional
Staples, optional
Hemoclips (assorted sizes)
Vessel loops, umbilical tapes
Chest drainage tube(s) (e.g., Argyle)
Connector, e.g., straight or large Y (if 2 tubes are
    used)
Sealed drainage unit (e.g., Pleurevac)

Special notes

Have the patient's x-ray films in the room.
Ascertain that blood is available as ordered.
Have second suction immediately available.
Weigh sponges.
Keep accurate record of irrigation fluid used.
Protective goggles may be worn.

WEDGE RESECTION OF THE LUNG

Definition

Excision of a small wedge-shaped section from the periphery of the lung.

Discussion

This procedure is performed to remove a benign lesion.

Procedure

The affected lung is usually exposed through a posterolateral thoracotomy. The lesion is identified. A wedge of peripheral lung tissue containing the lesion is excised over clamps (a linear stapler may be used). The lung tissue held in the clamps is sutured. The suture line is tested for air leaks. Additional sutures may be required to achieve hemostasis and check air leaks. A chest tube is inserted. The wound is closed in layers. The chest tube is connected to a sealed drainage unit.

Preparation of the patient, Skin preparation, Draping, Equipment, Instrumentation, Supplies, and Special Notes

See Segmental Resection of the Lung, p. 208.

PULMONARY LOBECTOMY

Definition

Excision of one or more lobes of the lung.

Discussion

This procedure is usually performed when the lesion is limited to the lobe.

Procedure

The affected lung is exposed through a postero-lateral incision. The diseased lobe is identified. The visceral pleura is dissected free from the hilus. The pulmonary artery and vein of the diseased lobe are ligated and divided. The bronchus is isolated, doubly clamped, and transsected; suctioning of the area prior to clamping prevents blood and fluid from entering the nonaffected space. The bronchial stump is sutured; more frequently a stapling device may be employed. The suture line is tested for air leaks. The pleural cavity is irrigated. Hemostasis is achieved. Chest tubes are inserted. The chest is closed in layers. Chest tubes are connected to a sealed drainage unit.

Preparation of the patient, Skin preparation, Draping, Equipment, Instrumentation, Supplies, and Special Notes

See Segmental Resection of the Lung, p. 208.

PNEUMONECTOMY

Definition

Removal of the lung.

Discussion

The chief indication for pneumonectomy is bronchogenic carcinoma; among other indications are extensive unilateral tuberculosis, some benign tumors, bronchiectasis, and multiple lung abscesses. At the completion of this procedure, the affected pleural cavity is empty and the mediastinal structures are liable to shift position causing central circulatory compromise. Special measures may be employed to stabilize the mediastinum at the end of the procedure.

Procedure

The affected lung is exposed through a postero-lateral thoracotomy. The chest is explored and the feasibility of the procedure is determined. Advanced metastases contraindicate resection, in which case chest tubes are inserted, the wound is closed, and chest tubes are connected to a sealed drainage unit. The mediastinal pleura is dissected free. The bronchus, pulmonary artery, and superior and inferior pulmonary veins are isolated. Care is taken to avoid injury to the vagus nerve. The pulmonary artery and veins are ligated. The bronchial stump is clamped, transsected, and sutured or stapled; suctioning prevents blood and fluid from entering the unaffected lung. Lymph-node-bearing tissues are excised as necessary. Hemostasis is achieved. The chest is closed in interrupted layers.

Preparation of the patient, Skin preparation, Draping, Equipment, Instrumentation, Supplies, and Special Notes

See Segmental Resection of the Lung, p. 208.

Special notes

Ask the surgeon if a chest tube or large syringe with a large bore needle will be necessary postoperatively to create a slightly negative pressure in the affected pleural space and stabilize the mediastinum.

DECORTICATION OF THE LUNG

Definition

The stripping of a restrictive membrane on the visceral pleura that interferes with respiration.

Discussion

Some indications for decortication of the lung are chronic empyema, clotted hemothorax, and tuberculosis.

Procedure

The affected lung is exposed through a posterolateral incision; rib resection may be indicated for adequate exposure. The fibrous membrane is carefully peeled away from the visceral pleura. Hemostasis may be difficult. Chest tubes are inserted. The wound is closed in layers. Chest tubes are connected to a sealed drainage unit.

Preparation of the patient, Skin preparation, Draping, Equipment, Instrumentation, Supplies, and Special Notes

See Segmental Resection of the Lung, p. 208.

INSERTION OF TRANSVENOUS ENDOCARDIAL PACEMAKER

Definition

Placing of an electrode lead in the endocardium through the cephalic, subclavian, or jugular vein and attaching the lead to a pulse generator.

Discussion

Permanent pacemakers are necessary when heart block exists.

Types

Asynchronous. Stimulates ventricular contraction when a specified rate of pacing is required.
Demand. Initiates ventricular contraction only when the heart rate falls below a preset rate.

Physiologic. Synchronizes atrial and ventricular activity to improve cardiodynamics.

Procedure

A cutdown is performed to expose the subclavian, cephalic, or external jugular vein; the right side is preferred. Through a venotomy a pacing electrode is inserted and advanced (under fluoroscopy) into the right ventricle. The electrode is attached to an external pacemaker for testing. An incision is made in the chest wall and deepened down to the fascia, creating a "pocket" for the pulse generator. A tunneling instrument is used to make a path for the electrode which is attached to the pulse generator. The pulse generator is placed in the "pocket." Both incisions may be irrigated with antibiotic solution and closed.

Preparation of the patient

The patient is supine; the head may be turned to the left. Usually the left arm is restrained at the side (check pressure point at the elbow) and the right arm is extended on an arm table. The procedure is often performed under local anesthesia. The patient is monitored continuously. An anesthetist is usually present. Apply electrosurgical dispersive pad.

Skin preparation

Begin cleansing the right chest, including right axilla, shoulder, and arm to the elbow. Extend preparation from chin to lower ribs; prepare well beyond the midline on the left border, and down to the table on the right side.

Draping

The hand is grasped in a tube or an impervious stockinette. A large sheet is draped over the hand table and tucked under the shoulder. Folded towels and a fenestrated sheet or individual drape sheets complete the draping.

Equipment

Electrosurgical unit
Hand table
Image intensifier and C-arm (x-ray department)
External pacemaker

Instrumentation

Pacemaker tray
Hemoclip appliers (small and medium)

Supplies

Basin set
Tube or impervious stockinette
Blades (2) No. 10, (1) No. 15, (1) No. 11
Needle magnet or counter
Electrosurgical pencil
Local syringe and needle (e.g., 10-ml control syringe, 25-gauge, 1½" needle)
Vessel loops
Antiobiotic irrigation and bulb syringe, optional

Special notes

Lead aprons are worn for protection during fluoroscopy.

Make the patient as comfortable as possible because the procedure may be lengthy.

Check with the surgeon regarding availability of the generator and leads (usually brought by a pacemaker company representative).

X-ray equipment can be set up in the room on the patient's left side.

The scrub person positions the back table on the patient's right side and assists the surgeon side-to-side.

Complete forms from the manufacturer. Chart serial numbers.

CORRECTION OF PECTUS EXCAVATUM

Definition

The correction of pectus excavatum, or funnel chest, refers to the straightening of a deformity of the anterior chest wall in which there is a depression of the sternum and costal cartilages.

Discussion

This procedure may be performed to alleviate circulatory or respiratory symptoms, although it is most frequently performed for cosmetic reasons. Variations of the procedure are performed according to the extent of the deformity. The patient is often a child.

Procedure

Approach is through a vertical presternal incision. The origins of the pectoral muscles are reflected. Rib cartilages are separated from the sternum. The xiphoid process is transsected from the sternum. An incision is made into the anterior mediastinum, and the pericardium is dissected from the sternum. According to the extent of the deformity, the sternum is reshaped by a wedge-shaped osteotomy, or reversed, and the sternum and costal cartilages are trimmed as necessary. The sternum is fixed in place with sutures. Previously detached muscles are resutured to their points of division. Drains are placed, or chest tubes are inserted if the pleural cavity has been entered. The wound is closed. Chest tubes, if used, are attached to a sealed drainage unit.

Preparation of the patient

The patient is supine and the chest is slightly elevated, for example, with a rolled sheet. Arms may be extended on armboards. Apply electrosurgical dispersive pad.

Skin preparation

Begin at the midline, extend from the chin, to below the umbilicus, and down to the table at the sides.

Draping

Folded towels and a laparotomy sheet

Equipment

Electrosurgical unit
Suction
Power source for saw (e.g., Stryker)

Instrumentation

Minor orthopedic procedures tray
Bone holding instruments tray
Thoracotomy tray and Vascular procedures tray
    (available)
Gigli saw set
Power saw, e.g., Stryker (with circular blade)
Lebsche sternal knife
Bone tenacula (2) single-hook
Awl with fenestration
Pliers

Supplies

Basin set
Blades (2) No. 10, (1) No. 15
Electrosurgical pencil
Suction tubing
Needle magnet or counter
Bone wax
Drains, optional

Special notes

Children require padded extremity restraints, smaller drapes and instruments, etc.; see p. 467 for Pediatric General Information.

THYMECTOMY

Definition

Removal of the thymus gland.

Discussion

This surgery is performed in an attempt to alleviate myasthenia gravis or to remove benign or malignant tumors. The thymus gland is largest in infancy and atrophies in adulthood.

When thymectomy is performed to treat myasthenia gravis the possibility of respiratory compromise must be anticipated. Prolonged endotracheal intubation or a tracheostomy may be necessary with the concomitant administration of neostigmine methyl sulfate (Prostigmin).

Procedure

Approach is usually through a sternal splitting incision. The mediastinal fat pad is incised and the thymus gland dissected from it and the underlying pericardium. Vascular attachments are ligated. Care is taken to avoid the great vessels and the parathyroid glands. Hemostasis is achieved. A drain may be inserted. If either pleural space has been entered, chest tube(s) and a sealed drainage unit may be necessary.

Preparation of the patient

The patient is supine; arms may be extended on armboards. Apply electrosurgical dispersive pad.

Skin preparation

Sternal splitting incision: Begin at the midline extending from the chin to below the umbilicus, and down to the table at the sides.

Draping

Folded towels and a fenestrated sheet

Equipment

Electrosurgical unit
Suction
Power source for saw (e.g., Stryker, Sarns)

Instrumentation

Thoracotomy procedures tray
Vascular procedures tray
Basic/Minor procedures tray
Tracheostomy tray (available)
Lebsche sternal knife
Mallet
Sternal saw (e.g., Stryker, Sarns)
Rake retractors (4- and 6-prong)

Supplies

Basin set
Blades (2) No. 10, (1) No. 15 adult; (2) No. 15 child
Electrosurgical pencil
Suction tubing
Drain, e.g., ¼" Penrose, optional
Umbilical tape (for retraction)
Dissectors (e.g., peanut)
Needle magnet or counter
Bone wax
Chest tube(s), connector, and sealed drainage unit
    (optional)

Special notes

Sternal sutures (e.g., wire) are available.

Chapter 14

CARDIOVASCULAR SURGERY

CAROTID ENDARTERECTOMY

Definition

Excision of intimal plaque from the carotid artery.

Discussion

This procedure is done to restore carotid artery blood flow and enhance cerebral circulation in order to relieve transient cerebral ischemia or prevent stroke.

Procedure

An incision is made along the anterior border of the sternomastoid muscle. The carotid sheath is exposed and incised. Care is taken to identify and prevent injury to cranial nerve branches. Proximal and distal control of the carotid artery and its bifurcation is achieved with vascular clamps and/or umbilical tapes and vessel loops. Arteriotomy is made with a No. 11 blade and Potts scissors. An intraluminal shunt

221

from the common carotid artery to the internal carotid artery may be inserted and secured with tourniquets or shunt clamps. Plaque is freed from the arterial wall. Care is taken to extract all plaque and debris to prevent subsequent embolization. If an intimal flap has developed, it is tacked to the vessel wall with fine sutures to prevent dissection when blood flow is restored. The arterial lumen may be flushed with heparin solution. The arteriotomy is closed primarily, or if the lumen appears stenotic a patch graft (autogenous or synthetic) may be employed. Prior to placement of final sutures the shunt, if used, is removed and the lumen is flushed to remove any residual debris or air bubbles. The wound is closed in layers. A drain may be employed.

Preparation of the patient

The patient is supine with the head slightly extended and turned toward the opposite side. Excessive rotation of the head and extension of the neck is avoided because this significantly decreases blood flow to the carotid-vertebral artery system. The head may be supported by a doughnut headrest. A rolled towel may be placed between the scapulas. Apply electrosurgical dispersive pad.

Skin preparation

Begin at the neck on the affected side extending from the infra-auricular border to the axilla, and down to the table at the sides.

Draping

Folded towels and a fenestrated sheet

Equipment

Headrest (e.g., doughnut)
Electrosurgical unit
Suction
Scales (weigh sponges)

Instrumentation

Basic/Minor procedures tray
Shunt tray
Hemoclip appliers, short (small and medium)

Supplies

Basin set
Blades (2) No. 10, (1) No. 15, (1) No. 11
Electrosurgical pencil
Suction tubing
Umbilical tapes, vessel loops
Dissectors (e.g., peanut)
Heparinized saline
Graduate and disposable syringe
Hemostatic agents (e.g., Avitene, Surgicel)
Hemoclips (small, medium)
Shunt (e.g., Javid)

Special notes

Have the patient's x-ray films in the room.

The anesthetist usually records the time the carotid artery is clamped.

Every effort is made by the surgical team to minimize the amount of time the carotid artery is clamped; organization of equipment, efficiency of movement, and attention to the wound site by the scrub person is extremely important.

Retractors must have dull teeth to avoid injury to blood vessels.

Moistened umbilical tapes and vessel loops are passed on a clamp (e.g., tonsil).

A shunt may be fashioned out of a 5- to 7.5-cm (2- to 3-inch) piece of vinyl tubing, or a commercially prepared shunt (e.g., Javid) may be used.

Check with blood bank that blood is available as ordered.

Weigh sponges.

Keep accurate record of irrigation used.

ABDOMINAL AORTIC PROCEDURES
(ABDOMINAL AORTIC ANEURYSMECTOMY,
ABDOMINAL AORTIC ENDARTERECTOMY)
WITH AORTOILIAC GRAFT

Definition

Aortic aneurysmectomy is the excision and/or internal bypass of an attenuated widening of the aortic wall (aneurysm) that requires the insertion of a prosthetic graft to reestablish vascular continuity; if the aortic bifurcation is involved an aortoiliac Y-graft is employed.

Aortic endarterectomy is the removal of intimal plaque with the insertion of a tubular graft or patch to restore the integrity of the aorta.

Discussion

These lesions most often result from arteriosclerosis. The aortic wall weakens and dilation occurs; thrombus fills most of the increased lumen, a potential source of emboli. Infection also may lead to weakening of the wall and aneurysm formation (mycotic aneurysm). In the absence of an aneurysm it may be possible to spare the aorta by resecting plaque and repairing the aorta and/or its major branches or by bypassing the diseased segment (aortoiliac or aortofemoral graft).

Aortic aneurysm surgery is usually performed as an elective procedure. If an aneurysm ruptures incompletely, dissection of the aortic wall by blood and clot will occur resulting in an acute surgical emergency.

Procedure

The abdominal aorta is approached by a long midline incision. The intestines are mobilized and packed out of the field. The posterior parietal peritoneum is incised, and the aorta is exposed taking care to protect the inferior vena cava and ureters.

When the aneurysm involves the inferior mesenteric artery, the artery may be sacrificed (or preserved if backflow is brisk). Proximal and distal control is obtained with vascular forceps. The aneurysm is opened and the clot evacuated. The lumbar vessels are suture-ligated leaving the posterior portion of the aneurysm in situ. The aorta and usually the common iliac arteries are transsected and anastomoses made using a prosthesis. When appropriate, the inferior mesenteric artery (distally), or renal artery (proximally), may require reimplantation. Special prostheses (grafts) are available. Control clamps are removed and the anastomoses tested for leakage. The shell of the aneurysm may be closed over the prosthesis for reinforcement. In endarterectomy the aorta and iliac vessels are incised, the plaque removed, and the vessels repaired with or without prosthetic patches. In aortic bypass, the aorta is connected to the iliac or femoral vessels according to their degree of patency, eliminating the need for extensive endarterectomy. Various combinations of these techniques can be employed. Local anticoagulation with heparinized saline may be used. Prior to closure of the anastomoses, clots are flushed out by the transient release of the control clamps. The posterior peritoneum is closed, and the wound is closed.

Preparation of the patient

The patient is supine with arms extended on armboards. Apply electrosurgical dispersive pad. Check with the surgeon regarding insertion of a Foley catheter.

Skin preparation

Begin at the midline extending from axillae to midthighs, and to the table at the sides.

Draping

Folded towel (in thirds lengthwise) over pubic area, folded towels around the operative site, sterile, plastic adhesive drapes (2) (optional), and a laparotomy sheet (which may be cut) or individual drape sheets

Equipment

Electrosurgical unit
Suction (2 units)
Scales (weigh sponges)
Headlight and fiberoptic light source, optional
Doppler, optional

Instrumentation

Major procedures tray
Vascular procedures tray
Balfour retractor
Weitlaner retractors (2)
Harrington retractors (2)
Extra towel clips
Hemoclip appliers (various sizes and lengths)

Supplies

Basin set
Blades (2) No. 10, (1) No. 15, (1) No. 11
Needle magnet or counter
Suction tubings (2)
Electrosurgical pencil
Penrose drains, umbilical tapes, vessel loops
Dissectors (e.g., peanut)
Hemostatic agent (e.g., Avitene, Surgicel, Thrombostat)
Needle 18-gauge (to vent, to prevent air embolus)
Graft (type and size of choice)
Hemoclips (various sizes)
Heparin (anticoagulant) and heparinized saline (diluted to preference)
Protamine sulfate (neutralizes heparin)
Antibiotic (intravenous or for irrigation), optional
Graduate and syringes

Special notes

Have the patient's x-ray films in the room.

Check with the surgeon regarding the type and size of graft and prepare the graft for use according to the surgeon's directions.

Mark pedal pulses before preparing the skin so that if a pulse check is requested, it can be found immediately.

Have a variety of Fogarty catheters (irrigation and embolectomy) in the room.

Check urinary output as requested.

Do *not* cut double-armed sutures.

Check with blood bank that blood is available as ordered.

Weigh sponges.

Keep accurate record of amount of irrigation used.

Moistened umbilical tapes and vessel loops are passed on a clamp (e.g., tonsil).

FEMOROPOPLITEAL BYPASS

Definition

The interposition of a graft from the common femoral artery to the popliteal artery in order to bypass an occluded segment of the superficial femoral artery.

Discussion

The graft may be the patient's own saphenous vein (autogenous) or a synthetic prosthesis. Patency of the popliteal artery must be determined prior to the surgery by angiography. When the popliteal artery is occluded, shunting the blood flow to a more distal artery becomes necessary.

Procedure

A vertical incision is made from above the inguinal ligament over the course of the greater saphenous vein; there may be several interruptions in the incision. The saphenous vein is harvested for a graft by dividing and ligating its multiple branches. The segment is flushed with a heparinized saline solution and tested for leakage. The common femoral artery and its bifurcation are exposed. The distal popliteal artery is exposed, retracting or excising the gastrocnemius and soleus muscles posteriorly and adductor muscles anteriorly. The posterior tibial nerve is protected. A tunneling instrument is used to make a passage from the femoral triangle to the popliteal space under the sartorius muscle. The femoral artery is controlled with a vascular clamp and heparinized. The graft is sutured to the common femoral artery making certain that the distal portion of the vein is used, that is, reversed anatomic position. Endarterectomy and patch angioplasty may be performed at the origin of the deep femoral artery. The graft is passed through the tunnel (avoiding kinking or tension) and anastomosed to the popliteal artery. Prior to placing the final sutures, the graft is flushed with blood controlled by pressure or further sutures. Intraoperative angiography may be done. The incisions are closed. If vessels distal to the popliteal artery are used similar maneuvers are performed.

Preparation of the patient

The patient is supine with the affected thigh externally rotated and abducted, and the knee flexed. Arms may be extended on armboards. Check with the surgeon regarding insertion of a Foley catheter. Apply electrosurgical dispersive pad.

Skin preparation

Both legs may be prepared for harvesting saphenous vein(s). Check with the surgeon.

Unilateral. Begin at the groin on the affected side extending from the umbilicus to the toes (including front and back of thigh, leg, and entire foot). Prepare down to the table on the affected side and well beyond the midline on the opposite side.

Bilateral. Prepare both groin regions extending from the umbilicus to the toes (including front and back of thighs, legs, and feet). Two persons are required to complete the preparation or a leg holder may be used.

Draping

Unilateral. The affected extremity is held up and abducted. A large sheet is draped over the end of the table. A towel (folded in thirds, lengthwise) is placed over the pubic area. A split sheet is draped under the thigh. Two towels are placed on the table, the foot is lowered onto the towels, and the towels are fashioned into a "boot" and clipped. A large sheet is draped over the top of the patient's body. The affected leg may be passed through a laparotomy sheet and lowered to the table, or individual drape sheets complete the draping.

Bilateral. The legs are held up and abducted. A large drape sheet is placed over the end of the table. A towel (folded in thirds, lengthwise) is placed over the pubic area. Sheets are draped along the sides of the patient and fastened. A large sheet is draped under the thighs. Two towels for each foot are placed on the table, the feet are lowered onto the towels, and the towels are fashioned into "boots" and clipped. Another large sheet is draped over the top of the patient.

Equipment

Leg holder, optional
Electrosurgical unit
Suction

Instrumentation

Basic/Minor procedures tray
Vascular procedures tray
Hemoclip appliers, short (small, medium, large)
Tunneling instrument

Supplies

Basin set
Suction tubing
Electrosurgical pencil
Blades (2) No. 10, (1) No. 15, (1) No. 11
Umbilical tapes, Penrose drains, vessel loops
Heparin and heparinized saline (diluted to surgeon's preference)
Protamine sulfate (neutralizes heparin)
Needle magnet or counter
Dissectors (e.g., peanut)
Antibiotic (intravenous or for irrigation), optional
Graduate and syringes
Hemostatic agents (e.g., Gelfoam, Surgicel, Thrombostat, Collastat, Oxycel, and Avitene)
Graft (type and size of choice)

Special notes

Have the patient's x-ray films in the room.

Check with the surgeon regarding the type and size of graft and its preparation.

Do *not* cut double-armed sutures.

The surgeon may choose to perform intraoperative angiography. Notify the x-ray department. Check with the surgeon for type of catheters needed; have available syringes and contrast medium. Observe x-ray safety precautions, see p. 20.

A glove may be placed over the distal portion of the foot instead of a "boot."

GREATER SAPHENOUS VEIN LIGATION AND STRIPPING

Definition

Excision of the greater saphenous vein and its tributaries.

Discussion

This procedure is indicated in patients with varicose vein disease secondary to venous valvular incompetence. Another indication is superficial thrombophlebitis of the lower extremities. The lesser saphenous vein system may also be excised as indicated.

Procedure

An oblique incision is made in the groin overlying the saphenofemoral junction. The superficial fascia is incised and the proximal portion of the saphenous vein is mobilized, divided, and ligated close to the saphenofemoral junction. Tributaries are divided and ligated as indicated. A transverse incision is made over the saphenous vein distally anterior to the medial malleolus; tributaries are exposed, divided, and ligated. The probe end of the internal stripper is inserted into the distal end of the saphenous vein and threaded proximally. A ligature is tied around the distal end securing the vein around the "acorn" end of the stripper. The stripper (with vein attached) is gently pulled out through the proximal incision as the assistant applies pressure with a folded towel over the course of the vein in the leg and thigh. The vein may be removed segmentally, or sections of it may be removed with external strippers. Saphenous vein branches and perforating veins (usually marked by the surgeon preoperatively) are stripped, excised, or ligated. This might entail numerous small incisions. The lesser saphenous vein (posterior aspect of the leg) may require similar treatment. All incisions are closed, dressed, and wrapped with an elastic bandage.

Preparation of the patient

The patient is supine; arms may be extended on armboards. The affected thigh is externally rotated and abducted, and the knee is flexed. The patient is secured to the table with the safety belt fastened over the unaffected thigh. Apply electrosurgical dispersive pad.

Skin preparation

Unilateral. Begin at the groin on the affected side extending from the umbilicus to the toes (including front and back of thigh, leg, and foot). Prepare down to the table on the affected side and well beyond the midline on the opposite side.

Bilateral. Prepare both groin regions extending from the umbilicus to the toes (including front and back of thighs, legs, and feet). Two persons are required to complete the preparation or a leg holder may be employed.

Draping

Unilateral. The affected extremity is held up and abducted. A large sheet is draped over the end of the table. A towel (folded in thirds, lengthwise) is placed over the pubic area. A split sheet is draped under the leg. Two towels are placed on the table, the foot is lowered onto the towels, and the towels are fashioned into a "boot" and clipped. A large sheet is draped over the top of the patient's body. The affected leg is passed through a laparotomy sheet and lowered to the table, or individual drape sheets may complete the draping.

Bilateral. The legs are held up and abducted. A large drape sheet is placed over the end of the table. A towel (folded in thirds, lengthwise) is placed over the pubic area. Sheets are draped along the sides of the patient and fastened. A large sheet is draped under the legs. Two towels for each foot are placed on the table, the feet are lowered onto the towels, and the towels are fashioned into "boots" and clipped. Another large sheet (or more) is draped over the top of the patient.

Equipment

Leg holder
Electrosurgical unit
Suction

Instrumentation

Basic/Minor procedures tray
Vascular procedures tray
Internal and external vein strippers
Hemoclip appliers, short (small, medium, large)
Weitlaner retractor, sharp

Supplies

Basin set
Marking pen
Blades (2) No. 10, (1) No. 15
Needle magnet or counter
Suction tubing
Electrosurgical pencil
Elastic bandages

Special notes

A glove may be placed over the distal portion of the foot instead of a "boot."

The scrub person should remove the vein from the internal stripper by cutting the suture in order to have it available for continued use.

PORTASYSTEMIC SHUNT

Definition

Diversion of portal venous blood to the systemic venous system.

Discussion

This procedure is performed to relieve elevated portal venous pressure (portal hypertension), which can result in bleeding from esophageal or gastric varices, ascites, and hepatic failure. The primary cause is cirrhosis. The portal blood may be shunted into the inferior vena cava from the portal vein (end-to-side or end-to-end), from the splenic vein (with splenectomy), from the distal splenic vein (retaining the spleen), or from the superior mesenteric vein (with or without an interposing prosthetic graft). The particular type of shunt is determined by the patient's condition and the surgeon's preference. Preoperative angiography (splenoportagram) is useful for diagnosis.

Procedure

A portacaval shunt will be described. A long right subcostal incision is usually employed; less often a thoracoabdominal incision is made. Careful dissection is performed because even minor vessels may bleed significantly. The duodenum is reflected exposing the inferior vena cava. The hepatoduodenal ligament is incised protecting the common bile duct and hepatic artery. The portal vein is exposed from the porta hepatis to the superior border of the pancreas. Portal pressure is measured for a reference through a needle inserted in a small mesenteric vein. Partial occlusion of the vena cava and the portal vein are obtained with vascular clamps. Anastomosis is made side-to-side after excising a generous window in either vein. For end-to-side anastomosis the portal vein is transsected at the porta hepatis ligating the proximal stump securely. The distal end is anastomosed to the side of the vena cava. Repeat manometry is done. The wound is closed in layers.

Preparation of the patient

The patient is supine with the right side elevated by a folded sheet; arms may be extended on armboards. Check with the surgeon regarding insertion of a Foley catheter. Apply electrosurgical dispersive pad.

Skin preparation

Begin in the subcostal region extending from the axillae to the upper thighs, and down to the table at the sides.

Draping

Folded towels and a laparotomy sheet

Equipment

Electrosurgical unit
Suction
Spinal manometer
Scale (for weighing sponges)

Instrumentation

Major procedures tray
Vascular procedures tray
Hemoclip appliers (assorted sizes and lengths)

Supplies

Basin set
Blades (2) No. 10, (1) No. 15, (1) No. 11
Electrosurgical pencil
Suction tubing

Needle magnet or counter
Three-way stopcock, polyethylene tubing (e.g., Angiocath), and syringe
Hemoclips (assorted sizes)

Special notes

To measure portal pressure, polyethylene tubing inserted into a jejunal mesenteric vein is attached to a three-way stopcock and a spinal manometer.

Portal pressure is measured again following the portacaval anastomosis to determine if the shunt is functioning.

Weigh sponges.

Measure irrigation fluids accurately.

Check with blood bank that blood is available as ordered.

ARTERIOVENOUS SHUNT—ARTERIOVENOUS FISTULA

Definition

Establishment of a communicating prosthetic loop (shunt) or a direct communication between an artery and vein (fistula).

Discussion

Arteriovenous shunt and arteriovenous fistula are usually performed under local anesthesia. The procedure is performed to provide easy access for venipuncture with large-bore needle for purposes of renal dialysis and infusion chemotherapy. Several varieties of arterial venous communication may be achieved employing a buried synthetic prosthesis, an arteriovenous fistula, or an external prosthesis (least often used).

Procedure

Incisions are made over selected arterial and venous sites (often the radial artery and cephalic vein of the proximal forearm). Use of the nondominant forearm is preferable; lower extremities can be used if forearm sites cannot be used because of previous surgery, etc. Vascular clamps or bulldog clamps control the vessels. An incision is made into the lumen of the artery, which may be dilated with coronary dilators. The venous side is ligated distally. A shunt (e.g., bovine artery prosthesis) is anastomosed to the artery and vein. Heparin solution is instilled into the graft. If a fistula is to be performed the selected artery is anastomosed to an adjacent vein. The wound is closed and a protective dressing placed.

Preparation of the patient

The patient is supine with the nondominant forearm extended on a hand table; the other arm may be extended on an armboard.

Skin preparation

Begin at the proposed site of the shunt on the forearm; include the entire forearm and hand from fingertips to several centimeters (inches) above the elbow.

Draping

The hand is held up in a tube or an impervious stockinette. A large cuffed sheet is draped over the table and under the arm. A folded towel is wrapped around the arm and clipped. A drape (or split) sheet is draped under the arm and clipped. A drape sheet covers the shoulder and is clipped under the arm. Either a fenestrated sheet or additional drape sheets completes the draping.

Equipment

Electrosurgical unit
Hand table
Loupes, optional
Sitting stools (2) surgeon and scrub person

Instrumentation

Shunt tray
Coronary artery dilators

Supplies

Basin set
Electrosurgical pencil
Needle magnet or counter
Blades (1) No. 10, (1) No. 15, (1) No. 11
Silastic cannula(s)
Teflon tips (2)
Shunt connector
Heparinized saline (diluted to surgeon's preference)
Graduate (for heparin solution) and syringe
Heparin
Shunt clamps (2)

Special notes

If an external shunt is performed two shunt
clamps are to be secured to the gauze dressing
when the procedure is completed. Should the cannula become separated from the connector, both
ends of the cannula must be clamped immediately.

CARDIAC PROCEDURES

Definition

Involves the correction of congenital anomalies, acquired diseases of the heart, pericardium, and great
vessels (including repair and replacement of dis-

eased valves, resection of ventricular aneurysm, pericardiectomy, pulmonary embolectomy, and replacement of segments of the great vessels, etc.) and the revascularization of ischemic myocardium.

Discussion

Three representative cardiac procedures will be described. Pediatric cardiac surgery, procedures to correct congenital anomalies, cardiac transplantation, and the employment of artificial cardiac devices will not be discussed. Insertion of an intraaortic balloon catheter will be covered briefly.

1. *Aortic valve replacement:* Involves the excision and replacement of the diseased aortic valve.
2. *Mitral valve replacement:* Involves the excision and replacement of the diseased mitral valve.
3. *Coronary artery bypass:* Refers to the grafting of the internal mammary artery or segments of autologous saphenous vein to bypass coronary artery obstruction.

Cardiac surgery often necessitates the use of cardiopulmonary bypass. To fully comprehend cardiac abnormalities and the function of cardiopulmonary bypass, knowledge of anatomy and the circulation is mandatory.

Cardiopulmonary Bypass. Cardiopulmonary bypass is the technique by which the patient's blood is diverted, oxygenated, and reperfused. This artificial means of oxygenating and circulating the blood is employed for intracardiac procedures, coronary artery bypass, and procedures on intrathoracic major vessels.

Prior to instituting cardiopulmonary bypass the patient is anticoagulated with heparin. This status is reversed following the procedure, using protamine sulfate.

Cardiopulmonary bypass may be either total or partial. For *total bypass* (used for intracardiac procedures such as valve replacements, septal defects, major anomalies, and ventricular aneurysm resection), all the blood is diverted from the heart, except intrinsic cardiac circulation, by completely occluding the vessels around the bypass cannulas. *Partial bypass* (used for coronary artery surgery, thoracic aortic aneurysms, etc.) allows a portion of the blood flow to pass through the heart by limiting the degree of occlusion around the cannulas.

There are several anatomic sites at which cardiopulmonary bypass can be established. The femoral vein, inferior vena cava, and right atrium are examples of sites from which blood is diverted from the patient to the pump. Blood is returned to the patient through the femoral artery, subclavian artery, or the ascending aorta. The preference of the surgeon, nature of the surgery, and condition of the vessels will determine the sites chosen for each patient.

A commonly used configuration is the cannulation of the right atrium by a single multi-holed cannula, the tip of which inserts into the inferior vena cava transporting the venous return from the patient to the pump. A cannula inserted in the ascending aorta returns blood to the patient from the pump.

During cardiac surgery the patient's hemodynamics and other physiologic functions are monitored continuously. In addition to those monitors employed for most major surgeries, such as the electrocardiogram, pulse oximeter, urimeter, etc., invasive hemodynamic catheters are placed. These include an arterial line to measure blood pressure directly and to serve as a ready access for blood gas determination sampling, and a central venous pressure (CVP) or Swan-Ganz line to measure intracardiac pressures. The electroencephalogram may be monitored.

Hypothermia and/or pharmacologic agents may be employed when it is necessary to slow or arrest the heart. Hypothermia can be induced by using a hypothermia mattress, the direct application of iced saline, and/or by cooling the blood being returned to the patient from the pump oxygenator. Pharmacologic agents used to produce cardioplegia contain a potassium solution that induces hyperkalemia, resulting in electromechanical cardiac arrest. Body temperature is restored, and the potassium preparation is flushed out, at the conclusion of the cardiac procedure. The heart beat may resume spontaneously, or electrical cardioversion may be employed to restore effective activity to the heart in its state of arrest or ventricular fibrillation. Pacemaker wires are often inserted at the completion of cardiopulmonary bypass.

Intra-aortic Balloon Catheter. An increasingly performed adjunct to cardiopulmonary bypass is the insertion of an intra-aortic balloon catheter. This procedure can also be performed independent of cardiopulmonary bypass following myocardial infarction. The purpose of the intra-aortic balloon catheter is to increase coronary artery flow and to assist peripheral perfusion. This procedure is indicated following myocardial infarction or cardiopulmonary bypass when left ventricular function is inadequate. The cylindrical balloon catheter, which is inserted through the femoral artery, is postioned in the descending aorta distal to the level of the left subclavian artery and attached to an intra-aortic balloon pump unit. The femoral arteriotomy site is reinforced with prosthetic graft material. The pump is coordinated with the patient's electrocardiogram so that the balloon inflates during diastole, forcing blood retrogradely to better perfuse the coronary arteries, and antegradely into the distal aorta and its branches. This improves oxygenation of the myocardium and increases peripheral blood flow, thus diminishing the workload of the heart. When counterpulsation assistance is no longer necessary, the catheter is removed by opening the arteriotomy site.

Procedures

Aortic Valve Replacement. Approach is through a median sternotomy. Cannulation for total cardiopulmonary bypass is achieved. The aorta is occluded distal to the valve. A cardioplegic solution is infused through the aortic root into the coronary arteries. Aortotomy is performed. The valve is excised. The annulus is measured and the appropriate size prosthesis is inserted and sutured into place. The aortotomy is closed. Air is vented from the left ventricle and the aorta. The aorta is unclamped. Cardiopulmonary bypass is discontinued. The wound may be irrigated with an antibiotic solution. Temporary pacemaker electrodes are sutured to the heart. Mediastinal drains are inserted. The wound is closed.

Mitral Valve Replacement. Approach is through a median sternotomy. Cannulation for total cardiopulmonary bypass is achieved. The ascending aorta is occluded. A cardioplegic solution is infused through the aortic root into the coronary arteries. A left atriotomy is performed to expose the mitral valve. The valve is excised, the annulus measured, and the appropriate prosthesis is inserted and sutured into place. The aortic cross-clamp is removed and air is aspirated from the aorta. Cardiopulmonary bypass is discontinued. The wound may be irrigated with an antibiotic solution. Temporary pacemaker electrodes are sutured to the heart. Mediastinal drains are inserted. The wound is closed. There are many types of cardiac valve prostheses available, including preserved biologic valves (porcine) or totally fabricated prostheses of various sizes, shapes, and mechanics. More than one valve may require replacement.

Coronary Artery Bypass Graft. Approach is through a median sternotomy. The internal mammary artery directly, free segments of the saphenous vein, or a combination of these will be grafted. The internal mammary artery is dissected to obtain maximal length and is evaluated for adequate blood flow. If saphenous vein segments are to be used, they are harvested and tested for leaks. Cannulation for partial cardiopulmonary bypass is achieved. The aorta is occluded and the cardioplegic solution is infused. A coronary artery is isolated and dilators may be inserted. The graft is anastomosed to the coronary artery and tested for leaks. Multiple grafts may be necessary. The grafts may be placed sequentially, that is, one graft segment can be anastomosed to more than one coronary artery. The aortic cross-clamp is released and a portion of the aorta is then occluded. The grafts are measured, cut, and anastomosed to the aorta. The clamp on the aorta is removed. (Some surgeons prefer to perform the aortic anastomoses on bypass prior to the coronary artery anastomoses. The sequence of anastomoses varies with each surgeon, particularly if multiple grafts are performed.) Grafts are again inspected for leaks. All sources of air bubble accumulation are vented. Cardiopulmonary bypass is discontinued. The wound may be irrigated with an antibiotic solution. Temporary pacemaker electrodes are sutured to the heart. Mediastinal drains are inserted. The wound is closed. Coronary artery bypass may be performed in conjunction with a valve replacement procedure.

Preparation of the patient

The patient is supine. (For coronary artery bypass a pillow is placed under the knees to maintain slight flexion, which provides access to the proximal greater saphenous veins.) After the vascular access lines are placed in the upper extremities, the arms are padded and tucked in at the patient's sides. A Foley catheter is inserted and connected to a urimeter. Apply electrosurgical dispersive pad.

Skin preparation

Valve Replacement. Begin at the midline of the chest extending from the chin to midthighs, and down to the table at the sides. The genitalia are prepared last.

Coronary Artery Bypass. The preparation is best performed by two persons, or a leg holder may be used. Begin at the midline of the chest extending from the chin to the pubic symphysis, and down to the table at the sides. The thighs and legs are prepared front and back including the feet. The genitalia are prepared last.

Draping

Valve Replacement. A drape sheet is placed over the end of the table. A towel (folded in thirds, lengthwise) is placed over the genitalia. A sheet is draped over the thighs and legs. Towels folded longitudinally are placed along the patient's sides and across the sternal notch. Sterile, adhesive plastic drapes may be applied across the chest and abdomen. Large drape sheets are placed at the sides and across the top of the patient.

Coronary Artery Bypass. Two circulators lift and abduct the legs as a large drape sheet is placed on the end of the table. A towel (folded in thirds, lengthwise) is placed over the genitalia. A split sheet is placed under and around both legs. Two towels for each foot are placed on the table. The feet are lowered onto the towels and the towels are fashioned into "boots" and clipped. Towels are folded longitudinally and placed along the patient's sides and across the sternal notch. Sterile, adhesive plastic drapes may be applied across the chest and abdomen. Large drape sheets are placed at the sides and across the top of the patient.

Equipment

Extra IV standards
Suctions (4)
Cell Saver
Hypothermia mattress
Temperature probe
Cardioverter
Electrosurgical unit

Instrumentation

Cardiac procedures tray
Oscillating saw (cordless or with cord, as available)
Hemoclip appliers (assorted sizes and lengths)

Supplies

Supplies for vascular lines, CVP and/or Swan-Ganz
    lines, and a cardioplegia administration set
Basin set
Knife blades (2) No. 10, (2) No. 15, (2) No. 11
Beaver blade
Large graduate pitchers (2)
Heparinized saline
Assorted syringes and needles
Sterile, adhesive plastic drapes (2)
Electrosurgical pencils (2) (1 spatula, 1 needle
    point)
Electrosurgical pencil holders (2), optional
Needle magnets or counters
Suction tubing
Cell Saver suction tubing
Asepto (or bulb) syringes (2)
Foley catheter tray
Urimeter
Hemostatic agents (e.g., Gelfoam or Surgicel)
Teflon felt strips and pledgets
Suture boots
Bone wax
Pacemaker wires
Elastic bandages (for saphenous vein grafts)
Mediastinal drains (2) with Y-connector
Intrapleural sealed drainage unit (e.g., Pleurevac)
Defibrillator paddles
Hemoclips (assorted sizes)

Special notes

    Circulator(s) and scrub person(s) must be thoroughly familiar with the routine of the surgeon and
the "open heart" team.
    Pad the patient's arms to protect hemodynamic
monitoring lines.
    The scrub person should keep instruments free
of blood clots, plaque, and tissue debris.
    A bag fashioned out of a Mayo stand cover may

be fastened to the head of the table for the defibrillator paddles.

Fibrin "glue" (mixture of thrombin, calcium, and cryoprecipitate) may be injected over bleeding site (i.e., graft site).

Several liters of iced saline may be needed when going on the pump.

Measure urine every 15 minutes while on the pump.

A separate tray of instruments may be used for saphenous vein removal.

Warm saline may be used coming off the pump.

Check with blood bank that blood is available as ordered.

Weigh sponges.

Keep track of irrigation fluid used so that an accurate blood loss can be determined.

Follow hospital policy regarding the insertion of a prosthesis for valve replacements.

Chapter 15

ORTHOPEDIC SURGERY

OPEN REDUCTION OF A CARPAL BONE FRACTURE

Definition

Realignment and fixation of fractures (or fracture-dislocation) of the bones of the wrist through an operative incision.

Discussion

Most fractures of the wrist are treated by closed reduction and immobilization (cast). Surgery is required when the fracture is displaced, dislocated, or when there is a nonunion. Fixation may be achieved with a number of devices including pins, wires, and a compression plate and screws. Persistent nonunion may necessitate a bone graft from a bone in the forearm or the iliac crest. More severe injuries may require excision of carpal bones and/or the radial or ulnar styloid process to prevent arthritis. Arthrodesis of the wrist may be preferable in patients who engage in manual labor. Numerous permutations of fractures and dislocations occur. The most common fracture is of the scaphoid (navicular) bone.

Procedure

The approach is determined by the fracture site and the preference of the surgeon. For fracture of the scaphoid, an incision may be made on the dorsum of the wrist distal to the radiocarpal joint. Tendons and nerve roots are protected. Small bone fragments are excised; larger fragments are aligned and fixed with wires or pins, or by bone graft pegs (obtained with a tubular gouge). If a graft is employed, an additional incision is made to expose the radial styloid from which a bone graft may be taken. In some cases of nonunion as necrosis, larger fragments or the entire bone may be excised. The wound is closed. A splint or cast is applied.

Preparation of the patient

The patient is supine with the affected arm extended on a hand table; the other arm may be extended on an armboard. Sheet wadding and a tourniquet are applied to the affected arm. Apply electrosurgical dispersive pad.

Skin preparation

Begin at the wrist and cleanse the hand (including fingers and interdigital spaces) and forearm (front and back), extending 5 to 7.5 cm (2 to 3 inches) beyond the elbow.

Draping

The extremity is held up in a tube (or impervious) stockinette; the hand table is covered with a drape sheet. A cuffed sheet is draped under the arm. A folded towel is wrapped around the arm and clipped. A drape (or split) sheet covers the shoulder and is clipped under the arm. A fenestrated sheet or additional drape sheets completes the draping.

Equipment

Suction
Electrosurgical unit
Tourniquet and insufflator
Sitting stools (3) (surgeon, assistant, scrub person)
Power source for power drill (available)
Cast cart

Instrumentation

Minor orthopedic procedures tray
Hand drill or power drill and cord, drill bits
Kirschner wires
Tubular gouge (for bone graft peg)

Supplies

Basin set
Sheet wadding (unsterile for tourniquet)
Esmarch bandage
Blades (1) No. 10, (2) No. 15
Tube or impervious stockinette
Needle magnet or counter
Bulb syringe
Graduate
Suction tubing
Electrosurgical pencil
Antibiotic irrigation, optional

Special notes

Have x-ray films ready in room.

Do not allow preparation solutions to pool under tourniquet.

Place tourniquet as high on the extremity as possible.

Wrap sheet wadding around the extremity smoothly. Tourniquet ends must overlap at least 5 cm (2 inches). Do not apply the tourniquet at the elbow. Setting for an adult is approximately 300 mm Hg for the upper extremity. Monitor tourniquet time and setting. Tourniquet must be released after 2 hours to avoid injury.

Be prepared to assist the surgeon in applying a splint or cast.

Protective goggles may be worn.

EXCISION OF A GANGLION

Definition

Removal of a cystic dilation of the capsule of a joint or tendon sheath that contains synovial fluid.

Discussion

The most frequent site of origin is the dorsum of the carpus. Careful complete excision makes recurrence rare.

Procedure

A transverse incision is made over the ganglion. Soft tissue dissection to expose the ganglion is done. Care is taken to avoid injury to nerve branches. The ganglion is mobilized and excised (including a generous border at its base). The wound may be irrigated. The tendon sheath is repaired as necessary. The wound is closed. An elastic bandage is applied.

Preparation of the patient, Skin preparation, and Draping

See Open Reduction of a Carpal Bone Fracture, p. 247.

Equipment

Electrosurgical unit
Tourniquet and insufflator
Suction (available)
Sitting stools (2) (surgeon and scrub person)

Instrumentation

Minor orthopedic tray
Hayes metacarpal retractors, pediatric Deaver retractor (available)

Supplies

Basin set
Sheet wadding (unsterile for tourniquet)
Blades (2) No. 15
Tube or impervious stockinette
Esmarch bandage
Needle magnet or counter
Bulb syringe
Electrosurgical pencil
Suction tubing (optional)
Elastic bandage

Special notes

For tourniquet precautions, see Open Reduction of a Carpal Bone Fracture, p. 247.

CARPAL TUNNEL RELEASE

Definition

Decompression of the median nerve on the volar surface of the wrist.

Discussion

Symptoms of carpal tunnel syndrome (compressed median nerve) such as numbness and tingling of fingers and weakness of intrinsic thumb muscles are usually relieved by division of the deep transverse carpal ligament.

Procedure

A curved incision is made parallel to the thenar crease and angled toward the ulnar side of the wrist. Care is taken to avoid injury to sensory branches of the median nerve. After the skin and subcutaneous tissue are excised and reflected, the transverse carpal ligament (flexor retinaculum) is divided. The skin is closed. A compression dressing and a splint may be applied.

Preparation of the patient

The patient is supine with the affected arm extended on a hand table; the other arm may be extended on an armboard. Sheet wadding and a tourniquet are applied to the affected arm. Apply electrosurgical dispersive pad.

Skin preparation

Cleanse the hand (begin at the palm, including fingers, nails, and interdigital spaces), the wrist, and the forearm (front and back) to the elbow.

Draping, Equipment, Instrumentation, and Supplies

See Excision of a Ganglion, p. 250.

Special notes

For tourniquet precautions see Open Reduction of a Carpal Bone Fracture, p. 247.

OPEN REDUCTION OF THE HUMERUS

Definition

Realignment and fixation of a fracture of the arm employing an operative incision.

Discussion

A variety of fractures of the humerus may occur. When closed reduction and immobilization are unsatisfactory or when there is a nonunion, fixation may be achieved with a number of devices including rods and a compression plate and screws.

Procedure

An appropriate incision is made over the fracture site avoiding neurovascular structures. If malunion has occurred osteotomy is performed to restore alignment. Generally the fracture is fixed with screws and a compression plate; for condylar fractures threaded Kirschner wires or screws may be employed. The wound is closed. The arm is immobilized.

Preparation of the patient

The patient is supine with the affected arm in a comfortable position (possibly across the chest); the other arm may be extended on an armboard. A sandbag or rolled sheet may be placed under the shoulder on the affected side. In distal fractures, a tourniquet may be used. Apply electrosurgical dispersive pad.

Skin preparation

Begin with the arm and hand; extend from the fingertips to the shoulder. Cleanse the axilla well; extend to the table posteriorly, beyond the midline of the chest anteriorly, and down to the level of the lower ribs.

Draping

The extremity is held up in a tube (or impervious) stockinette. A large drape sheet is tucked under the patient's shoulder. A towel is folded longitudinally and towel-clipped around the top of the arm (stockinette is brought up to the shoulder). A drape (or split) sheet is draped under the arm and clipped at the shoulder. A drape sheet covers the shoulder and is clipped under the arm. A fenestrated sheet or additional individual drape sheets completes the draping.

Equipment

Suction
Electrosurgical unit
Power source for drill
Tourniquet and insufflator (for distal fractures)
Cast cart

Instrumentation

Basic orthopedic procedures tray
Bone holding instruments tray
Bone hooks, drill bits, Bennett retractors
Fixation device, e.g., Rush rods (with awl, driver, and
    extractor), screws and plates, compression set
    (with drill sleeve), Steinmann pins
Power drill and cord

Supplies

Basin set
Sheet wadding (unsterile)
Blades (2) No. 10
Electrosurgical pencil
Suction tubing
Needle magnet or counter
Graduate
Bulb syringe
Tube or impervious stockinette
Esmarch bandage
Antibiotic irrigation, optional

Special notes

Have x-ray films in room.
Check level of gas in tank for power drill.

For tourniquet precautions see Open Reduction of a Carpal Bone Fracture, p. 247.

Be prepared to assist the surgeon in applying a cast or splint.

Protective goggles may be worn.

OPEN REDUCTION OF THE RADIUS AND/OR ULNA

Definition

Realignment and fixation of fractures of the forearm employing an operative incision.

Discussion

When closed reduction is unsatisfactory, or when a nonunion exists, fixation may be achieved with a variety of devices including rods, intramedullary nails, and long screws.

Procedure

An appropriate incision is made depending on the location of the fracture. Neurovascular structures are identified and protected. Radial head fractures (in adults) may require excision; all fragments and debris are removed including excess periosteum. A splint is applied. Radial shaft fractures are repaired with compression plates or a triangular medullary nail (Sage) is inserted via the radial styloid. Proximal ulna or olecranon fractures are treated by fixation with long screws or wires for smaller fragments. Fixation for distal wrist fractures may be achieved with screws, Kirschner wires, or specially shaped plates (e.g., T-plates) may be used. A splint or bivalve cast is applied.

Preparation of the patient

The patient is supine; the affected arm is positioned across the chest or extended on a hand table;

the other arm may be extended on an armboard. Sheet wadding and a tourniquet are applied to the affected arm. Apply electrosurgical dispersive pad.

Skin preparation

Begin with the forearm and include the hand, fingers, and interdigital spaces. Next scrub the elbow up to the level of the tourniquet.

Draping

The extremity is held up in a tube (or impervious) stockinette and a large drape sheet is draped under the arm (and over the hand table if one is used). A folded towel is wrapped around the arm and clipped, and the tube stockinette is brought up over the towel. A drape (or split) sheet is draped under the arm and clipped. A drape sheet covers the shoulder and is clipped under the arm. A fenestrated sheet or additional drape sheets completes the draping.

Equipment

Hand table, optional
Suction
Electrosurgical unit
Tourniquet and insufflator
Power source for drill
Cast cart

Instrumentation

Basic orthopedic procedures tray
Small bone holders, nail set, drill bits, awl
Power drill and cord
Fixation device, e.g., screws and plates, compression set (and drill sleeve), Steinmann pins, Kirschner wires, long screws, intramedullary nails, Rush rods (with awl, driver, and extractor)

Supplies

Basin set
Sheet wadding
Blades (2) No. 10
Tube (or impervious) stockinette
Esmarch bandage
Needle magnet or counter
Graduate
Bulb syringe
Suction tubing
Electrosurgical pencil
Antibiotic irrigation, optional

Special notes

See Open Reduction of the Humerus, p. 252.

OPEN REDUCTION OF AN OLECRANON PROCESS FRACTURE

Definition

Realignment and fixation of fractures of the elbow employing an operative incision.

Discussion

When fragments are separated open reduction and internal fixation are indicated. Small fragments may be removed and the triceps tendon reattached to the ulnar shaft. Large fragments may be fixed with a number of devices including a figure-of-eight wire loop, Kirschner wires, screws, and/or intramedullary pins (e.g., Steinmann).

Procedure

See Open Reduction of the Radius and/or Ulna, p. 255.

Preparation of the patient

The patient is supine with the affected extremity on a hand table or flexed across the chest; the other arm may be extended on an armboard. Sheet wadding and a tourniquet are applied to the affected arm. Apply electrosurgical dispersive pad.

Skin preparation

Begin at the elbow extending from the tourniquet to the fingertips (including fingers and interdigital spaces).

Draping and equipment

See Open Reduction of the Radius and/or Ulna, p. 255.

Instrumentation

Basic orthopedic procedures tray
Drill bits, awl
Hibbs and Bennett retractors
Fixation device: Wire and/or screws, Kirschner wires, intramedullary pins (e.g., Steinmann)
Wire tightener
Bone holders
Power drill and cord

Supplies

Basin set
Sheet wadding
Blades (2) No. 10
Tube stockinette
Esmarch bandage
Needle magnet or counter
Wire (e.g., No. 18-gauge or No. 20-gauge stainless steel)
Graduate
Bulb syringe

Suction tubing
Electrosurgical pencil
Penrose drain 1/4" (retraction for ulnar nerve)
Antibiotic irrigation, optional

Special notes

See Open Reduction of the Humerus, p. 252.

REPAIR OF RECURRENT ANTERIOR DISLOCATION OF THE SHOULDER

Definition

Strengthening of the anterior joint capsule and musculotendinous support of the shoulder.

Discussion

There are many procedures and modifications of procedures for the repair of recurrent anterior dislocation; posterior dislocations are rare.

Types
Bankart. The glenoid labrum and the anterior part of the capsule (which should cushion and support the humeral head) are reattached to the rim of the glenoid cavity.

Putti-Platt. The subscapularis tendon and the capsule are detached from the humerus and sutured laterally on the humeral neck in order to strengthen anterior supporting structures and to prevent excessive external rotation of the shoulder.

Bristow. The coracoid process and attached muscles are detached, inserted into the neck of the scapula, and fixed. The transferred muscular origins serve as a buttress across the anterior and inferior aspect of the joint, and also anchor the lower half of the subscapularis.

Procedure

An anterior incision is made over the pectoral groove. The joint capsule is exposed and the extent of the injury inspected. The coracoid process, with its muscular attachments, is osteotomized from the scapula. The subscapularis tendon is reattached to the coracoid process with a screw (or transferred to the anterior neck of the scapula). The lateral portion of the subscapularis tendon may be resutured to the joint capsule, and the medial edge of the subscapularis resutured to the rotator cuff or at the bicipital groove, overlapping the layers of the joint (Putti-Platt). The osteotomized coracoid tip may be transferred to the neck of the glenoid under the fibers of the subscapularis using a screw (Bristow). The soft tissues are repaired and the incision closed. A sling and swathe or a Velpeau dressing is applied.

Preparation of the patient

The patient is supine with the affected shoulder elevated with a sandbag or folded sheet. The arm on the affected side is flexed over the chest; the other arm may be extended on an armboard. Apply electrosurgical dispersive pad.

Skin preparation

Begin at the anterior aspect of the shoulder extending from the submandibular region to the inferior costal margin. Hold up and prepare the arm. Cleanse the axilla well. Prepare the back of the shoulder and the back of the arm down to the table. Cleanse forearm and hand.

Draping

The extremity is held up in a tube (or impervious) stockinette. A large, cuffed drape sheet is tucked under the patient's shoulder. The tube stockinette is brought up over the shoulder. A split sheet is draped under the arm and clipped. A large drape (or split) sheet is draped over the shoulder and clipped below. The arm may be passed through a fenestrated sheet, or individual drape sheets complete the draping.

Equipment

Sandbag or folded sheet (positioning)
Suction
Electrosurgical unit
Power source(s) for saw and drill

Instrumentation

Basic orthopedic procedures tray
Retractors (e.g., Hibbs, Bennett, Bankart)
Osteotomes
Steinmann pins
Power drill, cord, drill bits
Power saw and cord
Fixation devices: e.g., screws, staples (and instrumentation)

Supplies

Basin set
Blades (2) No. 10, (1) No. 15
Needle magnet or counter
Suction tubing
Electrosurgical pencil
Tube (or impervious) stockinette
Bulb syringe
Graduate
Antibiotic irrigation, optional
Sling and swathe or Velpeau dressing

Special notes

Have x-ray films in room.
Check levels in tanks for power equipment.

Do not allow preparation solution to pool under patient's shoulder.

Check with the surgeon regarding the immobilization of the shoulder following the procedure.

Protective goggles may be worn.

OPEN REDUCTION OF FRACTURE OF THE HUMERAL HEAD (INCLUDING HUMERAL HEAD PROSTHESIS)

Definition

Realignment and fixation of the humeral head through an operative incision.

Discussion

Most of these fractures are not treated surgically. They are often associated with dislocations, and in children the epiphyses may be involved. Fixation may be achieved with wire and/or special plates. A severely comminuted fracture may require replacement of the humeral head with a prosthesis.

Procedure

For an avulsion fracture of the tuberosities, a deltopectoral approach is used. The fracture fragment is repaired with wire. The soft tissue injury (e.g., rotator cuff) is repaired. When the humeral head is fractured as well, additional wire and a T compression plate may be required to achieve compression. Severely comminuted fractures may require a humeral head prosthesis. The deltoid muscle is detached. Attachments of major tendons are preserved with adequate bone fragments. Loose fragments and debris are irrigated away. The prosthesis is driven into the humeral shaft and the bone fragments attached to the prosthesis with wire sutures. Methylmethacrylate may be used in seating the prosthesis. The rotator cuff and soft tissues are closed over the wire sutures. The long head of the biceps tendon, previously detached, may be sutured to the repaired rotator cuff or implanted into the bicipital groove. The deltoid muscle is reattached. The incision is closed. A sling and swathe are placed.

Preparation of the patient

The patient is supine with arms extended on armboards. For insertion of a prosthesis the patient is supine with the knees over the lower break in the table. Following the administration of anesthesia, the sitting position is employed by raising the head of the table from the middle break. The foot of the table is lowered. A padded footboard supports the feet. The unaffected arm is placed on the patient's lap on a pillow secured with a padded restraint. The affected arm is usually supported by a sling. Apply electrosurgical dispersive pad.

Skin preparation

Begin at the anterior aspect of the shoulder extending from the submandibular region to the inferior costal margin. Hold up the arm and cleanse the axilla well. Prepare the back of the shoulder down to the table. Cleanse the arm, forearm and hand.

Draping

The extremity is held up in a tube (or impervious) stockinette. A large, cuffed drape sheet is tucked under the patient's shoulder. The tube stockinette is brought up over the shoulder. A drape (or split) sheet is draped under the arm and clipped. A large drape (or split) sheet is draped over the shoulder and clipped below. The arm may be passed through a fenestrated sheet or individual drape sheets complete the draping.

Equipment

Footboard (padded), padded arm restraint, pillow
Electrosurgical unit
Suction
Power sources for drill and saw

Instrumentation

Basic orthopedic procedures tray
Osteotomes, Bennett and Hibbs retractors, threaded
    pins, wire tightener
Power drill, cord, and drill bits
Power saw and cord, optional
Fixation devices, e.g., wire (stainless steel No. 20),
    T compression plate, screws
Prosthesis, with instrumentation, e.g., Neer I and Neer
    II (total shoulder joint replacement) and rasps,
    impactor, extractor, etc.

Supplies

Basin set
Blades (2) No. 10
Needle magnet or counter
Suction tubing
Electrosurgical pencil
Graduate
Bulb syringe
Tube (or impervious) stockinette
Methylmethacrylate kit
Antibiotic irrigation, optional
Sling and swathe

Special notes

Have x-ray films in room.
Check levels in tanks for power equipment.
Protective goggles may be worn.

INTERNAL FIXATION OF THE HIP

Definition

Stabilization of an intracapsular fracture of the femoral neck or an extracapsular fracture of the intertrochanteric region.

Discussion

The procedure is usually indicated in even the "poor risk" patient to enable early postoperative patient mobilization. The procedure can even be performed under local anesthesia in some instances. Fixation may be achieved with a nail, pin, or screw across the fracture site, sometimes in conjunction with a plate along the femoral shaft.

Procedure

A fracture table may be employed. After anesthesia is induced, the fracture is reduced and checked by x-ray in two planes. Following skin preparation and draping, a lateral (less often an anterior) incision is made exposing the fracture site. The appropriate nail with plate, threaded pins, or a compression screw is placed after guidewires are inserted temporarily to check alignment. A drill is used to facilitate placement of the plate screws. X-ray check again is performed. The wound may be irrigated with an antibiotic solution. The wound is closed.

Preparation of the patient

Determine if the fracture table is to be used. The patient is in the supine position either on the fracture table or the regular operating table (prepared for image intensifier). Adequate padding is needed to protect extremities and bony prominences. A sterile, plastic adhesive drape may be used to drape the perineum out of the field before preparing. Apply electrosurgical dispersive pad.

Skin preparation

Begin over the greater trochanter extending from the nipple to the toes. Prepare beyond the midline of the abdomen anteriorly, and down to the table on the affected side. The preparation should include the entire leg and foot, which are held up and abducted.

Draping

Fracture table: Folded towels, a sterile, plastic adhesive drape, and a laparotomy sheet. *Regular table:* The leg is abducted and the foot grasped in a towel (which is clipped) and then covered with a tube (or impervious) stockinette. A large, cuffed drape (or split) sheet is draped under the thigh. Towels are secured around the site of the incision. A large sheet is draped proximal to the inferior costal margin. The stockinette is rolled up over the extremity proximal to the iliac crest and fixed anteriorly and posteriorly. The leg is brought through a large fenestrated sheet. An opening is made in the stockinette over the site of the incision and is covered by a sterile, plastic adhesive drape.

Equipment

Fracture table (e.g., Stryker or Chick) or image intensifier extension
Electrosurgical unit
Suction
Power source for power drill

Instrumentation

Basic orthopedic procedures tray
Bone holding instruments tray
Hip retractors tray
Power drill, cord, and drill bits
Fixation device: Pins (e.g., Knowles, Deyerle, Hagie), nail (e.g., Jewett, Smith-Petersen), or Richards

sion screw (lag screw, barrel, plate) and instrumentation particular to each device
Guide pins

Supplies

Basin set
Suction tubing
Electrosurgical pencil
Blades (4) No. 10
Bulb syringes (2)
Graduate
Tube (or impervious) stockinette, if regular table is used
Sterile, plastic adhesive drapes (2), optional (for perineum and operative site)
Antibiotic irrigation, optional

Special notes

Have x-ray films in room.
Some surgeons prefer to double-glove and remove first pair following completion of draping.
Notify x-ray department when the patient is being positioned on the table. (Fluoroscopy will give views of fracture, guide pins, and position of nailing device.
Observe x-ray precautions; see p. 20.
Protective goggles may be worn.

FEMORAL HEAD PROSTHETIC REPLACEMENT

Definition

Substitution of the femoral head with a prosthesis made of Vitallium or similar inert metal.

Discussion

This procedure is indicated in nonunion of femoral neck fractures, avascular necrosis of the femoral head, degenerative changes of the hip postfracture, or from arthritis (primarily fractures that cannot be expected to heal retaining the femoral head). One advantage of this procedure is that immediate weight-bearing is permitted; it is more extensive and entails more risks than procedures retaining the femoral head. Several prostheses are used including Moore, Müller, Thompson, and Bateman.

Procedure

Several incisions and approaches are employed. A posterior incision may be made over the gluteus maximus superiorly and paralleling the proximal femur. The muscle fibers are split. The sciatic nerve is protected. The external rotators of the hip are freed from the femur, and the joint capsule is incised. Flexion, adduction, and internal rotation of the thigh are employed to dislocate the hip. The femoral head is removed and measured so that a similar-sized prosthetic head can be used. The medullary canal is reamed with a special rasp. The neck is shaped to receive the prosthesis without rotation, leaving enough of the calcar medially. After checking the size of the prosthesis in the actual acetabulum, the prosthesis is seated using special driving instruments for that particular prosthesis. Excess bone fragments are trimmed. Care is taken not to fracture the usually thinned femoral shaft. Methylmethacrylate may be used in seating the prosthesis into the femoral shaft. The incision is closed.

Preparation of the patient

Usually a posterior approach is used with the patient in the lateral position with sandbags, Vac Pac, or kidney rests supporting the torso. The arm on the unaffected side is extended on an armboard and the other arm is flexed over the chest, with a pillow between the arms, and secured by a padded restraint (or a double armboard may be used). The unaffected leg is extended and the affected leg is flexed over it (or both legs may be flexed). A pillow is placed between the legs. Adequate padding around feet, ankles, and bony prominences must be taken into consideration. The position is secured by wide adhesive tape at the shoulder anchored to the underside of the table and by the safety strap over the unaffected leg. A sterile, plastic adhesive drape may be used to drape the perineum out of the field. Apply electrosurgical dispersive pad.

Skin preparation

Begin over the greater trochanter extending from the nipple to the toes. Prepare beyond the midline of the abdomen anteriorly, and down to the table posteriorly. The preparation should include the entire leg and foot.

Draping

The leg is abducted and the foot is grasped in a towel (which is clipped) and then covered with a tube (or impervious) stockinette. A large sheet is draped over the end of the table. A large drape sheet (cuffed) or a split sheet is draped under the leg. Towels are secured around the site of the incision. A large sheet is draped proximal to the inferior costal margin. The stockinette is rolled up over the extremity proximal to the iliac crest and fixed anteriorly and posteriorly. The leg is brought through a fenestrated sheet. An opening is made in the stockinette over the site of the incision, and covered by a sterile, plastic adhesive drape.

Equipment

Sandbags, Vac Pac, pillows, kidney rests, and padded restraints (for positioning)
Electrosurgical unit
Suction
Power sources for power drill and saw
Pillows (for positioning postoperatively)

Instrumentation

Basic orthopedic procedures tray
Hip retractors tray
Osteotomes, bone hooks
Drill bits (including ¼″ and ½″)
Extra guide pins
Power drill and cord
Power saw and cord
Femoral head extractor, acetabular knife, hip skid, femoral rasps, caliper, driver
Prosthesis (e.g., Moore, Bateman) and specific instrumentation

Supplies

Basin set
Blades (3) No. 10
Needle magnet or counter
Suction tubing
Electrosurgical pencil
Sterile, plastic adhesive drapes (2) (perineum and operative site)
Bulb syringes (2)
Graduate
Tube (or impervious) stockinette
Methylmethacrylate kit, optional

Special notes

Have x-ray films in room.

Notify x-ray department of times films are to be taken.

Observe x-ray precautions; see p. 20.

Protect skin under adhesive tape with tincture of benzoin.

Some surgeons may prefer to double-glove and remove the first pair following draping.

Protective goggles should be worn.

Follow hospital policy for recording the insertion of a prosthesis.

TOTAL HIP REPLACEMENT

Definition

Substitution of the femoral head with a prosthesis and the reconstruction of the acetabulum with the placement of an acetabular cup, both of which may be fixed with methylmethacrylate.

Discussion

Disorders of the hip joint for which this procedure may be indicated are rheumatoid arthritis, degenerative disease (e.g., osteoarthritis, post-traumatic conditions), avascular necrosis, after an infection, and failed reconstruction. Numerous modifications of prostheses are employed, such as different alloys, porous coating, ceramics, and the use of a bipolar cup. Some, but not all of these, require methylmethacrylate to seat the prosthesis. Prostheses requiring methylmethacrylate to ensure stability include Bechtol, OPTI-FIX, Spectron, Charnley, Charnley-Müller, Aufranc-Turner, Harris Precoat, and Ob. The noncemented technique may be employed when the prosthesis can be tightly fitted into healthy strong bone (i.e., not usually for use in the elderly). The press-fit type (Judet, Lord), porous metal (Harris/Galante, Lanceford, Bias, Engh), bipolar cup (Bateman), and ceramic (Mittelmeir) are varieties of noncemented prostheses. The hip is weight-bearing within several days postoperatively when a cemented prosthesis is used. When a noncemented prosthesis is used the hip is not weight-bearing for up to 3 months. The noncemented prosthesis has the advantage, however, of relatively easy removal should it become necessary. The long-term efficacy of the noncemented type (versus cemented) has not yet been assessed. The "Charnley type" cemented total hip cup prosthesis remains the standard.

Procedure

One of several techniques may be employed. In the lateral approach a longitudinal incision is made proximal to the greater trochanter and distally along the proximal femoral shaft. The fascia is incised and the muscle fibers are separated. Scar tissue is freed. The insertions of the rotator muscles of the hip are divided (and tagged for later reapproximation). The hip joint capsule is exposed. By adduction and internal rotation the hip is dislocated as gently as possible. If this maneuver is difficult, scar tissue and/or additional tendons may be divided. The femoral neck is osteotomized and the femoral head extracted. The proximal femur is trimmed and the medullary canal reamed to accept the prosthesis. The acetabulum is then exposed, any remaining labrum is excised, and the capsule is detached from the anterior and inferior margins. Cartilage and soft tissues are curetted from the acetabulum. Acetabular reamers are employed to prepare the acetabulum to accept the cup prosthesis. Anchoring holes are drilled in the acetabulum. The proper position and angulation of the cup are determined. Methylmethacrylate is prepared and applied, and the cup positioned. Excess methylmethacrylate is trimmed. The femoral prosthesis is inserted, and test relocation is performed making any corrections to provide proper seating of the prosthesis. The prosthesis is then removed and seated again after methylmethacrylate has been placed in the medullary canal; excess methylmethacrylate is trimmed. When the methylmethacrylate is set the hip is relocated. The previously incised soft tissue and osteotomized (or tendon) attachments are replaced using nonabsorbable sutures. The wound is closed. A closed drainage system may be employed. Pillows are placed postoperatively to prevent adduction of the thighs.

Preparation of the patient, Skin preparation, and Draping

See Femoral Head Prosthetic Replacement, p. 267.

Equipment

Laminar airflow (if available)
Sandbags, Vac Pac, kidney rests, pillows, and/or padded restraints (for positioning)
Electrosurgical unit
Suction
Power sources for drill and saw
Scales (to weigh sponges)
Pillows (for positioning postoperatively)

Instrumentation

Basic orthopedic procedures tray
Hip retractors tray
Hip gouges, hip skid, rasps, femoral head extractor, acetabular reamer, acetabular knife, caliper
Extra guide pins
Osteotomes, curettes, bone hooks
Power drill, cord, and drill bits (including ¼" and ½")
Trial prosthesis
Total hip implant and specific instrumentation

Supplies

Basin set
Suction tubing
Electrosurgical pencil
Blades (4) No. 10
Needle magnet or counter
Asepto or bulb syringes (2)
Graduate
Tube (or impervious) stockinette
Sterile, plastic adhesive drapes (2) (perineum and operative site)
Gelfoam and thrombin (available)
Abduction pillow
Antibiotic irrigation, optional
Methylmethacrylate kit
Closed drainage unit (e.g., Hemovac)

Special notes

Have x-ray films in room.

Laminar airflow may be used.

Protect skin under adhesive tape with tincture of benzoin.

Have all instrumentation for specific prosthesis sterile.

Keep movement and conversation in the room to a minimum.

Some surgeons will double-glove and discard first pair after draping.

Keep accurate record of irrigation.

Check with blood bank that blood ordered is available.

Check levels in tanks for power drill and saw.

Notify x-ray department of time films will be needed.

Observe x-ray precautions, see p. 20.

Be prepared to change suction apparatus and tubing if it becomes clogged.

Follow hospital policy for recording the insertion of a prosthesis.

Protective goggles should be worn.

OPEN REDUCTION OF THE FEMORAL SHAFT

Definition

Realignment and fixation of a fracture of the femur through an operative incision.

Discussion

Surgical intervention may be indicated in certain fractures of the femur in the adult patient. Fractures of the femur in children and young adults are treated with traction followed by immobilization. Intramedullary nails include Hansen-Street, Küntscher, Lottes, Rush, Schneider, Enders, and Zickel. If a compression plate is used, it must have at least three holes above and below the fracture.

Procedure

Use of the fracture table is desirable. Temporary traction devices are removed prior to skin preparation. A posterolateral incision is made over the fracture site. The medullary canal is reamed with special medullary reamers. A guide pin is driven from the fracture site proximally to emerge subcutaneously just proximal to the greater trochanter. A small counterincision is made over the prominence of the emerging guide pin. The cortical opening can be enlarged with a drill. An appropriate length and diameter Küntscher rod is seated over the guide pin with the extractor eye oriented posterolaterally. The rod is then introduced into the now reduced distal segment and seated securely into the condylar region. The proximal end should protrude no more than 2.5 cm. If the fracture site is comminuted, wire loops are placed around the fragments. X-ray control is used as necessary to avoid creating false passages, malalignment, or fracture of the nail. The wound is closed.

Preparation of the patient

The patient is usually positioned on the fracture table in the lateral position. The arm on the unaffected side is extended on an armboard and the other arm is flexed across the chest; it may be positioned on a Mayo stand padded with a pillow (or a double armboard may be used). Adequate padding around feet, ankles, and bony prominences must be taken into consideration, particularly because the fracture table is very hard. If the fracture table is not used, the unaffected leg is extended and the affected leg is flexed over it. A pillow is placed between the legs, and the feet and ankles are padded. The patient is held in position by wide adhesive tape at the shoulders and by the safety strap over the unaffected thigh. A sterile, plastic adhesive drape may be used to drape the perineum out of the field before skin preparation. Apply electrosurgical dispersive pad.

Skin preparation

Begin over the fracture site extending from the umbilicus to below the knee, well beyond the midline anteriorly (or to the sterile, plastic adhesive drape), and down to the table posteriorly. If the leg is draped free (i.e., the fracture table is not used), the leg and foot are completely prepared. A leg holder may be used.

Draping

The incisional site is draped with folded towels and a sterile, plastic adhesive drape (optional). Four sheets may be draped around the perimeter of the site; a fenestrated sheet covers the field. If the fracture table is not employed, see Femoral Head Prosthetic Replacement, p. 267.

Equipment

Fracture table (e.g., Stryker, Chick, as requested)
Leg holder, optional
Suction
Electrosurgical unit
Power source for drill

Instrumentation

Basic orthopedic procedures tray
Hip retractors tray
Bone holding instruments tray
Drill bits, including ¼" gauge
Power drill and cord
Extra guide pins, screw set
Fixation device: Rods or nails (e.g., Hansen-Street, Küntscher, Rush) or compression set and instrumentation particular to that device

Supplies

Basin set
Suction tubing

Electrosurgical pencil
Needle magnet or counter
Sterile, plastic adhesive drapes (2) (perineum and
    operative site)
Blades (2) No. 10
Asepto or bulb syringes (2)
Graduate
Tube (or impervious) stockinette, 6" (if fracture table
    not used)

Special notes

Have x-ray films in room.
Protect skin under adhesive tape with tincture of
benzoin.
Some surgeons prefer to double-glove and re-
move first pair following completion of draping.
Notify x-ray department when patient is being
positioned on the table for preliminary films.
Observe x-ray precautions, see p. 20.
Protective goggles may be worn.

ARTHROTOMY OF THE KNEE

Definition

Incision into the knee joint.

Discussion

A variety of injuries can occur about the knee joint.
These include fractures, meniscal tears, and ligamentous injuries related to torsion or tearing of the
ligaments. Synovectomy may be performed for
chronic synovitis, post-trauma or after infectious conditions, in addition to rheumatoid arthritis, hemangioma, and villonodular changes. Arthroscopy may
be employed for some presentations of these conditions. Others require arthrotomy; there is a wide variety of procedures. Some of these include:
   ***Open Reduction of Femoral Condyle and Tib-
ial Plateau Fractures.*** Alignment and stabilization

of the articular surfaces of the distal femur and proximal tibia to provide joint stability.

Meniscectomy. Excision of a torn meniscus and either or both semilunar fibrocartilages.

Patellectomy. Excision of all or a portion of the patella.

Synovectomy. Excision of all or a portion of the synovial membrane of the knee.

Collateral or Cruciate Ligament Repair. Repair of damaged ligaments of the knee, restoring them as closely as possible to the original anatomy.

Procedure

Open Reduction of Fractures of the Femoral Condyles and Tibial Plateau. A longitudinal incision is made exposing the fracture site. Debris and minor bone fragments are irrigated out. Temporary reduction may be achieved with Kirschner wires, which are removed following the insertion of Knowles pins, cancellous bone screws or bolts, etc. with penetration of the opposite cortex. "T" fractures of the femoral condyles may be stabilized with a plate or screws. In tibial plateau fractures the joint is explored after reflecting the iliotibial band and/or additional muscular attachments. Ligamentous and cartilaginous injuries are repaired. The fracture is reduced and fixed with hardware, as above. Cancellous bone from the proximal tibia may be packed into the fracture site. The wound is closed. A posterior splint may be applied.

Lateral Meniscectomy. An anterolateral incision is made from the level of the patella to the upper tibia. The quadriceps aponeurosis and joint capsule are incised. The meniscus is grasped and excised taking care to avoid injury to the popliteal tendon, fibular collateral ligament, and vascular structures. A secondary posterolateral incision may be necessary to visualize and excise the posterior horn of the meniscus. The incisions are closed. A bulky compression dressing is applied.

Open Reduction of Fractures of the Patella

and Patellectomy. A transverse prepatellar incision is made. The patellar tendon and joint are explored (and suture-repaired during closure). The fracture site is exposed. Debris and small fragments are irrigated from the joint. Major fracture fragments are approximated and repaired through a variety of techniques using wire and/or screws. Lesser fragments and the severely comminuted entire patella can be excised with shortening of the patellar tendon. The wound is closed, and a splint is applied.

Synovectomy. An anteromedial incision is made. The synovial membrane is excised from the medial, lateral, and anterior aspect of the joint including prepatellar fat pad and menisci (if they are degenerated). Using a sponge or curette, pannus is removed from the femoral condyles. By flexing the knee posterior synovium is excised. Optimal hemostasis is achieved. The wound is closed over a suction drain. The leg is immobilized.

Medial Collateral Ligament Repair. A medial longitudinal incision is made. The greater saphenous vein and sensory branches of the saphenous nerve are protected. The deep fascia is incised, and the sartorius muscle is retracted with the knee flexed. The tibial insertion of the medial collateral ligament is inspected. The joint capsule is incised and the cruciate ligaments, menisci, and adjacent articular surfaces are inspected. Capsular tears and other ligamentous injuries are repaired; menisci, if injured, are excised. The joint is closed, and the medial collateral ligament and posterior oblique ligament are repaired by sutures in their midportion or by staples or sutures to bone at their origins or insertions. Tendons may be transferred if further strengthening is required. Hemostasis is achieved. A long leg cast is applied.

Preparation of the patient

The patient is supine with the knees over the lower break in the table; arms may be extended on armboards. The patient is secured with the safety belt over the thigh of the unaffected extremity. Sheet wadding and a tourniquet are applied to the top of the thigh of the operative leg. Apply electrosurgical dispersive pad.

Skin preparation

Begin at the knee extending from immediately below the tourniquet (on the thigh) to the toes.

Draping

The leg is abducted and held up in a tube (or impervious) stockinette. A sheet is draped over the end of the table. A drape sheet (cuffed) or a split sheet is draped under the thigh. A folded towel (in thirds, lengthwise) is wrapped around the top of the thigh, and the tube stockinette is brought up over the folded towel. A drape (or split) sheet is draped proximal to the knee and clipped below. Either a fenestrated sheet or individual drape sheets complete the draping. An additional sheet will be necessary if the foot of the table is lowered (in order to flex the knee) during the procedure.

Equipment

Suction
Electrosurgical unit
Tourniquet and insufflator
Power source for drill (for fracture of patella)
Cast cart

Instrumentation

Basic orthopedic procedures tray
Knee arthrotomy tray
Power drill, cord, drill bits (fracture of patella)
Staples and instrumentation (ligament repair)
Kirschner wires
Fixation devices and instrumentation (as required)

Supplies

Sheet wadding
Basin set
Blades (2) No. 10, (1) No. 15
Wire, e.g., stainless steel No. 18 (fracture of patella)
Suction tubing
Electrosurgical pencil
Needle magnet or counter
Asepto or bulb syringe
Tube (or impervious) stockinette, 6"
Esmarch bandage

Special notes

Have x-ray films in room.

Protective goggles may be worn.

Be sure knees are over the lower break in the table.

Do not allow preparation solution to pool under the tourniquet.

Place tourniquet as high on the extremity as possible.

Wrap sheet wadding around the extremity smoothly. Tourniquet ends should overlap about 7.5 cm (3 inches).

Setting for an adult is approximately 400 mm Hg for the lower extremity.

Monitor tourniquet time and setting.

Tourniquet must be released after 2 hours to avoid injury.

ARTHROSCOPY OF THE KNEE

Definition

Endoscopic visualization of the knee joint.

Discussion

By direct visualization of the intra-articular structures, diagnoses, as well as specific surgeries such as meniscectomy, synovectomy, shaving of the patella, excision of loose bodies, and transcutaneous suture repair of ligaments, can be performed.

Procedure

The knee joint is distended with saline via a needle inserted laterally into the suprapatellar pouch near the superior pole of the patella. A trocar and sheath are inserted through a stab wound at a point predetermined according to the disease process. When the trocar penetrates the capsule, the capsule and synovium form a tight seal around the sheath. An obturator replaces the trocar in the sheath, and the obturator is advanced into the joint. The obturator is removed and replaced by the arthroscope. Inflow and outflow irrigation tubing are attached to the sheath. The outflow irrigation tubing is attached to suction. The knee joint is thoroughly examined. Procedures such as meniscectomy or synovectomy may be performed. Instruments such as probes, scissors, and hooks can be employed using a separate skin incision (or the side channel of some operating arthroscopes). The patella may be smoothed with a power shaver. A carbon dioxide laser may be employed with some arthroscopes; see Appendix, p. 572 for laser precautions. A video camera may be attached to the eyepiece as the view is projected on a television monitor. Following completion of the procedure, the saline is aspirated. The scope is withdrawn. The wound or wounds are closed and a compression bandage is applied.

Preparation of the patient

The patient is supine with knees over the lower break in the table; arms may be extended on armboards. The patient is secured to the table with a safety belt over the thigh of the unaffected extremity. Usually the surgeon will drop the foot of the table for the procedure; for this a leg-holding device may be used. Apply sheet wadding and a tourniquet to the thigh of the operative leg. Apply electrosurgical dispersive pad (if arthrotomy is to follow).

Skin preparation and Draping

See Arthrotomy of the Knee, p. 277.

Equipment

Suction (large collector containers, multiunit, if available) with trap (for specimen)
Electrosurgical unit (if arthrotomy is to follow)
Leg holder (for preparation)
Leg-holding device (table attachment)
Tourniquet and insufflator
Light source for fiberoptic telescope
Intra-articular shaver power unit and foot pedal (for patella shaving), optional
Camera, screen, and articulated viewing device for video arthroscopy, optional
Meniscutome power unit and foot pedal (for meniscectomy), optional
Arthroplasty power unit and foot pedal, optional

Instrumentation

Knee or ankle arthroscopy tray
Have available:
Fat pad retractor
Acuflex 90° rotary basket forceps
Hook basket forceps
Oretorp meniscectomy knife with blades and sheath
Magnetic rod (to retrieve broken instrument parts)
Beaver blade handle
Video camera
Intra-articular shaver with obturators, cannulas, and cord
Meniscutome, sheath and outer blade, inner blade, and cord
Arthroplasty instruments
Arthroplasty power instrumentation and cord

Supplies

Sheet wadding
Basin set
Blade (1) No. 15, (1) No. 11
Smillie Beaver blade (available)
Needle magnet or counter
Tube (or impervious) stockinette, 6"
Esmarch bandage
Suction tubing
Irrigation tubing (multiple lines, disposable, if available)
Saline irrigation (several 2000-ml or 3000-ml bags)
Large-bore needle (e.g., 16- or 18-gauge)

Special notes

Have x-ray films in room.

Be sure the patient's knees are over the break in the table.

For tourniquet precautions, see Arthrotomy of the Knee, p. 277.

Room lights are dimmed; x-ray viewing-box lights may be used.

Ethylene oxide sterilization and aeration of the arthroscope is recommended; however, disinfection with activated glutaraldehyde solution according to manufacturer's instructions may be performed.

If arthrotomy is to follow arthroscopy, the patient must be reprepared and redraped, and a change of gowns, gloves, and instruments is required.

Many bags of irrigation solution may be used.

Be prepared to change suction collection devices frequently.

A sterile cover is required for articulated viewing device from camera during video arthroscopy.

When an instrument is broken, the irrigation is immediately turned off.

Protective goggles may be worn.

EXCISION OF POPLITEAL (BAKER'S) CYST

Definition

Excision of a cyst located in the popliteal space.

Discussion

These cysts are formed by the herniation of synovial membrane or the escape of synovial fluid of the knee joint with the accumulation in one of several bursae in the popliteal space. The cysts also occur in rheumatoid arthritis. Other conditions affecting the knee may be associated (e.g., torn meniscus). Arthrography may be used to delineate the cyst and to distinguish it from other lesions such as tumors and popliteal artery aneurysm.

Procedure

An oblique incision is made over the mass. Deep fascia is incised exposing the sac that is then dissected free, tracing its attachment to the posterior aspect of the knee joint capsule. The pedicle is ligated, and the cyst excised. Tendon bundles may be used to reinforce the closure. The wound is closed. A splint is applied.

Preparation of the patient

The patient is prone with chest rolls under the thorax and a roll in front of the ankles. The arms are positioned on armboards angled toward the head of the table with the hands pronated. If a tourniquet is used, it is applied on the thigh of the affected leg. A safety strap is secured across the unaffected thigh. Apply electrosurgical dispersive pad.

Skin preparation

A leg holder may be used. Begin at the back of

the knee and include the entire thigh (up to tourniquet, if used), knee, leg, and foot.

Draping

The leg is abducted and the foot is held up in a tube (or impervious) stockinette. A large sheet is draped over the end of the table. A folded towel (lengthwise) is wrapped around the top of the thigh and clipped; the stockinette is brought up over the towel. A drape (or split) sheet is draped under the thigh and clipped. A large drape (or split) sheet is draped over the thigh and clipped underneath. The field is covered with additional drape sheets, or the leg is passed through a fenestrated sheet.

Equipment

Leg holder
Electrosurgical unit
Chest rolls, an ankle roll, pillows, padding (as necessary for positioning)
Tourniquet and insufflator (available)
Cast cart

Instrumentation

Basic/Minor procedures tray
Basic orthopedic procedures tray
Knee arthrotomy tray (available)

Supplies

Basin set
Blades (2) No. 10, (1) No. 15
Electrosurgical pencil
Needle magnet or counter
Tube (or impervious) stockinette, 6"
Bulb syringe
Esmarch bandage

Special notes

In the adult patient, a popliteal cyst may be indicative of intra-articular disease; arthrotomy may be necessary.

Adequate padding is required for female breasts and male genitalia.

For tourniquet precautions, see Arthrotomy of the Knee, p. 277.

Protective goggles may be worn.

TOTAL KNEE REPLACEMENT

Definition

Replacement of the articular surfaces of the knee joint by prostheses.

Discussion

The procedure is performed for pain, deformity, and instability secondary to rheumatoid arthritis, osteoarthritis, and post-traumatic conditions. The articular surfaces of the femoral condyles, tibial plateau, anterior trochlear surface of the femur, and articular surface of the patella are trimmed to accept the prostheses. The prostheses are bonded to the bone with methylmethacrylate.

On occasion a single component of the knee's articular surface (e.g., medial femoral and tibial condyles), needs to be replaced (unicompartmental). More commonly the entire or total surface requires replacement (tricompartmental).

There are four categories of total knee systems:
1. *Constrained (hinged):* A hinge joint, infrequently used. Examples are Walldius, Guepar, Shiers, and St. Georg prostheses.
2. *Nonhinged Constrained:* Spherocentric, allows motion that nearly duplicates that of the normal knee. Examples are Attenborough and Sheehan prostheses.

3. *Nonconstrained:* Provides full coverage of the articular surfaces, but adds little stability. Examples are Marmor, Savastano, Oxford, Porous Coated Anatomic (PCA), Bias, Mod II Unicompartmental, TRICON-M, and TRICON-C prostheses.
4. *Partially Constrained:* Provides stability as well as providing full coverage of the articular surface. Examples include Richards Maximum Contact (RMC), Insall-Burstein, Kinematic II, and Freeman-Swanson prostheses.

Procedure

A longitudinal incision extends from over the patella to the tibial tuberosity. The quadriceps tendon is incised superiorly and the knee joint entered. The capsule is incised, the knee is flexed, and the knee joint exposed. The anterior portions of menisci, any osteophytes, and hyperplastic synovium are excised. Soft tissues (if any) are released. Jigs, templates, and spacers of varying sizes for each prosthetic type are employed. Lines may be marked with methylene blue dye and appropriate bone excised (as are the cruciate ligaments and remaining posterior aspect of the menisci). Slots or holes are cut or drilled to accept the prostheses. Methylmethacrylate is used to seat the prosthesis; the excess is removed. The patella may be replaced by a prosthesis as well. A check is made of stability, alignment, and range of motion. Realignment of the quadriceps mechanism and patella tendon is carefully performed. Hemostasis is achieved when the tourniquet is released. Suction drains are placed in the joint, and the wound layers are closed in partial flexion (to avoid tension or closure). A bulky dressing is applied. The extremity may be placed in a continuous passive motion (CPM) device when the patient reaches the recovery room, or several days postoperatively. (The CPM device may also be used for other postoperative conditions of the knee, hip, shoulder, and elbow.)

Preparation of the patient

The patient is supine with the knees over the lower break in the table; arms may be extended on armboards. The patient is secured with a safety strap over the thigh of the unaffected extremity. Sheet wadding and a tourniquet are applied to the top of the thigh of the operative extremity. Apply electrosurgical dispersive pad.

Skin preparation

A foot holder may be used. Begin at the knee extending from immediately below the tourniquet (on the thigh) to the toes.

Draping

The leg is held up and abducted, and the foot is grasped in a tube (or impervious) stockinette. A large sheet is draped over the end of the table. A drape sheet (cuffed) or a split sheet is draped under the thigh. A folded towel (in thirds, lengthwise) is wrapped around the top of the thigh and clipped; the tube stockinette is brought up over the towel. A drape (or split) sheet is draped over the top of the thigh and clipped underneath. Either a fenestrated sheet or individual drape sheets complete the draping. An additional drape sheet will be needed when the dropped end of the table is returned to normal position.

Equipment

Laminar airflow (if available)
Foot holder
Suction
Electrosurgical unit
Tourniquet and insufflator
Power sources for drill and saw

Instrumentation

Basic orthopedic procedures tray
Knee arthrotomy tray
Osteotomes, gouges
Trial prosthesis, total knee prosthesis, and necessary
    instrumentation
Power drill and cord
Power oscillating saw with jigs and templates and
    cord

Supplies

Basin set
Electrosurgical pencil
Suction tubing
Blades (3) No. 10, (1) No. 15
Graduate
Bulb syringes (2)
Tube (or impervious) stockinette, 6″
Esmarch bandage
Needle magnet or counter
Methylmethacrylate kit
Antibiotic irrigation
Closed drainage system (e.g., Hemovac), optional
Methylene blue dye, optional

Special notes

Laminar airflow may be used.

Have x-ray films in room.

Have prosthesis and all necessary instrumentation sterile.

Keep conversation and movement in the room
to a minimum.

Check levels in tanks for power equipment.

For tourniquet precautions see Arthrotomy of the
Knee, p. 277.

Protective goggles may be worn.

Follow hospital policy for recording the insertion
of a prosthesis.

OPEN REDUCTION OF THE TIBIAL SHAFT

Definition

Realignment and fixation of the tibia through an operative incision.

Discussion

The type of fixation device is determined by the anatomic considerations of the fracture (i.e., comminuted). Severely comminuted fractures may have to be treated with prolonged traction rather than fixation.

Procedure

The fracture is exposed. Transverse bone screws or plates (including compression plates) are applied to the reduced fracture fragments. When an intramedullary nail is employed (e.g., Lottes, Rush, Enders, Schneider), an incision over the tibial tuberosity is made. A drill reamer penetrates the medullary canal. The measured nail is inserted, aligning it to avoid malrotation. It is then driven past the fracture site into the distal portion until the threaded end remains exposed (for later extraction). A counterincision over the fracture site may be needed to effect reduction. Care is taken during the driving of the nail to avoid injury to the shaft. The wound is closed.

Preparation of the patient

The patient is supine; arms may be extended on armboards. The safety strap is applied to the unaffected thigh. Sheet wadding and a tourniquet are applied to the thigh of the operative leg. Apply electrosurgical dispersive pad.

Skin preparation

Preparation is best performed by two people to prevent further injury to the bone. Begin at the fracture site; cleanse the leg, thigh (up to the tourniquet), and foot (including interdigital spaces and nails).

Draping

The leg is abducted and the foot is held up in a tube (or impervious) stockinette. A large sheet is draped over the end of the table. A folded towel (in thirds, lengthwise) is wrapped around the top of the thigh and clipped; the stockinette is brought up over the towel. A drape (or split) sheet is draped under the leg. A large drape (or split) sheet is draped over the thigh and clipped underneath. The leg is passed through a fenestrated sheet or additional drape sheets complete the draping.

Equipment

Suction
Electrosurgical unit
Tourniquet and insufflator
Power source for drill

Instrumentation

Basic orthopedic procedures tray
Bone holding instruments tray
Fixation device (and necessary instrumentation)
Power drill, cord, and drill bits

Supplies

Basin set
Sheet wadding
Blades (2) No. 10
Tube (or impervious) stockinette
Esmarch bandage
Needle magnet or counter
Graduate
Bulb syringe
Suction tubing

Electrosurgical pencil
Antibiotic irrigation, optional

Special notes

Have x-ray films in room.
Check pressure level in tank for power drill.
For tourniquet precautions see Arthrotomy of the Knee, p. 277.
Protective goggles may be worn.

OPEN REDUCTION OF THE ANKLE

Definition

Realignment and fixation of fractures of the medial malleolus (tibia), lateral malleolus (fibula), and/or posterior "malleolus" (posterior aspect of the distal tibia).

Discussion

This procedure is performed for acute fractures or nonunion of fractures. Many anatomic variations of ankle fractures and dislocations occur.

Procedure

For fracture of the lateral malleolus, an anterolateral incision is made over the fracture site avoiding the sural nerve. The malleolus is exposed and the fracture is fixed with screws engaging the opposite cortex. Care is taken not to compromise the tendon sheaths. After the incision is closed a short leg cast is applied.

Preparation of the patient

The patient is supine; arms may be extended on armboards and the safety belt is secured over the unaffected extremity. Apply sheet wadding and a tourniquet to the thigh of the operative leg. Apply electrosurgical dispersive pad.

Skin preparation

The preparation is performed by two people or a knee holder may be employed. Begin at the ankles and continue to foot (including interdigital spaces and nails). Next prepare the leg (including the knee).

Draping

The leg is abducted and the foot is held up in a tube (or impervious) stockinette. A large sheet is draped over the end of the table. A folded towel (in thirds, lengthwise) is wrapped around the top of the thigh and clipped; the tube stockinette is brought up over the towel. A drape (or split) sheet is draped under the leg. A large drape (or split) sheet is draped over the thigh and clipped underneath. The extremity is passed through a fenestrated sheet, or additional drape sheets cover the field.

Equipment

Leg holder, optional
Suction
Electrosurgical unit
Tourniquet and insufflator
Power source for drill
Cast cart

Instrumentation

Basic orthopedic procedures tray
Power drill, cord, and drill bits
Kirschner wires and Steinmann pins
Fixation device with instrumentation (e.g., Rush rods
    or compression plate and screw sets)

Supplies

Sheet wadding
Basin set
Blades (2) No. 10, (1) No. 15
Needle magnet or counter
Suction tubing
Tube (or impervious) stockinette
Esmarch bandage
Bulb syringe
Graduate
Electrosurgical pencil
Antibiotic irrigation, optional

Special notes

Have x-ray films in room.
For tourniquet precautions see Arthrotomy of the Knee, p. 277.
Protective goggles may be worn.
Be prepared for the application of a cast.

TRIPLE ARTHRODESIS OF THE ANKLE

Definition

Fusion of the talocalcaneal (subtalar), talonavicular, and the calcaneocuboid joints.

Discussion

Arthrodesis is performed to relieve pain, provide stability, and arrest a joint-destroying disease process. Multiple combinations of ankle joint arthrodeses and techniques may be employed which are classified as intra-articular, extra-articular, or a combination of the two.

Procedure

An incision is made from the dorsal prominence of the lateral aspect of the foot to the midportion of the calcaneus. Tendons are retracted exposing the floor of the sinus tarsi. The periosteum of the calcaneus is exposed and the calcaneocuboid joint capsule is incised. The articular surfaces are excised; the bone fragments are saved. The talonavicular joint capsule is incised and the head of the talus is excised. The proximal articular surface of the navicular is removed. The subtalar joint is incised and the articular surface removed with that of the sustenaculum tali and anterior facet of the talus. Bony surfaces are trimmed to correct deformity and to provide for maximum contact. An accessory medial incision may be required. Bone chips are packed into the defect. Soft tissues are sutured to fill the sinus tarsi obliterating dead space. Kirschner wires may be used to maintain alignment. A long leg cast is carefully applied, molding the foot to correct shape and aligning the malleoli. Ten to fourteen days postoperatively remanipulation of the foot under anesthesia may be necessary.

Preparation of the patient, Skin preparation, Draping, Equipment, and Supplies

See Open Reduction of the Ankle, p. 293.

Instrumentation

Basic orthopedic procedures tray
Power drill, cord, drill bits
Osteotomes, curette gouges
Steinmann pins, Kirschner wires
Fixation device and instrumentation (e.g., screws, staples)
Vertebral spreader (small)

Special notes

See Open Reduction of the Ankle, p. 293.

TOTAL ANKLE JOINT REPLACEMENT

Definition

Substitution of the articular surfaces of the distal tibia and the talus with high-density polyethylene and metal components that are fixed with methylmethacrylate.

Discussion

Indications for this procedure include traumatic, degenerative, and rheumatoid arthritis. In general, younger, more active patients will have better ankle function with fusion (arthrodesis). Elderly, less active patients are usually better candidates for joint replacement. The prostheses are classified as: constrained (restricted motion), semiconstrained (semirestricted motion), or nonconstrained (unrestricted motion).

Procedure

An anterolateral incision is made. Tendons and neurovascular structures are retracted. The tibiotalar joint and dome of the talus are exposed. Using special templates, osteotomy incisions for the tibia and talus are outlined and made with an oscillating saw. Care is taken to avoid injury to the posteromedial neurovascular bundle and the anterior talofibular ligament. A template is used to cut a section of tibia to accept the stem of the prosthesis. Holes are made in the talus with a curette to provide fixation points for the cement. Trial insertion of the prosthesis is made and range of motion is determined. The metallic tibial prosthesis is permanently seated after prepared methylmethacrylate is applied. Similarly, the polyethylene talar prosthesis is seated; excess methylmethacrylate is trimmed. The wound is irrigated. The incision is closed over suction drains. A splint is applied over a bulky dressing.

Preparation of the patient, Skin preparation, and Draping

See Open Reduction of the Ankle, p. 293.

Equipment

Laminar airflow (if available)
Suction
Electrosurgical unit
Tourniquet and insufflator
Cast cart

Instrumentation

Basic orthopedic procedures tray
Osteotomes, curettes
Power oscillating saw with jigs, templates, and cord
Trial prosthesis, total ankle prosthesis, and specific
    instrumentation
Power burr set (available)

Supplies

Basin set
Tube (or impervious) stockinette
Esmarch bandage
Needle magnet or counter
Blades (2) No. 10, (1) No. 15
Suction tubing
Electrosurgical pencil
Bulb syringes
Graduate
Methylmethacrylate kit
Antibiotic irrigation, optional
Closed drainage system (e.g., Hemovac)

Special notes

Laminar airflow may be used.
Keep conversation and movement in the room
to a minimum.

Have x-ray films in room.

Check pressure level in tanks for power equipment.

For tourniquet precautions, see Arthrotomy of the Knee, p. 277.

Have prosthesis and all necessary instrumentation sterile.

Protective goggles may be worn.

Follow hospital policy for recording the insertion of a prothesis.

BUNIONECTOMY

Definition

Excision of a soft tissue and/or bony mass at the medial aspect of the first metatarsal head.

Discussion

Correction may be achieved by a variety of procedures. Excision of exostosis, realignment of the great toe, transfer of tendons and/or osteotomy of the first metatarsal shaft may be performed. A frequently performed procedure is the Keller; others include the McBride and Silvers.

Procedure

Keller Procedure. A curved incision is made dorsally along the medial aspect of the first metatarsophalangeal joint. Care is taken to preserve the cutaneous nerves. The capsule and periosteum at the base of the proximal phalanx are incised and retracted. The metatarsal head is dislocated. The proximal half of the phalanx is resected. Exostosis and osteophytes are excised. The sesamoids are excised if they are enlarged, deformed, or arthritic. A Kirschner wire is inserted aligning the toe and the metatarsal head or the resected joint surfaces may be replaced by Silastic prosthesis. A figure-of-eight suture is placed in the capsule and periosteum to cover the end of the phalanx. The wound is closed.

Preparation of the patient

The patient is supine; arms may be extended on armboards and the safety belt is secured over the unaffected extremity. Sheet wadding and a tourniquet are applied to the thigh of the operative leg. Apply electrosurgical dispersive pad.

Skin preparation

A leg holder may be used. Begin with the great toe and prepare all nails, and interdigital spaces. Cleanse foot and leg extending up to the knee.

Draping

The leg is abducted and the foot is grasped in a tube (or impervious) stockinette. A large sheet is draped over the end of the table. A folded towel (in thirds, lengthwise) is wrapped around the top of the leg and clipped; the tube stockinette is brought up over the towel. A drape (or split) sheet is draped under the leg and clipped. A large drape (or split) sheet is draped over the thigh and clipped underneath. The extremity is passed through a fenestrated sheet, or additional drape sheets cover the field.

Equipment

Leg holder, optional
Electrosurgical unit
Tourniquet and insufflator
Power sources for drill and saw

Instrumentation

Minor orthopedic procedures tray
Osteotomes
Kirschner wires

Power saw and cord
Small power drill, cord, and drill bits

Supplies

Basin set
Sheet wadding
Tube (or impervious) stockinette, 6"
Blades (2) No. 10, (1) No. 15
Needle magnet or counter
Esmarch bandage
Bulb syringe
Graduate
Electrosurgical pencil
Antibiotic solution, optional

Special notes

Have x-ray films in room.
Check pressure levels of tanks for drill and saw.
For tourniquet precautions see Arthrotomy of the Knee, p. 277.
Protective goggles may be worn.

CORRECTION OF HAMMER TOE DEFORMITY WITH INTERPHALANGEAL FUSION

Definition

Resection and fixation of the proximal interphalangeal joint.

Discussion

The procedure corrects the deformity and prevents its recurrence. Corns are not disturbed because they disappear following the procedure.

Procedure

A longitudinal incision is made over the dorsum of the proximal interphalangeal joint. The extensor tendon is split and retracted exposing the joint. The base of the middle phalanx and the head of the proximal phalanx are excised. The remaining parts of the proximal and middle phalanges are fixed with a Kirschner wire drilled through the distal phalanx and out through the skin. A dorsal capsulotomy may be performed through a second incision to release a contracture. The wounds are closed. The wires may be capped.

Preparation of the patient, Skin preparation, Draping, Equipment, Instrumentation, Supplies, and Special notes

See Bunionectomy, p. 299.

METATARSAL HEAD RESECTION

Definition

Excision of the metatarsal head(s).

Discussion

The procedure is indicated in patients with pain related to the prominence of the metatarsal heads; it is often performed on patients with rheumatoid arthritis and dorsally dislocated toes.

Procedure

A longitudinal incision is made in the interspace adjacent to the particular metatarsal head to be excised. The metatarsal head and neck, as well as the articular surface of the phalanges, are freed of soft tissue and resected. Contracted soft tissue is released. The end of the metatarsal is smoothed with a bone rasp. A Kirschner wire is inserted through the medullary canal of the metatarsal stump, aligning it in proper relation to the appropriate toe. The wound is closed. A bulky pressure dressing is applied. The wire may be capped.

Preparation of the patient, Skin preparation, Draping, Equipment, Instrumentation, Supplies, and Special notes

See Bunionectomy, p. 299.

PROCEDURE FOR CORRECTION OF SCOLIOSIS

Definition

The insertion of various rods, frames, and other fixation devices that act as internal splints until the vertebrae involved in the curvature fuse in an improved position.

Discussion

Surgical treatment of scoliosis is performed when musculoskeletal and respiratory functions become compromised or for cosmetic purposes. A variety of systems (each requiring its own instrumentation) employing compression and distraction rods, hooks, spring hooks, buttons, wires, etc. are in use. The need for a plaster cast or jacket postoperatively varies with the procedure and individual patient requirements. Younger patients are more amenable to corrections. In the Harrington rod procedure a longitudinal compression rod is placed along the convex aspect of the curvature, and a distraction rod is placed on the concave side. Appropriate hooks are attached to the rods that when tightened diminish the curvature.

A variation of this technique using the Cotrel-DuBousset system employs transverse rods (in addition to the longitudinal rods) that apply corrective forces to segmental areas of the curvature, as well as the full length of the curvature.

Correction can also be accomplished with the Luque system of L-shaped rods and wires, which distributes the corrective forces to vertebral levels rather than the entire length of the deformity.

In the Wisconsin compression rod system Keene

hooks are applied to multiple transverse processes or laminae.

An alternative anterior approach (by anterolateral thoracotomy) for a thoracolumbar deformity uses the Dwyer system. A cable is placed through special screws that also anchor special staples placed in the vertebral bodies on the convex side of the curvature. The involved invertebral discs are removed and the cable tightened. Bone grafts (from a rib) are used.

Procedure

Harrington Rod. Incision is made over the spinous processes of the involved segments; by staying in the midline blood loss is minimized. The vertebral levels are identified using radiography as necessary. Muscular and ligamentous structures are reflected using elevators (Cobb) and curettes about the area to be fused. Bleeding is controlled with cautery and bone wax. Distraction hooks are placed on the concave side of the curvature avoiding penetration into the medullary cavity. Bone slots may be cut to accept the hooks. The distraction rod is then placed. Hooks for the compression rod are placed. Bone grafts from the posterior iliac crests are obtained and kept moist; the iliac wound is closed. The concave vertebral facets are obliterated, and decortication of the laminae and transverse processes is performed. Spinal fusion is achieved with bone grafts packed in predominantly on the concave side. Suction drains are placed and the wound closed. Casting or replacement of a preoperative bivalved cast may be employed, but usually not until several days postoperatively.

Preparation of the patient

The patient is prone on the Andrews or Wilson frame or on the operating room table with arms on armboards angled toward the head of the table and the hands pronated. Chest rolls are placed under the thorax and abdomen, and a roll is placed in front of the ankles. All pressure points require adequate padding, for example, elbows and knees. A sterile, plastic adhesive drape may be used to drape buttocks out of the field before preparing the skin. Apply electrosurgical dispersive pad.

Skin preparation

Begin at the midline of the back extending from the base of the skull to the midthighs and down to the table at the sides. (Particular attention is paid to the area above the iliac crests).

Draping

Folded towels are placed around the site of the incision and the iliac crests. A sterile, adhesive plastic drape may be used. Four drape sheets may be used to drape the head, foot, and sides of the table. A laparotomy sheet, which is cut over the iliac crest(s), completes the draping.

Equipment

Special frame (e.g., Andrews or Wilson), optional
Chest rolls, ankle roll, pillows, padding (for positioning)
Suctions (2)
Scales (for weighing sponges)
Electrosurgical unit
Fiberoptic headlight and light source, available
Cell Saver, available
Cast cart

Instrumentation

Laminectomy tray
Kerrison rongeurs and Pituitary forceps tray
Spinal fixation device and specific instrumentation (e.g., Harrington rod: distraction and compression rods and hooks, hook clamps, rod clamps,

spreader, drivers, wrench, outrigger distraction unit, Harrington elevator, sacral rod, nut and eyelet)
Self-retaining retractors (e.g., Weitlaner, Beckman)
Large bone cutter, large pin cutter, Steinmann pins, and protractor

Supplies

Basin set
Blades (2) No. 10, (1) No. 15
Suction tubings (2)
Electrosurgical pencil
Needle magnet or counter
Bone wax
Cottonoids (assorted sizes)
Gelfoam (usually soaked in thrombin 1000 units in 10 ml saline)
Sterile, plastic adhesive drapes (2) (buttocks and operative site)
Stainless steel wire, 16- or 18-gauge (for Wisconsin, Luque)
Graduate
Bulb syringes (2)
Antibiotic irrigation, optional
Closed drainage system (e.g., Hemovac)

Special notes

Have x-ray films in room.
Check with blood bank that all blood ordered is available.
Weigh sponges.
Measure blood loss accurately.
Skin and subcutaneous tissues may be injected with a vasoconstricting agent such as epinephrine (advise anesthetist accordingly).
Have additional suction collection devices ready.
Protective goggles may be worn.

AMPUTATION OF LOWER EXTREMITY

Definition

Severance of a thigh, leg, foot, digit(s), or portions thereof.

Discussion

Amputation may be necessitated by gangrene secondary to diabetes, vascular insufficiency, malignancy, severe trauma, etc. Commonly performed amputations include above the knee (AK), below the knee (BK), and transmetatarsal (TM).

Procedure

For an above the knee amputation the incision is made creating musculocutaneous flaps for better coverage of the femoral stump. The distal adductor canal is entered and the neurovascular bundle (superficial femoral artery and vein and saphenous nerve) are ligated and divided. Muscles are further transsected circumferentially. The sciatic nerve is ligated and divided. The femoral periosteum is incised and the bone transsected with a saw. Bone edges are smoothed with a rasp. Hemostasis is achieved and the wound is closed. A closed suction unit may be employed. A bulky dressing can be applied, but preferably a plaster cast or temporary prosthesis is used to minimize postoperative edema and to prepare the stump for a permanent prosthesis later on.

Preparation of the patient

The patient is supine; arms may be extended on armboards and the safety belt is secured over the unaffected extremity. Apply electrosurgical dispersive pad.

Skin preparation

At the surgeon's discretion, a grossly septic distal part need not be prepared. The extremity may be isolated by covering it with a Mayo stand cover or a sterile, plastic adhesive drape.

Transmetatarsal: Begin at the ankle extending up to the knee and down to the foot and toes (as directed).

Below the knee: Begin below the knee, include the thigh and extend distally to include leg, foot, and toes (as directed).

Above the knee: Begin at the thigh extending distally to include the knee, leg, foot, and toes (as directed).

Draping

The distal portion of the extremity may be wrapped in a Mayo stand cover or a sterile, plastic adhesive drape before the preparation or immediately following the preparation. The extremity is abducted and the foot is grasped in a tube (or impervious) stockinette. A large sheet is draped over the end of the table. A drape (or split) sheet is draped under the thigh and clipped. A folded towel (in thirds, lengthwise) is wrapped around the thigh and clipped. A sheet is draped proximal to the thigh and clipped underneath. The extremity is passed through a fenestrated sheet, which covers the field. During surgery an extra Mayo cover may be used to hold the amputated part.

Equipment

Electrosurgical unit
Power source for power saw, optional
Cast cart, optional

Instrumentation

Basic orthopedic procedures tray

Amputation saw and knife, bone hook
Oscillating power saw and cord, optional

Supplies

Basin set
Tube (or impervious) stockinette, 6"
Blades (2 to 4) No. 10
Needle magnet or counter
Bulb syringe
Graduate
Electrosurgical pencil
Culture tubes, aerobic and anaerobic
Antibiotic irrigation, optional
Closed suction unit (e.g., Hemovac)

Special notes

When preparing, begin with the cleanest area and work toward the dirtiest area (gangrenous part). Do not use sponges from a "dirty" area on a "clean" area.

Dispatch aerobic and anaerobic cultures promptly.

Protective goggles may be worn.

Ask the surgeon if a bulky dressing, plaster cast, or temporary prosthesis will be applied at the conclusion of the procedure.

Determine where the amputated part is to be sent (e.g., laboratory, morgue). Be certain it is well wrapped and labeled correctly.

Chapter 16

NEUROLOGICAL SURGERY

CRANIOTOMY

Definition

Opening of the skull.

Discussion

The most basic form of craniotomy is the burr hole, a limited opening through which blood or fluid may be evacuated, or instruments inserted, to divide neural tracts (as in prefrontal lobotomy).

Burr holes also may be employed as a preliminary to other procedures, serving as points that are connected, for example, when a bone flap is raised. When bone is excised to permit better exposure or because it is involved in a disease process it is referred to as a *craniectomy*. Trephination may refer to larger burr holes.

Numerous neurosurgical conditions are treated by craniotomy. Some of those commonly encountered and their treatments are as follows.

Intracranial Aneurysm. An arterial dilation

secondary to muscular weakness in a vessel wall prone to rupture (hemorrhage). The patient's blood pressure is controlled and the aneurysm isolated by the application of clips, or the aneurysm can be coated with methylmethacrylate or a cyanoacrylate used to strengthen the aneurysm wall or provide external support.

Arteriovenous Malformation. The capillary bed is bypassed, thus making the veins more prone to rupture. The feeding vessels may be clipped, coagulated, or treated by laser.

Occluded Intracranial Vessel. The superficial temporal artery may be microsurgically anastomosed to the middle cerebral artery distal to the occlusion. The superficial temporal artery is dissected free for an appropriate distance and then passed intracranially through a frontotemporal burr hole preparatory to anastomosis.

Tumors Near the Pituitary. The tumor (e.g., optic glioma, craniopharyngioma, suprasellar, and parasellar) is resected; sometimes complete resection is not possible. These tumors are resected by a frontal or frontotemporal approach (see Transsphenoidal Hypophysectomy, p. 321).

Cerebrospinal Fluid Otorrhea or Rhinorrhea. A skull fracture with a tear in the dura mater and the leakage of cerebrospinal fluid from the ear (otorrhea) or the nose (rhinorrhea). The approach for repair of a dural tear with cerebrospinal otorrhea is temporal or suboccipital. Frontal craniotomy may be performed for cerebrospinal rhinorrhea.

Subdural or Epidural Hematoma (Acute, Subacute, or Chronic). The evacuation of blood, clots, and membranes; the elevation and debridement of associated depressed fractures; and the excision of devitalized brain.

Acoustic Neuroma. Excision of the tumor (without damaging the facial nerve) by a posterior fossa approach. Removal of the bony superior wall of the auditory canal may be necessary to expose the tumor. Some small tumors may be removed by drilling directly through the temporal bone. A nerve stimulator, microscope, and a high-speed power drill may be used.

Neurologic Disorders. Examples are trigeminal neuralgia for which rhizotomy is performed or absolute alcohol injected; for Parkinson's disease, a cryoprobe is inserted under stereotaxic control into the globus pallidus through a burr hole producing a destructive lesion.

Hydrocephalus. Treated by insertion of a ventriculoperitoneal or ventriculoatrial shunt (see Ventricular Shunts, p. 325).

Congenital Abnormalities. Premature closure of the sutures is an example; these sutures are resected and the edges covered with Silastic sheeting to prevent healing of the suture lines.

Procedure

The incision may be marked. The layers of the scalp are incised and scalp clips are applied. The scalp is covered with a moist sponge and reflected. Burr holes are made and the dura mater is carefully separated from the skull. A craniotome may be used to remove the bone, or a bone flap that is hinged on the adjacent periosteum and musculature is made. Bleeding is controlled with electrosurgical forceps, gelatin sponge, and bone wax. If the bone flap is to be replaced at the end of the operation, drill holes are made in the periphery of the skull; the dura and brain are protected. Matching holes are drilled in the bone flap. The dura mater is incised, vessels in the dural margins are coagulated or ligated with Hemoclips, and the dura mater may be tacked up to the pericranium. Moist cottonoids are placed as necessary; the brain is continually moistened by saline irrigation or moist cottonoids to prevent cortical injury caused by drying. Lumbar drainage of cerebrospinal fluid and intravenous administration of mannitol or urea and steroids may be done to decrease cerebral edema before any cortical incision is made. A subcortical mass is approached by the most direct route except when this is through a vital region such as a motor or speech area. In these cases, the incision is made in a less important area and continued obliquely. Care is taken to cover areas adjacent to the incision with moist cottonoids. Blood vessels are electrocoagulated or clipped. The pia mater and gray matter are usually incised with a knife. The white matter is divided by a dissector or suction tip. Moist cottonoids and cotton balls are employed to restrict capillary oozing or to tamponade blood vessels. During the resection of a brain tumor, the center of the neoplasm may be evacuated or a neoplastic cyst aspirated to facilitate dissection and exposure. Tumor removal may be completed with curettes, pituitary forceps, and a brain spoon. When cerebral resection is completed, the wound is irrigated and hemostasis is ensured. The dural flap is closed, making the suture line watertight. If the dural defect is too large to be closed, a dural graft may be inserted (using temporalis fascia, periosteum, fascia lata, or an artificial dural substitute). The dura mater may be left open after operations in the posterior fossa (if there is adequate closure of the nuchal muscles), beneath simple burr holes, and following subtemporal craniectomy for subdural hematoma. The bone flap is wired back. Burr holes may be covered with silicone rubber buttons, methylmethacrylate, or autogenous bone chips. As the scalp is closed, the skin clips are removed. The wound is dressed and the head is wrapped in a turbanlike gauze bandage.

Preparation of the patient

The patient's hair may be partially or completely removed following the patient's arrival in the surgery department. A cubicle in the preoperative area or the recovery room can be screened off to maintain the patient's privacy. The hair is cut with electric clippers and the scalp is carefully shaved with disposable razors and warm soapy water. The patient's hair is saved in a bag labeled with the patient's identification and returned to him or her postoperatively. A hypothermia mattress may be put on the table. The patient's temperature is monitored. A Foley catheter is often inserted in the bladder. Elastic bandages or antiembolic hose may be applied from the toes to the groin to prevent venous stasis and to help maintain blood pressure. A right atrial or central venous pressure line may be inserted. Hypotension may be induced by drugs injected intravenously. The surgeon may mark the site of the incision with an indelible marking pen. The position of the patient depends on the location of the lesion and the preference of the surgeon. After the patient is positioned, apply electrosurgical dispersive pad.

Supine, sitting, and prone positions are described.

Supine. The patient is supine with arms extended on armboards or tucked in at the patient's sides; the head may be stabilized by the insertion of the sterile pins from a headrest attachment to the table, or it may simply be positioned on a doughnut headrest.

Sitting. The patient is supine with the knees over the lower break, the table is raised from the middle break, and the foot of the table is lowered. A padded footboard supports the feet. The arms are placed in the patient's lap on a pillow and secured with padded restraints. The safety strap is secured across the thighs. The head may be stabilized by the insertion of the sterile pins of a headrest attachment to the table.

Prone. The patient is intubated on the gurney and carefully rolled over to the prone position onto the table. The arms are extended on armboards (angled toward the head of the table) with the hands pronated. Chest rolls are placed under the patient from the acromioclavicular joints to the iliac crests to facilitate breathing. A pillow or roll is placed in front of the ankles. Padding is placed under the elbows and knees. Female breasts and male genitalia are protected from pressure. The safety strap is secured across the patient's thighs.

Skin preparation

Check with the surgeon regarding the type of solution to be used and the area to be prepared. Care is taken to avoid getting preparation solution in the eyes. Antibiotic ointment may be put in the eyes and nonirritating tape may be used to tape the lids shut. Small cotton pledgets are helpful in preventing solution from pooling in the ears.

Draping

The surgeon usually prefers to do the draping. Folded towels are placed around the operative site and secured by towel clips or sutures. To suture towels in place heavy silk suture on a cutting needle, a needle holder, toothed forceps, and suture scissors are needed. A sterile, plastic adhesive drape may be used; the prepared area must be dry or the adhesive drape will not stick. If an overhead table (e.g., Mayfield) is used, a large drape sheet, fanfolded at the front edge of the table, is used. The fanfolded sheet is brought down toward the operative site and secured; this covers the space between the unsterile area under the table and the operative field. A disposable craniotomy sheet eliminates the need for multiple drape sheets; otherwise, individual drape sheets cover the field.

Equipment

Headrest clamp (e.g., Mayfield, Crutchfield, Gardner)
Overhead table (e.g., Mayfield)
Hypothermia/Hyperthermia mattress, optional
Pillows, chest rolls, padded restraints, etc. (for positioning)
Suction (2)
Electrosurgical unit (monopolar)
Electrosurgical unit (bipolar)
Temperature monitoring device
Fiberoptic light source for retractors, optional

Power sources for power drill and saw
Loupes and/or microscope (e.g., Zeiss)
Blood warming units
Blood pumps (for infusion of blood)
Footstools (6 to 8)
Scales
Cell Saver (available)
Carbon dioxide laser (available, depending on procedure): see Appendix, p. 572, for precautions

Instrumentation

Craniotomy tray
Microsurgical instruments, optional (e.g., micro forceps, scissors, needle holders, curettes, suction tips, bayonet bipolar electrosurgical forceps, dissectors, elevators)
Power saw and/or drill (optional)
Aneurysm clips, and appliers, assorted (e.g., Heifetz, Yasargil, Sundt-Kees, Mayfield, Keer, Olivecrona) for aneurysm, arteriovenous malformation, and pituitary tumors

Supplies

Basin set
Blades (2) No. 10, (1) No. 15, (1) No. 11
Needle magnet or counter
Sterile, plastic adhesive drape
Suction tubing
Needle and local anesthesia with epinephrine (to inject site of incision for hemostasis)
Nerve stimulator (locator)
Bulb syringes (2)
Graduate
Electrosurgical pencil
Telfa (for specimens)
Cottonoids, assorted (e.g., ½″ × ½″, 1″ × 1″, 1″ × 3″, ½″ × 3″)
Bone wax, 2 packages
Hemostatic agents (e.g., Surgicel, Gelfoam and thrombin, Avitene)

Cotton balls

Hemoclips (small, medium)

Scalp clips (e.g., Raney, Michel)

Drain (e.g., Hemovac), optional

Antibiotic irrigation, optional

Medications

Sodium nitroprusside (Nipride) to induce hypotension. *Note*: Nipride when mixed in solution for intravenous use is unstable in light. Cover bottle and tubing with aluminum foil.

Dexamethasone (Decadron), a synthetic steroid, to decrease inflammation

Mannitol, 20% with filter, to reduce intracranial pressure

Methylmethacrylate kit, optional

Special notes

Planning prior to bringing the patient to the operating room is essential. Consider equipment, special physical needs of the patient, surgical approach, position, instrumentation, supplies and medications.

Headrest clamps attached to the table headrest attachment (e.g., Mayfield, Crutchfield, or Gardner) secure the skull by two or three sterile fixation pins. Insertion sites for the pins are prepared with preparation solution.

Have x-ray and CT scan films in the room.

Check with blood bank that blood is available as ordered.

Extra care is taken to be certain that all bony prominences are padded (these procedures can be lengthy) to avoid damage to skin and nerves.

An electrosurgical dispersive pad is necessary if the monopolar electrosurgical unit is used.

Have a second suction unit available.

Have all equipment (electrosurgical unit, suction, microscope, drills, etc.) connected and ready before the skin incision is made.

A kickbucket may be used to catch irrigation and blood below the head of the table (gather drapes to form a funnel) if a special craniotomy sheet is unavailable.

Towels around the operative site may be secured with suture; have heavy suture, cutting needle, needle holder, and forceps with teeth ready.

If the lines of the incision are marked, methylene blue is *never* used because it produces an inflammatory reaction in nervous tissue.

Keep both (bulb or Asepto) syringes filled at all times.

Measure irrigation used accurately.

Place moistened cottonoids, cotton balls, and bone wax within the surgeon's view on a neurosurgical sponge ("pattie") plate.

Record the number of cotton balls used, in addition to sponges and cottonoids.

Saline or Ringer's lactate solution is used during bipolar coagulation to minimize tissue heating.

Drill sites or saw incisions into the cranium are irrigated with saline to minimize the heat (produced by friction).

Aneurysm clips are applied with clip appliers only and should be discarded after being compressed.

If methylmethacrylate is used to coat a blood vessel, all surrounding tissues are protected with moistened cottonoids.

Protective goggles may be worn.

CRANIOPLASTY

Definition

Repair of a cranial defect.

Discussion

Cranial defects may result from fractures, infections, surgical procedures (e.g., cranial bone biopsy, craniectomy), or a congenital deformity. Indications for the procedure include protection from external trauma, pain, seizures, and cosmesis. The artificial cranium may be fashioned from autogenous bone grafts, metal (e.g., tantalum) or acrylic material (e.g., methylmethacrylate). Methylmethacrylate is the preferred material for cranioplasty, except in cases of wound infection, in which autogenous grafts are better accepted.

Procedure

The scalp is incised over the defect. The defect may be trimmed as necessary. Methylmethacrylate is mixed according to manufacturer's directions (i.e., until doughlike, put in a polyethylene bag, and rolled flat). The surgeon then molds the material to fit the defect. Acrylic is removed from the polyethylene bag and allowed to harden. Excess material may be trimmed with rongeurs or a power saw. A craniotome may be used to smooth rough spots. Holes are drilled in the periphery of the acrylic plate and the cranial defect. The plate is placed over the defect and secured by stainless steel wire passed through the poles. The wound is irrigated and closed.

Preparation of the patient

The hair over the area of the defect must be removed. Complete hair removal may be indicated; check with the surgeon. The patient's hair is removed, saved in a bag, and labeled with the patient's identification prior to entering the operating room and returned to him or her postoperatively. See Craniotomy, Preparation of the Patient, p. 313. The position of the patient depends on the area of the defect. Apply electrosurgical dispersive pad.

Skin preparation

Check with the surgeon regarding the type of solution to be used and the area to be prepared.

Care is taken to avoid getting preparation solution in the eyes. Antibiotic ointment may be instilled in the eyes and a nonirritating tape may be used to tape the lids shut. Small cotton pledgets may be used to prevent solution from pooling in the ears.

Draping

The surgeon usually prefers to do the draping. Folded towels are placed around the operative site and secured by towel clips or sutures. A sterile, plastic adhesive drape may be used; the prepared area must be dry or the adhesive drape will not stick. The patient is covered with a craniotomy sheet, or individual drape sheets may be used.

Equipment

Suctions (2)
Electrosurgical unit
Power sources for power saw and power drill

Instrumentation

Craniotomy tray
Power saw or craniotome and cord
Power drill, burrs, and cord

Supplies

Basin set
Blades (2) No. 10
Needle magnet or counter
Sterile, plastic adhesive drape
Suction tubing
Asepto or bulb syringes (2)
Graduate
Electrosurgical pencil
Bone wax
Scalp clips (e.g., Raney, Michel)
Cranioplasty kit (methylmethacrylate, polyethylene bag, roller, mixing bowl, and spoon)

Stainless steel wire
Cottonoids, large (e.g., 1" × 3")
Antibiotic irrigation, optional

Special notes

If suture is used to secure the towels, have ready heavy silk suture on a cutting needle, needle holder, toothed forceps, and suture scissors.

Methylmethacrylate is mixed by adding one volume of liquid monomer to one volume of powdered polymer. When mass is doughy, put in plastic bag and roll flat. The surgeon will then mold the plate. When cool, excess material will be sawed or cut off with rongeurs. The process from mixing to hardening takes 7 minutes.

TRANSSPHENOIDAL HYPOPHYSECTOMY

Definition

Excision or destruction of all or a portion of the pituitary gland.

Discussion

Hypophysectomy is performed for endocrine disorders, primary tumors of the pituitary, some presentations of diabetic retinopathy, and hormonally dependent metastatic breast and prostatic carcinoma. Its use in control of other malignancies is controversial (e.g., malignant melanoma, hypernephroma, and thyroid cancer). A side effect of hypophysectomy is the production of diabetes insipidus, which can be controlled by vasopressin (Pitressin) replacement. More than 90% removal of the gland is usually necessary to effect the desired results. Radiotherapy to ablate the pituitary by either interstitial radiation (placed by stereotaxic approaches) or external beam radiation gives less than favorable results. Open craniotomy presents greater stress and risk to these often frail patients.

Stereotaxic hypophysectomy, a modality which can be performed under local anesthesia, employs an integrated system controlled by computer. The patient's head is secured in a stereotaxic frame. Preoperatively the patient undergoes computerized axial tomography, tomographic pneumoencephalography, and vascular angiography. Using coordinates thus established, the surgeon places the patient in the same frame for surgery, the patient is anesthetized and, under computerized control, checked by fluoroscopy. After a drill is used to perforate the sphenoid sinus and the floor of the sella turcica, a cryoprobe is placed in the sella turcica (position predetermined) via cannula. Cryodestruction is then performed. On removal of the probe a silicone plug is placed in the sellar opening to prevent cerebrospinal fluid leakage. This procedure is usually performed in a specially designed radiology suite.

Procedure

General anesthesia is administered by endotracheal tube. The nasal cavity and gums are infiltrated with a local anesthetic containing epinephrine to minimize blood loss and aid in elevation of the mucosa. A horizontal incision is made under the upper lip and extended over the maxilla into the nasal cavity. The mucosa is elevated and a portion of the cartilaginous septum is excised and saved in a saline-soaked sponge. Using a bivalve nasal speculum the floor of the sphenoidal sinus is exposed and incised by rongeur. The boundaries of the sella are determined by direct vision with a microscope and by fluoroscopy. The sella is entered in the midline; a sphenoidal punch is used to enlarge the opening exposing the dura of the pituitary fossa. The dura is incised avoiding entry into the pituitary capsule. The gland is dissected extracapsularly and the stalk is identified. Care is taken not to penetrate the posterior wall of the sella. Again, fluoroscopy confirms the position of the instruments. A sickle knife or scissors may be used to sever the stalk. Further dissection, with a specifically designed blunt dissector, frees the remainder of the gland from its dural attachments and the gland is delivered intact. Gelfoam soaked in thrombin can be used to control oozing.

A patch of fascia lata and muscle is excised from the previously prepared thigh and packed into the empty sella. A segment of previously excised cartilaginous nasal septum is used to seal the muscle plug to the floor of the sella, "snapping" it into place. Antibiotics may be instilled. Nasal packing reapproximates the nasal mucosa. The gingival incision is closed with absorbable suture. The thigh incision (donor site) is closed.

Preparation of the patient

The patient may be supine with arms tucked in at the sides; the head may be supported by a headrest. One leg (usually the right) is not restrained by the safety belt to provide access for the muscle tissue graft.

The procedure is usually performed under general anesthesia with endotracheal intubation. The nasal cavity and gums are infiltrated with local anesthesia containing epinephrine. Apply electrosurgical dispersive pad.

Skin preparation

The thigh is prepared from the knee to the groin, and down to the table at the sides. Check with the surgeon for type of solution to be used and the area to be prepared; the area may include the face, and oral and nasal cavities (the surgeon may do this preparation). In addition to the standard preparation tray include bayonet forceps, nasal speculum, long cotton-tipped applicators, and hemostat.

Draping

The patient's face is draped with folded towels, as is the prepared thigh. The patient may be covered with a disposable fenestrated sheet (an opening can be cut for access to the thigh). A drape is necessary for the image intensifier and the microscope.

Equipment

Headrest (e.g., Richards, doughnut, Shea)
Suction
Electrosurgical unit (bipolar)
Microscope
Image intensifier (with C-arm) and TV monitor
Fiberoptic headlight and light source (available)

Instrumentation

Craniotomy tray
Limited procedure tray (muscle tissue graft)
Bayonet bipolar electrocoagulating forceps, micro tip
Bivalve nasal speculum (long blades), punch forceps, small ring currettes (angled), Hardy's enucleator (angled), pituitary spoon (angled), micro scissors (straight, curved, angled), micro dissectors (angled), (sickle) knife (angled)

Supplies

Basin set
Blades (1) No. 10, (2) No. 15, (1) No. 12
Needle magnet or counter
Electrosurgical pencil
Suction tubing
Bulb syringes (2)
Cottonoids (e.g., ½" × ½", ½" × 1" frequently used)
Syringe (e.g., 10-ml Luer-lock control) long needle; local anesthesia with epinephrine
Bone wax
Nasal packing (e.g., ½" petrolatum-impregnated gauze)
Hemostatic agents (e.g., Gelfoam and thrombin, Surgicel, Avitene)
Antibiotic irrigation, optional

Special notes

Lead aprons are worn during fluoroscopy.

A second Mayo stand may be used for taking the muscle tissue graft.

Have materials available for aerobic and anaerobic cultures.

VENTRICULAR SHUNTS

Definition

Refers to the insertion of a valve system to divert the flow of cerebrospinal fluid from the ventricular system.

Discussion

Shunting the ventricular fluid to a body cavity outside the cranium is performed to treat hydrocephalus (congenital, neoplastic, traumatic, and infectious). The distal end of the shunt is placed in the peritoneal cavity unless contraindicated by intraperitoneal disease. If peritoneal placement cannot be performed, the shunt may be indirectly placed in the right atrium by way of the internal jugular vein, or directly placed in the atrium by thoracotomy. The advantages of peritoneal over atrial placement of the distal catheter are avoidance of vascular and cardiopulmonary complications, faster and simpler placement of the distal catheter, space to place a longer distal catheter (prolonging the interval before revision), and easier replacement of the distal catheter.

Procedure

Ventriculoperitoneal Shunt for Hydrocephalus
Lines are marked for a right-sided shunt incision (several centimeters above and posterior to the ear), and a transverse right-upper-quadrant incision of the abdomen. The scalp is incised and reflected

on its base. Bleeding is controlled by electrocoagulation. The burr hole site in the periosteum is electrocoagulated and a self-retaining retractor is placed. The periosteum is incised, and a burr hole is made and enlarged as necessary to accommodate the reservoir. The dura is electrocoagulated and the outer layer incised. Bipolar electrocautery is used to seal the dura to the pia and cortex. A straight ventricular catheter is passed into the posterior aspect of the lateral ventricle, the stylet is removed, and the opening pressure recorded. A premeasured length of catheter is advanced anterior to the foramen of Munro. Air (5 to 10 cc) is injected and an x-ray film is taken to confirm the position of catheter placement.

The transverse abdominal incision is carried down to the anterior rectus sheath. A distal catheter is passed from the scalp incision to the abdominal incision subcutaneously. The reservoir is attached to the proximal end of the valve with a connector and suture. The reservoir is attached to the ventricular catheter with suture. The valve mechanism is placed in the subgaleal space behind the ear. A longitudinal incision is made in the anterior rectus sheath. The rectus abdominis muscle is split. An incision is made in the posterior rectus sheath and transversalis fascia. The peritoneum is grasped and incised (1 mm). The peritoneal catheter, passed intraperitoneally, is attached to the reservoir. Wounds may be irrigated with antibiotic solution. The abdominal wound is closed. An antibiotic may be injected into the ventricle through the reservoir after compression of the valve. The scalp incision is closed.

Preparation of the patient

The patient is supine with the right arm tucked in at the patient's side and the left arm extended on an armboard. The patient's head is slightly elevated and turned to the left; a headrest may be used. See Pediatric General Information, p. 467, for measures to maintain the pediatric patient's body temperature, to restrain the extremities, and so on. Fluoroscopy or x-rays may be employed to determine correct placement of the catheter.

Skin preparation

Check with the surgeon regarding preparation and the solution to be used. In pediatric patients, hair is shaved in the operating room prior to the skin preparation. The area to be prepared may include the exposed scalp and the right side of the face extending from the forehead to the shoulder (including the lateral aspect of the face to the orbital rim and the neck), and down to the table at the sides.

Draping

The surgeon usually does the draping. Folded towels are placed around the operative site. The superior tip of the ear may be sutured forward to the skin (to keep it out of the field). A sterile, plastic adhesive drape may be used. A fenestrated sheet may be used to cover the field.

Equipment

Suction
Electrosurgical unit (bipolar)
Headrest (e.g., doughnut), optional
Restraints, soft-padded (pediatric)
Power source for power drill
Scale, optional
Body heat maintenance equipment (e.g., heating lamps, warming mattress)

Instrumentation

Craniotomy tray
Power drill (e.g., micro Stryker) and cord
Shunt, ventricular catheter, peritoneal catheter
Small bulldog clamp
Uterine packing forceps or a long passing instrument

Supplies

Basin set
Blades (2) No. 15
Needle magnet or counter
Sterile, plastic adhesive drape, optional
Suction tubing
Plastic syringe (3 ml) and blunt needle (e.g., 18 gauge) to pump through shunt reservoir and tubing
Shunt (e.g., Rickham reservoir, Holter valve, and catheter)
Cottonoids (e.g., ½" × ½")
Gelfoam and thrombin
Bulb syringe
Graduate
Antibiotic irrigation, optional

Special notes

Take extra precautions to correctly identify the pediatric patient.

Check with the surgeon and anesthetist regarding measures to be employed to prevent loss of body heat such as heating lamps, warming mattress, wrapping the extremities, etc. Use warmed solutions.

Determine the area to be prepared. Do not allow solution to pool under the patient. Do not allow solution to run into eyes or pool in the ear. Ask if the patient's head is to be shaved partially or completely.

Employ measures to protect the eyes, for example, eye ointment and hypoallergenic tape (to tape eyes shut).

Notify x-ray department before the surgery starts regarding the necessity for equipment such as a portable x-ray machine or fluoroscopy unit.

Ask if sponges are to be weighed.

Follow hospital policy for recording the insertion of an implant.

Regarding the implant:

A reservoir such as the Rickham reservoir

  may be inserted into the system between the valve and the catheter.

  Check valve patency and pressure with normal saline before use.

  Flush unit with saline or Ringer's solution (surgeon's preference); do *not* allow air into the unit.

  Observe x-ray precautions; see p. 20.

Regarding the shunt unit:

  Handle the unit only as much as absolutely necessary. Avoid contact with lint or other foreign materials; do not place on gauze sponges. Always place the unit in a basin. The valve must be properly oriented to allow a one-way passage of fluid only.

  Antibiotic solution may be used for irrigation.

LAMINECTOMY

Definition

Laminectomy is the removal of one or more vertebral laminae.

Discussion

Indications for laminectomy, hemilaminectomy, and an interlaminar procedure include herniated disc, compression fracture, dislocation, and spinal cord tumor. Other procedures may be performed in conjunction with laminectomy such as cordotomy, the division of the anterolateral tracts of the spinal column for intractable pain; and rhizotomy, the interruption of spinal (sensory) nerve roots for relief of spasm or intractable pain.

Procedure

Laminectomy for Herniated Intervertebral Disc

A midline vertical incision may be used. The wound is deepened with a knife, or more frequently an electrosurgical pencil is used. Self-retaining retractors are placed and the fascia is incised. The paraspinous muscles and periosteum are reflected (this may be done unilaterally on the side of the involved disc). Sponges are packed along the vertebrae with a periosteal elevator to aid in blunt dissection and effect hemostasis. A larger retractor (e.g., Beckman, Taylor, or Scoville) is placed for exposure. Small portions of the laminae overlying the herniated disc are removed with a Kerrison rongeur; portions of vertebral spines and intervertebral facets may also be excised. Hemostasis is achieved with bone wax. The ligamenta flava are incised; care is taken to avoid injury to the epidural veins. If the electrosurgical pencil is used, the vein is held away from the dura to prevent thermal injury to neural tissues. Moistened cottonoids are placed to protect the dura. Additional ligament or bone may be removed to provide adequate exposure. Nerve roots are cautiously retracted exposing the herniated disc, which is removed with a pituitary rongeur and curettes; care is exercised anteriorly to avoid the aorta and vena cava. The wound is irrigated. The area is examined to ensure that all protruding disc has been removed. Hemostasis is achieved. The wound is closed in layers.

Preparation of the patient

Check with the surgeon regarding removal of the patient's hair. The position of the patient depends on the type of laminectomy to be performed and the surgeon's preference. Cervical laminectomy is most frequently performed in the sitting position. Thoracic and lumbar laminectomies are most frequently performed in the prone or a modified knee-chest position. Occasionally, the lateral position is used for thoracic or lumbar laminectomy. Antiembolic hose or woven elastic bandages (e.g., Ace) may be applied to the legs to prevent venous stasis and to help maintain blood pressure.

Sitting. The patient is supine with knees over the lower break of the table. The head of the table is raised from the middle break. The foot of the table is lowered; a padded footboard supports the feet. The arms are placed in the patient's lap on a pillow and secured with padded restraints. The safety strap is secured above the knees. The Mayfield (skull) clamp is attached to a headrest table attachment. Preparation solution is applied to the insertion sites of the pins; some hair will need to be shaved.

Prone. Following placement of an intravenous line, the administration of general anesthesia, and the insertion of an endotracheal tube (while the patient is on the gurney or the hospital bed), the patient is carefully rolled over to the prone position onto the table. The arms are extended on armboards angled toward the head of the table with the hands pronated. Chest rolls are placed under the patient from the acromioclavicular joint to the level of the iliac crests to facilitate breathing. A pillow or roll is placed in front of the ankles. Pads are placed under the elbows and knees. Female breasts and male genitalia are protected from pressure. The safety strap is secured across the patient's thighs. A sterile, plastic adhesive drape may be put on the buttocks at this time to seal the rectal area out of the field.

Modified Knee-Chest. Following placement of an intravenous line, the administration of general anesthesia, and the insertion of an endotracheal tube (while the patient is on the gurney), the patient is carefully rolled over to the prone position onto the table. Adjust the patient's position so the hips are over the middle break in the table. The foot of the table is lowered and a padded extension is added on perpendicular to the table. The arms are extended on armboards angled toward the head of the table with the hands pronated. Chest rolls are placed under the patient from the acromioclavicular joint to the level of the iliac crests to facilitate breathing. Pads are placed under the elbows and knees. Female breasts and male genitalia are protected from pressure. Pillows are placed in front of the ankles and under the feet. The patient's position is secured with the safety strap or 7.5-cm- or 3-inch-wide adhesive tape across the thighs. A sterile, plastic adhesive drape may be put on the buttocks at this time to seal the rectal area out of the field. After the patient is positioned, apply electrosurgical dispersive pad.

For cervical laminectomy, hair on the lower portion of the scalp (supra-auricular border) and the neck is removed after the patient has arrived in the surgery department, but before entering the operating room. Hair on the top of the head need not be removed. Long hair is secured at the top of the head. The hair to be removed is clipped with electric clippers. The area is then shaved with warm soapy water and disposable razors.

For thoracic or lumbar laminectomy, hair present on the dorsal thorax is shaved in the operating room.

Skin preparation

Check with the surgeon regarding the area to be prepared.

Cervical: Begin cleaning at the midline extending from the supra-auricular border to the level of the axillae, and down to the table at the neck and shoulders.

Thoracic: Begin cleansing at the midline extending from the base of the skull to the level of the waist, and down to the table at the neck and sides.

Lumbar: Begin cleansing at the midline extending from the shoulders to the coccyx (or the adhesive drape), and down to the table at the sides.

Draping

The surgeon usually prefers to do the draping. Folded towels are placed around the operative site and secured with towel clips or sutures. To suture towels, heavy silk sutures on a cutting needle, needle holder, toothed forceps, and suture scissors are needed. A sterile, plastic adhesive drape may be used. The field is covered with a craniotomy sheet or a sheet with a moderate-sized fenestration for a cervical procedure. For a thoracic or lumbar procedure, the field may be covered with a laparotomy sheet.

Equipment

Suction
Electrosurgical unit (monopolar)
Electrosurgical unit (bipolar)
Power source for power drill, optional
Fiberoptic headlight and light source
Pillows and pads for elbows and knees, chest rolls
    (for prone or modified knee-chest position)
Pillows and padded arm restraints (for sitting position)
    sition)
Headrest, e.g., Mayfield (for cervical approach)
Scales (to weigh sponges)

Instrumentation

Laminectomy tray
Kerrison rongeurs and pituitary forceps tray
Power drill (e.g., micro Stryker), drill bits, cord (optional)
    tional)

Supplies

Basin set
Suction tubing
Blade (3 or 4) No. 10, (1) No. 15
Sterile, plastic adhesive drapes (2)
Needle magnet or counter
Bone wax
Bulb or Asepto syringes (2)
Electrosurgical pencil
Gelfoam and thrombin (e.g., 5000 units)
Roller gauze 2" (to hold retractor)
Cottonoids (e.g., ½" × ½", 1" × 1")
Antibiotic irrigation, optional

Special notes

Have x-ray films in room.

Check with blood bank that blood is available as ordered.

Save patient's hair in a bag labeled with the patient's identification.

Utmost care must be taken when moving the patient from the gurney to the table. Have adequate assistance.

In positioning, protect bony prominences from pressure to prevent skin and nerve damage.

Protect the eyes from injury (e.g., eye ointment and taping lids shut).

Have all equipment (e.g., suction, electrosurgical unit) ready before the incision is made.

Keep both bulb or Asepto syringes filled at all times.

Irrigation temperature should be tepid.

Place moistened cottonoids and bone wax within the surgeon's view on a neurosurgical sponge ("pattie") plate.

Saline or Ringer's lactate solution is used during bipolar coagulation to minimize tissue heating.

When a Taylor retractor is used, after it has been appropriately placed the surgeon wraps the roller gauze around the tail of the retractor, and drops the roll to the circulator, who secures it to the table.

EXCISION OF A CERVICAL INTERVERTEBRAL DISC WITH FUSION, ANTERIOR APPROACH

Definition

Excision of a herniated intervertebral disc with the stabilization of the cervical spine.

Discussion

The procedure is indicated when nerve deficits and pain caused by spondylosis or herniated disc persist, despite conservative treatment by bed rest and traction. The anterior approach is preferred when spondylotic bars compromise the cord or the nerve root; the posterior approach is employed when multiple nerve roots must be decompressed. Fusion is accomplished with a bone graft, usually obtained from the iliac crest.

Procedure

A transverse incision is made at the level of the cricoid cartilage. The incision is deepened, usually to the right of the midline, retracting the carotid sheath and prevertebral muscles laterally, and the trachea and esophagus medially to expose the spine. Care is taken to avoid injury to the carotid sheath contents, vertebral vessels, and recurrent laryngeal nerve. The anterior longitudinal ligament is incised exposing the intervertebral disc. The disc level may be confirmed by x-ray (using a needle as a marker). A bone graft may be taken from the iliac crest using either an osteotome (after the periosteum has been reflected) or a dowel cutter. All bone chips are kept moist and saved for later packing of the fusion site. The iliac crest wound is closed after hemostasis is achieved. The diseased disc is incised and removed piecemeal with rongeurs. Bony spurs compressing the nerve roots or dura are excised with small rongeurs and/or burrs. The intervertebral space is packed with the bone graft (and chips). A depth gauge may be used to determine the size to use for the bone plug. After hemostasis is achieved the cervical wound is closed in layers.

Preparation of the patient

The patient is supine with the head turned to the left and the right hip elevated (e.g., with a folded sheet).

Skin preparation

For cervical incisin: Begin at the neck extending from the infra-auricular border to the nipples, and down to the table at the sides of the neck and shoulders.

For donor site incision (e.g., iliac crest): Begin cleansing the iliac crest area extending from the midthorax to the upper thigh, down to the table on the right side, and well beyond the midline on the left side.

Draping

The patient is draped with four folded towels at the neck and four folded towels at the hip; towel clips or suture may be used to secure the towels. A sterile, plastic adhesive drape may be used. A sheet with a small fenestration is used for the cervical incision; a laparotomy sheet is used for the donor graft incision.

Equipment

Suction
Electrosurgical unit (bipolar)
Fiberoptic headlight and power source
Power source for power drill, optional
Loupes or microscope (optional)

Instrumentation

Laminectomy tray
Kerrison rongeurs and pituitary forceps tray
Cervical fusion instruments (e.g., Cloward self-retaining retractors, drill guards, drills, dowel cutters, bone graft holder, impactor, vertebral spreaders)
Hudson brace, mallet, depth gauge
Power drill (e.g., Stryker), small burrs, and cord (optional)
Hemoclip appliers (short, medium)

Supplies

Basin set
Suction tubing

Blades (2) No. 10, (1) No. 15, (1) No. 11
Bayonet bipolar electrocoagulating forceps
Needle (inserted into disc space to determine level)
Cassette drape
Gelfoam
Thrombin (e.g., 5000 units)
Cottonoids (e.g., ½" × ½")
Graduate
Bulb syringes (2)
Hemoclips (small, medium)
Microscope drape, optional
Sterile, plastic adhesive drape, optional

Special notes

Have x-ray films in room.

Notify x-ray department regarding portable films to be taken.

Observe x-ray precautions; see p. 20.

The site of the donor graft is covered with a towel until the surgeon is ready to take the graft.

A Stryker drill with a small burr may be used on the vertebrae to facilitate access to the disc.

The cervical incision is covered with a towel while the graft is taken from the donor site (e.g., iliac crest).

Chapter 17

PLASTIC SURGERY

CLEFT LIP REPAIR

Definition

Correction of a congenital deformity of the lips and face.

Discussion

Cleft lip results from a fusion failure during the embryonic processes. Each cleft lip deformity varies. There are four categories:

1. Unilateral incomplete cleft with nasal deformity
2. Unilateral complete cleft with nasal deformity
3. Bilateral incomplete cleft with or without adequate columella
4. Bilateral complete cleft on one side and incomplete on the other side.

The cleft lip can be closed in the neonate, but repair at 3 months of age is preferable, because growth of the tissues facilitates the initial detailed surgery. Palatal and alveolar deformities may also be present.

Procedures

General anesthesia is administered and an endotracheal tube is inserted. In addition, a local anesthetic containing epinephrine is infiltrated locally to aid in hemostasis. Simple closure does not usually suffice, but may render subsequent stages easier. More often, any of several flaps are isolated and advanced. Proper restoration of the philtrum and shape of the bow of the lip is sought. Secondary repairs are performed according to individual situations even months or years later. Similarly, palatal and alveolar deformities are repaired in due time commensurate with the patient's feeding requirements and tissue growth. Postoperatively, the child's arms are restrained. The incision is protected with antibiotic ointment and the cheeks are splinted with a Logan's bow (to counter the effects of crying).

Preparation of the patient

The patient is supine. The head should be at the top edge of the table; a headrest or support may be used. Following induction of general anesthesia, the table is usually turned so that the surgeon may stand or sit at the head of the table and the anesthetist is at the patient's side. For the pediatric patient special measures must be taken to prepare the room, restrain the patient, and maintain the patient's body temperature. Refer to Pediatric General Information, p. 467.

Skin preparation

Check with the surgeon regarding choice of preparation solution. Begin at the upper lip, cleanse the face extending from the hairline to the shoulders, and down to the table at the sides of the neck.

Draping

The patient is usually draped with a head drape (drape sheet and two towels under the head with the uppermost towel wrapped around the head and clipped). A split (or drape) sheet covers the patient's body.

Equipment

Padded restraints
Headrest (e.g., doughnut), optional
Warming mattress or heat lamps, optional
Suction
Electrosurgical unit (bipolar)
Sitting stools, optional

Instrumentation

Basic plastic procedures tray
Lip clamp
Beaver knife handle

Supplies

Basin set
Bayonet bipolar electrocoagulating forceps
Blades (1) No. 15, (1) No. 11
Beaver blades (1) No. 64, (1) No. 65
Marking pen or methylene blue
Needle magnet or counter
Syringes (2) Luer-lock control, and needles (2) 25- or 27-gauge
Local anesthetic with epinephrine
Suction tubing
Antibiotic ointment
Logan's bow

Special notes

Do not allow preparation solution to pool in or around the eyes.

CLEFT PALATE REPAIR

Definition

Correction of congenital defects in the palate.

Discussion

The defects result from lack of embryonic development of elements of the prepalate (face, lips, premaxilla, and incisors) and the palate (hard and soft palate, uvula, and additional maxillary teeth). Multiple combinations and defects exist. In severe defects nursing and respiratory problems may be present. To minimize speech difficulties, repair is desirable prior to age 2. Mobilization of lateral tissue (by undermining) allows for midline closure. Anterior detachment of the hard and soft palate allows "push back" of the whole palate. Secondary repairs are performed to correct a residual fistula, to correct speech problems, and to facilitate dental restoration.

Procedure

General anesthesia is administered and an endotracheal tube is inserted. In addition, a local anesthetic containing epinephrine is infiltrated locally to aid hemostasis. For repair of a complete unilateral (prepalatal and palatal) defect, soft palate margins are incised. Layers for oral mucosa, muscle, and nasal mucosa are developed. The pterygoid hamulus is fractured and mucoperiosteal flaps are elevated. Nasal mucosal flaps are freed and sutured. The nasal mucosa of the soft palate is sutured. The greater palatine vessels are preserved. Holes may be drilled in the hard palate for suture placement. Bone grafts may be employed. Muscle layers and the oral mucosa are sutured.

Preparation of the patient

The patient is supine with the head at the foot of the table. The table may be in slight reverse Trendelenburg position. For the pediatric patient special measures must be taken to prepare the room, restrain the patient, and maintain the patient's body temperature. Refer to Pediatric General Information, p. 467.

Skin preparation

Check with the surgeon regarding choice of preparation solution. Begin at the upper lip, cleanse the face extending from the hairline to the shoulders, and down to the table at the sides of the neck.

Draping

See Cleft Lip Repair, p. 338.

Equipment

Padded restraints
Warming mattress or heating lamps (optional)
Suction
Electrosurgical unit (bipolar)
Sitting stools, optional
Power source for power drill

Instrumentation

Basic plastic procedures tray
Power drill (small), cord, and drill bits (fine)

Supplies

Basin set
Bayonet bipolar electrocoagulating forceps
Blades (1) No. 15, (1) No. 11, (1) No. 12
Syringes (2) Luer-lock control, and needles (2) 25- or 27-gauge
Local anesthetic with epinephrine
Suction tubing
Needle magnet or counter

Special notes

Some surgeons may allow the patient's head to extend over the edge of the table, supporting it in the surgeon's lap. The surgeon's lap is covered with a drape sheet clipped to the table.

The table may be turned to facilitate access.

REDUCTION OF A NASAL FRACTURE

Definition

Molding and realignment of the nasal bones and septum.

Discussion

Fractures of the nasal bones, cartilage, septum, and frontal processes of the maxilla occur in multiple combinations. Most often reduction is accomplished by the closed method.

Procedure

A forceps (e.g., Asch) is placed to provide traction under the nasal bones. External digital manipulation reduces the fracture. Nasal packing is inserted and a nasal splint is applied. If the results of closed reduction are unsatisfactory, open reduction exposing the septum and portions of the nasal bones may be required. Modified rhinoplastic techniques are necessary to realign malpositioned bony and cartilaginous fragments, which may be stabilized by intranasal sutures. Nasal packing is inserted and an external nasal splint is applied.

Preparation of the patient

The patient is supine; arms may be tucked in at the patient's side and secured with padded restraints. The procedure may be performed under local anesthesia. The surgeon usually does a preliminary nasal preparation. If an anesthetist is not in attendance, see circulator responsibilities, p. 31.

Preliminary nasal preparation (on a "clean" tray):

Packing (e.g., ½" plain gauze or cotton)
Cotton-tipped applicators (long; wood or metal)
Medicine cups (2)
Topical anesthetic (e.g., cocaine 4% or 5%)
Local anesthetic with epinephrine
Syringes (2) Luer-lock control, and needles (2) 25- or
    27-gauge
Atomizer
Scissors (e.g., straight Mayo)
Bayonet forceps

Skin preparation

None is required for closed reduction.
Open reduction: Check with the surgeon regarding the type of preparation solution. Begin at the nose, cleanse the face and neck extending from the hairline to the shoulders, and down to the table at the sides of the neck.

Draping

None is required for closed reduction; the patient's body may be covered with a drape sheet. The Mayo stand is draped. Gloves are worn.
Open reduction: See Cleft Lip Repair, p. 338.

Equipment

Restraints, padded
Suction
Fiberoptic headlight and light source

Instrumentation

Closed: Frazier suction tip, bayonet forceps, Asch forceps (or rubber-shod Crile forceps, straight)
Open: Nasal procedures tray

Supplies

Closed:
Suction tubing
Small basin
Nasal splint
Nasal packing

Open:
Basin set
Blades (2) No. 15
Suction tubing
Needle magnet or counter
Antibiotic ointment, optional
Nasal packing
Nasal splint

Special notes

Do not allow preparation solution to pool in or around the eyes.
The table may be turned for easier access.
The table may be flexed for patient's comfort.

REDUCTION OF A MANDIBULAR FRACTURE

Definition

Correction of malocclusion resulting from a fracture of the lower jaw.

Discussion

Numerous presentations occur; all should be reduced and fixed as soon as possible after the injury.

When the fracture is anterior (so that teeth are on either side of the fracture), intermaxillary fixation may suffice. For fractures posterior to the teeth, intermaxillary fixation and open reduction are necessary.

Procedure

Closed Reduction. For closed reduction an arch bar is bent to conform to the teeth and the dental arch. Fine wire encircles the necks of the teeth, attaching the teeth to the bars. The maxillary and mandibular bars may be placed in occlusion or multiple small latex bands may be attached to the bars, which also produce occlusion.

Open Reduction. In open reduction an incision (one or more) is made below the inferior border of the mandible. The fracture site(s) is(are) exposed and the periosteum reflected. The fracture is reduced. Holes may be drilled into the mandible on both sides of the fracture. Wires passed through the holes maintain alignment. The fracture site may be stabilized with bone fragments. The wound(s) is(are) closed in layers. A small drain may be placed. Arch bars may be applied prior to or following the open reduction.

Preparation of the patient

The patient is supine; arms may be tucked in at the patient's sides and secured with padded restraints. The head may be positioned on a headrest. Apply electrosurgical dispersive pad for open reduction.

Skin preparation

Closed reduction: None is required.
Open reduction: Check with the surgeon regarding choice of preparation solution. Cleanse face, ears, and neck (including the sides and back of the neck) extending from hairline to shoulders. Some surgeons prepare the inside of the mouth with swabs saturated in preparation solution.

Draping

Closed reduction: None is required; however, a Mayo stand cover and a drape sheet (for back table) are necessary. A sheet may be draped over the patient's body and a towel placed over the eyes. This procedure is "clean", not sterile. Gloves (only) are required.

Open reduction: See Open Reduction of a Carpal Bone Fracture, p. 247.

Equipment

Headrest (e.g., Richards, Shea, doughnut)
Restraints, padded
Suction
Electrosurgical unit
Power source for power drill
Fiberoptic headlight and light source

Instrumentation

Closed Reduction and Application of Intermaxillary Wiring:
Suction tip (e.g., Yankauer)
Arch bars and latex bands (or other intermaxillary wiring device)
Wire cutters, Freer septal elevator, Weider tongue depressors (large and small), Heaney needle holders
Minor orthopedic procedures tray (available)

Open Reduction:
Minor orthopedic procedures tray
Weider tongue depressors (large and small)
Power drill (e.g., Mini Stryker or Hall II), cord, drill bits

Supplies

Closed Reduction:
Small basin
Suction tubing
Stainless steel wire (25- or 26-gauge)

Open Reduction:
Basin set
Suction tubing
Stainless steel wire (25-, 26-, or 28-gauge)
Blades (2) No. 15
Marking pen
Electrosurgical pencil
Bulb syringe
Drain (e.g., Penrose ¼"), optional
Local anesthetic with epinephrine (hemostasis),
    syringes (2) Luer-lock control, and needles
    (2) 25- or 27-gauge (optional)
Nerve stimulator (locator) (e.g., Concept), optional

Special notes

The table may be turned to facilitate access.

Do not allow preparation solution to pool in or around eyes or ears.

If arch bars (or other intermaxillary wiring devices) are applied first, a separate setup is required for the open reduction.

The surgeon may request the scrub person to irrigate (slow trickle of saline) over the drill point to prevent buildup of heat from the friction of the power drill.

Protective goggles may be worn.

Always have (disposable) wire cutters accompany patient on leaving the operating room.

REDUCTION OF A ZYGOMATIC FRACTURE

Definition

Correction of fracture(s) of the cheek (zygoma or malar bone).

Discussion

The two most common zygomatic fractures are depressed fractures of the arch and trimalar fractures.

Closed reduction is the treatment for zygomatic arch fractures. Trimalar fractures are treated by open reduction and internal fixation.

Procedure

Small, access incisions to the fracture fragments are made in the lateral third of the eyebrow and in the infraorbital region. Holes are drilled in the fragments, through which stainless steel wires are passed. The fragments are realigned and the position is maintained by the wires. The incisions are closed.

Preparation of the patient

The patient is supine; arms may be tucked in at the patient's sides and secured with padded restraints. The head may be positioned on a headrest. Apply electrosurgical dispersive pad if monopolar electrosurgical unit is used.

Skin preparation

Closed reduction: None is usually required. Check with the surgeon.

Open reduction: Check with the surgeon regarding the type of preparation solution. Begin cleansing the affected cheek. Cleanse the face and neck from the hairline to the shoulders; include the ear on the affected side.

Draping

None is usually required for *closed reduction;* the patient's body may be covered with a drape sheet. If instrumentation is used, the Mayo stand and back table are draped.

For *open reduction,* see Cleft Lip Repair, p. 338.

Equipment

Restraints, padded

Open Reduction:
Headrest (e.g., Richards, Shea, doughnut)
Suction
Power source for power drill
Electrosurgical unit, monopolar or bipolar

Instrumentation

Closed Reduction. Check with the surgeon.

Open Reduction:
Limited procedure tray
Minor orthopedic procedures tray (available)
Kerrison rongeurs, bone hook
Power drill, cord, and drill bits
Wire cutter

Supplies (open reduction)

Basin set
Blades (2) No. 15
Marking pen
Electrosurgical pencil or bayonet bipolar electro-
    coagulating forceps
Suction tubing
Bulb syringe
Stainless steel wire (e.g., 25-, 26-, or 28-gauge)
Local anesthetic with epinephrine (hemostasis), sy-
    ringes (2) Luer-lock control, and needles (2) 25-
    or 27-gauge

Special notes

Do not allow preparation solution to pool in or
around eyes and ears.
The table may be turned to facilitate access.
The table may be flexed for the patient's
comfort.

OPEN REDUCTION OF AN ORBITAL FLOOR FRACTURE

Definition

Elevation and restoration of the integrity of the thin bone that supports the eye and periorbital tissues.

Discussion

Orbital floor fractures often occur in combination with other facial fractures (maxillary and zygomatic). "Blowout" fracture refers to an isolated depressed fracture of the orbital floor (with the infraorbital rim intact), often with the orbital contents protruding into the maxillary sinus. Various structures including the infraorbital nerve and extraocular muscles must be recognized and protected. Repair should be done promptly.

Procedure

An incision is made over the infraorbital rim (avoiding injury medially to the orbicularis oculi muscle) and continued down to the periosteum. The periosteum is incised and reflected over the fracture site. Debris is removed from the fracture site. The defect may be covered with a synthetic material (e.g., a Teflon or Silastic sheet), autogenous cartilage, or bone. The globe is rotated to test the security of the implant and to make certain the inferior rectus muscle is not trapped. The periosteum is sutured back to its site of origin, as are the orbicularis oculi muscle and skin. An ice pack may be applied following the application of an antibiotic eye ointment and an eye patch.

Preparation of the patient

The patient is supine; arms may be tucked in at the patient's sides. The head may be positioned on a headrest. Apply electrosurgical dispersive pad if the monopolar electrosurgical unit is used.

Skin preparation

Check with the surgeon regarding the type of preparation solution to be used. Begin cleansing the operative eyelid; cleanse the face and neck from the hairline to the shoulders; include the ear on the affected side.

Draping

See Cleft Lip Repair, p. 338.

Equipment

Headrest (e.g., doughnut)
Electrosurgical unit, monopolar or bipolar
Power source for power drill (optional)
Suction
Fiberoptic headlight and light source (optional)
Sitting stools, optional

Instrumentation

Basic eye procedures tray
Globe and orbit procedures tray
Minor orthopedic procedures tray (available for bone graft)
Bone hook
Power drill, cord, and drill bits (for implant)

Supplies

Basin set
Needle magnet or counter
Blades (2) No. 15
Marking pen
Bulb syringe
Suction tubing
Electrosurgical pencil with needle tip or bipolar electrocoagulating forceps
Orbital floor implant material (Teflon or Silastic sheet), available

Local anesthetic with epinephrine (for hemostasis),
   syringes (2) Luer-lock control, and needles (2)
   25- or 27-gauge
Cotton-tipped applicators or cellulose sponges
Antibiotic ophthalmic ointment
Ice pack (available)

Special notes

The procedure may be performed by a plastic
surgeon, ophthalmologist, or otorhinolaryngologist;
equipment, instrumentation, and supplies particular
to that specialty must be taken into consideration
when setting up.

The table may be turned to facilitate access.

Do not allow preparation solution to pool in or
around eyes and ears. Irrigate eyes from inner to
outer canthus.

If cartilage or bone is to be taken for an autogenous graft, check with the surgeon regarding donor
site.

RHINOPLASTY

Definition

Correction of the external appearance of the nose.

Discussion

In addition to cosmetic considerations this procedure is performed to alleviate nasal airway problems caused by a deviated septum and nasal
trauma not relieved by closed reduction. Four inter-
related steps may be employed: tip remodeling,
hump removal, narrowing, and septoplasty. Rhinoplasty is modified according to each patient's needs.
The surgeon must endeavor to maintain proper
shape, symmetry, and proportion. Mentoplasty
Augmentation (see p. 356) is often performed in
conjunction with rhinoplasty to achieve a more balanced appearance.

Procedure

Through the nostril an intercartilaginous incision is made along the rim of the upper lateral cartilage bilaterally, and connected, freeing the skin from over the dorsal septum and anteriorly, freeing the columella. Prominent septal, lateral, and alar cartilage are excised and after reassessment are retrimmed as necessary. The nasal bones are then osteotomized laterally, medially (and horizontally, if necessary), and compressed to infracture the bones creating a more normal contour. Rasping smooths any irregularity. Alignment of the septum is achieved. The anterior septum and columella are sutured; alar incisions and marginal (rim) incisions of the lower lateral cartilages are sutured as well. Intranasal packing is inserted and an external splint is applied.

Preparation of the patient

The patient is supine; arms may be tucked in at the patient's sides and secured by padded restraints. The patient's head may be supported on a headrest. The procedure is usually performed under local anesthesia. The surgeon often does a preliminary nasal preparation before the skin preparation. If anesthetist is not in attendance, see circulator responsibilities, p. 31.

Preliminary nasal preparation (on a "clean" tray)

Packing (e.g., ½" plain gauze or cotton balls)
Cotton-tipped applicators (long; wood or metal)
Medicine cups (2)
Topical anesthetic (e.g., cocaine 4% or 5%)
Local anesthetic with epinephrine
Syringes (2) Luer-lock control, and needles (2) 25- or 27-gauge
Atomizer
Scissors (e.g., straight Mayo)
Bayonet forceps

Skin preparation

Check with the surgeon regarding the type of preparation solution to be used. Begin at the nose, cleanse the face and neck extending from the hairline to the shoulders, and down to the table at the sides of the neck.

Draping

See Cleft Lip Repair, p. 338.

Equipment

Headrest (e.g., doughnut, Shea, Richards)
Restraints, padded
Suction
Fiberoptic headlight and light source

Instrumentation

Nasal procedures tray
Beaver knife handle

Supplies

Basin set
Blades (4) No. 15
Beaver blade (e.g., No. 64)
Needle magnet or counter
Suction tubing
Syringes (2) Luer-lock control, and needles (2) 25- or
    27-gauge
Syringe, disposable (for cleaning suction tip)
Long cotton-tipped applicators
Nasal packing
Antiobiotic ointment, optional
Nasal splint

Special notes

Do not allow preparation solution to pool in and around eyes or ears.

The table may be turned for easier access.

The table may be slightly flexed for the patient's comfort.

MENTOPLASTY AUGMENTATION

Definition

Correction of micrognathia with the insertion of a chin prosthesis.

Discussion

The indication for this procedure is to improve the cosmetic appearance of the chin. The approach is submental or intraoral.

Procedure

A short transverse incision is made in the submental region or in the labial sulcus. A supraperiosteal pocket is created just large enough to accommodate the prosthesis. The implant may be fixed with a deep mattress suture. The wound is closed. A bulky pressure dressing is applied.

Preparation of the patient

The patient is supine; arms may be tucked in at the patient's sides and secured with padded restraints. Apply electrosurgical dispersive pad if the monopolar electrosurgical unit is used. The procedure is usually performed under local anesthesia; see circulator responsibilities, p. 31.

Skin preparation

Check with the surgeon regarding the type of preparation solution to be used. Begin at the chin, cleanse the face extending from the hairline to the shoulders, and down to the table at the side of the neck.

Draping

See Cleft Lip Repair, p. 338.

Equipment

Electrosurgical unit, monopolar or bipolar

Instrumentation

Basic plastic procedures tray

Supplies

Small basin
Electrosurgical pencil with needle tip or bipolar electrocoagulating forceps
Marking pen
Blades (2) No. 15
Needle magnet or counter
Local anesthetic with epinephrine
Syringes (2) Luer-lock control, and needles (2) 25- or 27-gauge
Implant (e.g., Silicone)

Special notes

Do not allow preparation solution to pool in and around the eyes.

The table may be turned for easier access.

The table may be slightly flexed for the patient's comfort.

BLEPHAROPLASTY

Definition

Excision of a protrusion of intraorbital fat and resection of excessive redundant skin of the eyelids.

Discussion

The amount of skin resected depends on the severity of the deformity and the age of the patient.

Procedure

An elliptical incision is made in the recess of the orbitopalpebral fold of the upper lid according to previously placed markings. The orbicularis oculi muscle is incised parallel to its fibers at the apex of the bulge. The fat protrudes through the incision and is excised. The upper lid incisions may be covered with moist saline sponges while resection of a portion of the lower lids is done. The skin is undermined. The orbicularis oculi muscle is split. Fat compartments are isolated; the fat is delivered, clamped at its base, and resected. The upper lids are checked for bleeding; hemostasis is obtained. Incisions in the upper lids are closed with fine interrupted sutures. The procedure is repeated for the lower lids. An occlusive (not pressure) dressing is applied.

Preparation of the patient

The patient is supine; arms may be tucked in at the patient's sides and secured with padded restraints. The surgeon may mark the eyelids prior to skin preparation and injection of the anesthetic. The procedure may be performed under general anesthesia, but local anesthesia is preferred; see p. 31 for circulator responsibilities regarding local anesthesia.

Skin preparation

Check with the surgeon regarding the type of preparation solution to be used. Begin at the eyelids; cleanse the face extending from the hairline to the shoulders, and down to the table at the sides of the neck.

Draping

See Cleft Lip Repair, p. 338.

Equipment

Restraints, padded
Electrosurgical unit (bipolar)
Sitting stools, 2 (surgeon and scrub person)
Fiberoptic headlight and light source (available)

Instrumentation

Basic plastic procedures tray

Supplies

Basin set
Bayonet bipolar electrocoagulating forceps
Marking pen
Blades (3 or 4) No. 15
Needle magnet or counter
Cotton-tipped applicators or cellulose sponges
Local anesthetic with epinephrine
Syringes (2) Luer-lock control, and needles (2) 25- or
    27 gauge

Special notes

Do not allow preparation solution to pool in or
around the eyes.

The table may be turned for easier access.

The table may be slightly flexed for the patient's
comfort.

RHYTIDECTOMY

Definition

Mobilization and excision of excessive facial skin
folds and subcutaneous tissue in order to minimize
wrinkles and excessive fatty deposits.

Discussion

Rhytidectomy is often combined with blepharoplasty
(see p. 357).

Procedure

The incision follows previously made markings, which follow the anterior contour of the ear extending superiorly into the scalp, inferiorly curving around the posterior aspect of the ear, and extending posteriorly to the scalp. The skin and subcutaneous tissue are mobilized by undermining. Care is taken to avoid injury to nerves (e.g., the facial nerve branches, the greater auricular nerve). After hemostasis is secured, plication sutures are placed in the musculofascial tissues. Tension is placed on the flap, directing it superiorly and posteriorly as anchoring sutures are placed. Excess skin is trimmed. Wound closure is completed with fine interrupted sutures. Care is exerted not to distort the ear. A closed suction drainage unit may be placed. A pressure dressing is applied taking care to pad the ears.

Preparation of the patient

The patient is supine with the back slightly elevated; arms may be extended on armboards or tucked in at the patient's sides, and secured with padded restraints. The head may be positioned on a headrest. The surgeon usually marks the face prior to skin preparation and injection of the anesthetic. The procedure may be performed under general anesthesia, but local anesthesia is preferred; see p. 31 for circulator responsibilities regarding local anesthesia. Hair is rarely shaved, but the surgeon may request the hair around the hairline to be secured.

Skin preparation

Check with the surgeon regarding the type of preparation solution to be used. The patient's face, ears, and neck are cleansed extending from the hairline to the shoulders, and down to the table at the sides of the neck.

Draping

See Cleft Lip Repair, p. 338.

Equipment

Headrest (e.g., doughnut, Shea, Richards), optional
Restraints, padded
Electrosurgical unit (bipolar)
Sitting stools, 2 (surgeon and scrub person)

Instrumentation

Basic plastic procedures tray
Deaver retractors (2) 1"

Supplies

Basin set
Bayonet bipolar electrocoagulating forceps
Marking pen
Blades (4 to 6) No. 15
Needle magnet or counter
Local anesthetic with epinephrine
Syringes (2) Luer-lock control, and needles (2) 25- or
    27-gauge
Cotton-tipped applicators
Drain (e.g., Hemovac, Jackson-Pratt), optional

Special notes

See Blepharoplasty, p. 357.

DERMABRASION

Definition

Sanding of the skin to smooth scars and surface ir-
regularities.

Discussion

This procedure removes or minimizes scars (e.g., from facial acne vulgaris and chickenpox). Dermabrasion may also be employed to remove tattoos. Fine wrinkling around the mouth can be temporarily improved with dermabrasion.

Procedure

The skin is stretched by hand and the epidermis is abraded by means of a motor-driven sanding cylinder and/or a wire brush. The area is irrigated copiously with saline during (and following) the procedure. The wound may be dressed with nonadherent gauze (e.g., Owens gauze) and gauze sponges moistened with saline. A compression bandage may be applied.

Preparation of the patient

The patient is supine; arms may be extended on armboards or tucked in at the patient's sides, and secured by padded restraints. The head may be positioned on a headrest. Anesthesia is achieved by infiltration with a local anesthetic. For circulator responsibilities regarding local anesthesia, see p. 31. The surgeon may mark the scars prior to skin preparation.

Skin preparation

Check with the surgeon regarding the type of preparation solution to be used. Begin with the area to be dermabraded. Cleanse the face, ears, and neck extending from the hairline to the shoulders, and down to the table at the sides of the neck.

Draping

See Cleft Lip Repair, p. 338.

Equipment

Headrest (e.g., doughnut)
Restraints, padded
Power unit (for dermabrader)

Instrumentation

Adson forceps
Straight Mayo scissors
Dermabrader (with wire brush and sanding cylinder) and cord, e.g., Stryker

Supplies

Basin set
Local anesthetic with epinephrine
Syringes (2) Luer-lock control, and needles (2) 25- or 27-gauge
Marking pen

Special notes

Do not allow preparation solution to pool in or around the eyes and ears.

The table may be turned to facilitate access.

The table may be slightly flexed for the patient's comfort.

This is a delicate procedure; keep distractions in the room to a minimum.

Do not leave loose sponges near the dermabrader because they may get caught in the mechanism.

OTOPLASTY

Definition

Most commonly refers to correction of a prominent ear that protrudes unduly from the side of the head;

it may also refer to the correction of microtia and other congenital deformities of the ears.

Discussion

The procedure is usually performed bilaterally. The ideal time for the correction of prominent ears is 4 years of age or before the child enters school.

Procedure

A planned skin excision is marked. A new antihelical fold is marked. Several diagonal lines are marked on corresponding sides of the elliptical incision. An incision is made on the distal side and a flap is undermined. The anterior surface of the cartilage is exposed. The anterior cartilage surface is abraded with a rasp to reduce the perichondrium, thereby subsequently reducing forward curling of the ear. A predetermined wedge may be excised and sutured with nonabsorbable suture. Mattress sutures are inserted through the previously made markings. Overlapping skin is excised. Wound closure is completed with interrupted sutures. A compression dressing is applied.

Preparation of the patient

The patient is supine; arms may be tucked in at the patient's sides and secured with padded restraints. If the procedure is unilateral, the patient's head may be positioned on a headrest with the operative side up; adequately pad lowermost ear. For bilateral procedure the surgeon will position the head as necessary. Apply electrosurgical dispersive pad. For the pediatric patient see Pediatric General Information, p. 467.

Skin preparation

Check with the surgeon regarding the type of preparation solution to be used.

Unilateral: Begin cleansing the external ear; extend preparation from the hairline to the shoulders, beyond the midline of the face, and down to the table at the neck of the affected side.

Bilateral: Cleanse each ear; extend preparation from the hairline to the shoulders, and down to the table at the sides.

Draping

The patient is draped with a head drape with the ears exposed (drape sheet and two towels under the head with the uppermost towel wrapped around the head and clipped). A split (or drape) sheet covers the body. An additional drape sheet may be needed to cover the foot of the table.

Equipment

Headrest (e.g., Shea, doughnut), optional
Restraints, padded
Electrosurgical unit

Instrumentation

Basic plastic procedures tray
Small rasp

Supplies

Basin set
Blades (2) No. 15
Marking pen or methylene blue
Needle magnet or counter
Electrosurgical pencil with needle tip
Bunnell needles
Local anesthetic with epinephrine
Syringes (2), e.g., Luer-lock control, and needles (2)
    25- or 27-gauge
Cotton pledgets

Special notes

For a unilateral procedure keep lowermost ear well padded to avoid pressure injury.

The table may be turned for easier access.

Do not allow preparation solution to pool in or around the ears or eyes; a sterile cotton pledget may be placed in the ear during preparation and removed following preparation.

REPAIR OF SYNDACTYLY

Definition

Separation of webbed or fused digits.

Discussion

Syndactyly most often occurs in the hand and is commonly found bilaterally. The middle and ring finger are the most frequently webbed. Toe syndactyly does not always require surgical intervention, because the movement of the toes individually is not necessary for walking. Fused digits may exist with only skin involvement, but also may occur with other digital anomalies. If webbing involves many digits, full-thickness skin grafts may be done.

Procedure

Zig-zag or Z-plasty incisions are made in the interdigital space(s) to avoid contractures and provide flaps for the webspace reconstruction. The neurovascular bundles are protected. Bony and ligamentous defects, if present, are corrected. The incisions are closed. Full-thickness grafts (e.g., skin from the abdomen or the medial aspect of the arm or the thigh) may be required to close the defects. Stents are sutured over the grafts. A bulky dressing and splint are applied.

Preparation of the patient

For *syndactyly of the hand,* the patient is supine; the arm on the unaffected side may be extended on an armboard and the affected hand may be extended on a hand table. Sheet wadding and a (pediatric) tourniquet are applied to the arm on the affected side.

For *syndactyly of the foot,* the patient is supine; arms may be extended on armboards. The patient is secured to the table with the safety belt over the unaffected extremity. Sheet wadding and a tourniquet (adult or pediatric) are applied to the thigh of the affected side.

The surgeon may mark the skin prior to the skin preparation. Apply electrosurgical dispersive pad (adult or pediatric).

Skin preparation

Syndactyly of the hand: Begin at the area(s) of syndactyly and cleanse the hand (including interdigital spaces and nails). Extend preparation from fingertips to the arm (include the elbow).

Syndactyly of the foot: Begin at the area(s) of syndactyly and cleanse the foot (including interdigital spaces and nails). Extend preparation from the toes to the leg (include the knee).

Draping

Syndactyly of the hand: The hand is held up in a tube (or impervious) stockinette as a sheet is draped over the hand table. A cuffed drape (or split) sheet is draped under the arm. A towel is folded (in thirds, longitudinally), wrapped around the arm, and clipped. A drape (or split) sheet is draped over the arm and shoulder, and clipped under the arm. A fenestrated sheet or individual drape sheets completes the draping.

Syndactyly of the foot: The foot is held up in a tube (or impervious) stockinette as a sheet is draped over the foot of the table. A cuffed drape (or split) sheet is draped under the leg. A towel is folded (in thirds, longitudinally), wrapped around the thigh, and clipped. A drape (or split) sheet is draped over the thigh and clipped underneath. A fenestrated sheet or individual drape sheets complete the draping.

Equipment

Hand table
Tourniquet (adult or pediatric) and insufflator
Electrosurgical unit
Sitting stools, 2 to 3 (surgeon, scrub person, assistant
    surgeon)
Cast cart

Instrumentation

Minor orthopedic procedures tray

Supplies

Basin set
Sheet wadding
Esmarch bandage
Blades (2) No. 15
Electrosurgical pencil with needle tip
Needle magnet or counter
Bulb syringe
Marking pen
Stents, optional

Special notes

Have x-ray films in room.
Regarding tourniquet precautions, see Open Reduction of a Carpal Bone Fracture, p. 247, for syndactyly of the hand, and Arthrotomy of the Knee, p. 277, for syndactyly of the foot.
If skin graft is needed, check with the surgeon regarding the donor site.

DIGITAL FLEXOR TENDON REPAIR

Definition

Approximation of severed ends of a tendon caused by injury or a failed previous tendon repair.

Discussion

When a large gap exists, a graft is employed, often the palmaris longus tendon. Tendons to the digits may be severed from the forearm to the base of the distal phalanx. Injuries between the distal palmar crease and proximal interphalangeal joint should be repaired initially, and treated by a tendon graft at a later time. Avoidance of tension, meticulous handling of tissue, good hemostasis, fine nonreactive sutures, and dynamic immobilization are important for success.

Procedure

The incision is made according to the site of injury. Midlateral digital incisions are often employed. Care is taken to avoid injury to the neurovascular bundle. Pulleys are preserved when possible. The proximal tendon end is retrieved. If length is not sufficient, a graft (e.g., from the palmaris longus tendon) is prepared. The tendon ends are approximated. If the tendon insertion is involved, suture to the bone may be facilitated using fine drill holes. The suture fixing the tendon graft to the insertion is tied over a button on the dorsum of the distal phalanx to prevent soft tissue necrosis. The wound is closed. A splint is applied.

Preparation of the patient

The patient is supine; the unaffected arm may be extended on an armboard and the arm on the affected side may be extended on a hand table. Sheet wadding and a tourniquet are applied to the affected arm. Apply electrosurgical dispersive pad.

Skin preparation

Begin at the repair site; cleanse the hand (including interdigital spaces and nails), extending from the fingertips to the level of the tourniquet.

Draping

The extremity is held up in a tube (or impervious) stockinette as a sheet is draped over the end of the hand table. A cuffed drape (or split) sheet is draped under the arm. A towel is folded (in thirds, longitudinally), wrapped around the arm, and clipped. A sheet is draped over the arm and shoulder and clipped under the arm. A fenestrated sheet or individual drape sheets completes the draping. If a microscope is used, a microscope drape is necessary.

Equipment

Tourniquet and insufflator
Electrosurgical unit
Hand table
Sitting stools, 2 to 3 (surgeon, scrub person, and assistant surgeon)
Loupes or microscope (available)
Cast cart
Power source for power drill, optional

Instrumentation

Basic plastic procedures tray
Power drill and fine drill points, optional
Micro instrumentation; see Peripheral Nerve Repair, p. 371

Supplies

Basin set
Sheet wadding
Esmarch bandage

Tube (or impervious) stockinette
Marking pen
Blades (2) No. 15
Needle magnet or counter
Bulb syringe
Electrosurgical pencil with needle tip
Straight Keith needle and button

Special notes

For tourniquet precautions, see Open Reduction of a Carpal Bone Fracture, p. 247.

If a graft is to be taken, check with the surgeon regarding donor site.

PERIPHERAL NERVE REPAIR

Definition

Refers to the anastomosis of a peripheral nerve in the hand, wrist, or forearm or the foot, ankle, or leg by direct approximation of the nerve or by a nerve graft.

Discussion

The procedure is performed to correct loss of sensation and/or motor function. If a nerve graft is used, it is often obtained along the posterolateral aspect of the leg.

Procedure

An adequate incision is made over the appropriate area. In secondary repairs knowledge of the original nerve injury may suggest the need for a nerve graft, in which case, incisions can be made over the proximal and distal stumps creating an intervening tunnel through which a graft can be placed. Under magnification the nerve fascicles (fibers) are identified; scar and irregular edges are excised. Epineural sutures approximate the fascicles or groups of fascicles. To avoid tension, a graft may be necessary. Following closure of the wound(s) a splint is applied.

Preparation of the patient

The patient is supine; for *upper extremity peripheral nerve repair,* the unaffected arm may be extended on the armboard and the affected arm may be extended on a hand table. Sheet wadding and a tourniquet are applied to the affected arm.

For *lower extremity peripheral nerve repair,* a tourniquet is applied to the affected extremity and the safety strap is secured over the thigh of the unaffected extremity.

Apply electrosurgical dispersive pad.

Skin preparation

Upper extremity peripheral nerve repair: Begin at the repair site; cleanse the hand (including nails and interdigital spaces), extending from the fingertips to the level of the tourniquet.

Lower extremity peripheral nerve repair: Begin at the repair site; cleanse the foot (including nails and interdigital spaces), extending from the fingertips to the level of the tourniquet.

Draping

See Digital Flexor Tendon Repair, p. 369. If a microscope is used a microscope drape is required.

Equipment

Hand table (upper extremity repair)
Tourniquet and insufflator
Electrosurgical unit
Cast cart
Loupes and micrscope (available)

Instrumentation

Basic plastic procedures tray
Micro instrumentation, e.g., Castroviejo needle
holder without lock, Castroviejo needle holder
with lock, von Graefe muscle hook, jewelers' forceps and Castroviejo-Vannas scissors

Supplies

Basin set
Sheet wadding
Tube (or impervious) stockinette
Esmarch bandage
Electrosurgical pencil with needle tip
Blades (2) No. 15
Needle magnet or counter
Marking pen
Nerve stimulator (locator), e.g., Concept
Bulb syringe

Special notes

For tourniquet precautions, see Open Reduction
of a Carpal Bone Fracture, p. 247.

When a nerve graft is to be taken, check with
the surgeon regarding donor site. If another site is
used for the nerve graft, that extremity may have a
tourniquet, and the extremity must be prepared and
draped.

PALMAR FASCIECTOMY

Definition

Excision of the fascia (partial or total) of the palm.

Discussion

Dupuytren's contracture is a hereditary condition
caused by hyperplasia of fibrous tissue in the pal-

mar subcutaneous tissues with nodules fixed to the palmar fascia. Subsequent contracture results in deformity and/or contractures of the dermis or digits. The condition may also affect the plantar surface of the foot. The extent of this process is variable and does not always require surgical intervention.

Procedure

For less involved presentations, a short longitudinal palmar incision is made adjacent to the restrictive band, which is resected. For more extensive disease a longer incision with a Z-plasty arrangement is employed resecting the palmar fascia distally. Care is taken to avoid injury to digital nerves and flexor tendons. A more extensive presentation requires excision of more tissue. Wound closure may be done by primary suture or full-thickness free skin graft (which may be taken from the medial aspect of the arm). An anterior splint is applied.

Preparation of the patient, Skin preparation, and Draping

See Digital Flexor Tendon Repair, p. 369.

Equipment

Hand table
Tourniquet and insufflator
Electrosurgical unit
Sitting stools, 2 to 3 (surgeon, scrub person, assistant surgeon)

Instrumentation

Basic plastic procedures tray
Basin set
Sheet wadding
Tube (or impervious) stockinette
Esmarch bandage
Electrosurgical pencil with needle tip

Blades (2) No. 15
Needle magnet or counter
Marking pen

Special notes

For tourniquet precautions, see Open Reduction of a Carpal Bone Fracture, p. 247.

When a skin graft is to be taken, check with the surgeon regarding donor site.

REDUCTION MAMMOPLASTY

Definition

Excision of excessive breast tissue and reconstruction of the breasts.

Discussion

The principal indication for this procedure is alleviation of symptoms associated with breast weight (greater than 0.45 kg or approximately 1 pound). The technique employed is determined by the size of the breast and the surgeon's preference. Proper symmetry including nipple and areolar position must be maintained. Two categories of procedures are performed: lateralizing, in which no scar is left medially; and procedures that result in an inverted T scar. The nipple is usually transplanted as a pedicle, but may (with the areola) be reapplied as a free graft.

Procedure

The incisions are marked. An incision circumscribes the areola, which is usually left attached to underlying tissue as a pedicle graft. Flaps are developed excising a wedge of excessive (breast) skin and adipose tissue inferiorly; a Freeman areola marker may be used. The breast is reconstructed by approximating the medial and lateral breast tissue with skin flaps inferior to the nipple site, and transversely, in the inframammary fold (creating an inverted T). A closed suction unit may be employed. A bulky dressing and a surgical bra may be applied.

Preparation of the patient

The patient is either supine or in modified sitting position with arms extended on armboards and the feet supported by a padded footrest. Apply electrosurgical dispersive pad.

Skin preparation

Cleanse both breasts beginning at the nipples; extend preparation from the neckline to the umbilicus. Cleanse the axilla well and prepare down to the table at the sides.

Draping

Folded towels and a transverse sheet (which may be cut) or individual drape sheets

Equipment

Padded footrest (modified sitting position)
Electrosurgical unit
Scales (for weighing breast tissue)
Fiberoptic headlight and light source

Instrumentation

Basic/Minor procedures tray
Freeman areola marker

Supplies

Basin set
Blades (4 to 6) No. 10
Marking pen

Electrosurgical pencil
Needle magnet or counter
Drainage unit (e.g., Hemovac), optional
Surgical bra, optional

Special notes

Keep tissue removed from each breast separate.
Weigh and record the amount of tissue taken from each breast.
The surgeon may request a surgical bra over the dressing; the nipples are left undressed for observation of viability.

AUGMENTATION MAMMOPLASTY

Definition

Implantation of breast prostheses for the purpose of enlarging the breasts.

Discussion

Indications for this procedure are micromastia (unilateral or bilateral), postpartum involution of the breasts, ptosis, and postsurgical deformity. The approach may be inframammary, periareolar, or transaxillary. The silicone rubber prostheses can be gel filled, inflatable, or filled with gel and saline.

Procedure

Inframammary. The line of the incision is marked. A 3- to 4-cm incision is placed just above the inframammary crease. A percutaneous flap is developed inferiorly to the pectoralis fascia. A plane is developed between the pectoralis fascia and the posterior capsule of the breast. A pocket is created by blunt dissection to accommodate the implant. Care is taken to avoid intercostal nerve damage. Meticulous hemostasis is obtained; a fiberoptic lighted retractor may be employed. The implant is inserted. The subcutaneous flap is approximated. The skin may be closed using a running subcuticular closure.

Periareolar. The line of the incision is marked circumferentially. The incision is made along the inferior border of the areola. The subcutaneous tissue is dissected to the inferior border of the breast. The retromammary space is enlarged by blunt dissection to accommodate the prosthesis. Hemostasis is accomplished; a fiberoptic lighted retractor may be employed for better visualization. The prosthesis is inserted. The inferior border of the breast tissue is sutured to the pectoralis fascia. The periareolar incision may be closed with a subcuticular suture.

Transaxillary. The line of the incision is marked in the axilla. The vertical or oblique incision is carried down through the subcutaneous tissue. Using blunt dissection, a pocket over the upper pole of the sternum is dissected. Hemostasis is achieved; a fiberoptic lighted retractor may be employed. The prosthesis is inserted. The wound is closed in layers.

Preparation of the patient

The patient is supine with arms extended on armboards. Apply electrosurgical dispersive pad.

Skin preparation

Cleanse both breasts beginning at incisional sites (areolar, transaxillary, or inframammary). Extend preparation from the neckline to the lower ribs; cleanse the axilla down to the table at the sides.

Draping

Folded towels and a transverse sheet

Equipment

Electrosurgical unit
Fiberoptic headlight and light source (optional)

Fiberoptic light source (for lighted retractor, optional)

Instrumentation

Basic/Minor procedures tray
Fiberoptic lighted retractor and cord (optional)

Supplies

Basin set
Blades (2) No. 10, (2) No. 15
Marking pen
Electrosurgical pencil
Needle magnet or counter
Skin closure strips, optional
Surgical bra, optional

Special notes

The surgeon may request a surgical bra over the dressing; the nipples are left undressed for observation of viability.

ABDOMINOPLASTY/ABDOMINAL LIPECTOMY

Definition

Removal of loose, redundant abdominal skin and underlying subcutaneous fat, and the repair of the rectus muscle as necessary.

Discussion

There are variations in technique according to fat distribution and the surgeon's preference.

Procedure

A W-shaped incision approximately 2.5 cm (1 inch) above the inguinal folds may be used. The umbilicus is incised in a diamond shape and preserved for later replacement under the flap. Dissection is begun at the lower portion of the W-incision and progresses upward leaving a fine layer of areolar tissue over the fascia. Each lateral branch of tissue is excised. The amount of tissue excised is carefully estimated before removal so that the defect can be closed with moderate tension. If there is diastasis of the rectus abdominis muscle, it is plicated. Large ventral hernias may be repaired with synthetic mesh. The wound is closed with heavy absorbable suture in the deep fat; the skin is closed with a subcuticular running suture. The vertical branch of the incision is closed first. The umbilicus is located in the vertical scar. Drains may be employed.

Preparation of the patient

The patient is supine with arms extended on armboards. Check with the surgeon regarding slight flexion of the hips. Apply electrosurgical dispersive pad.

Skin preparation

Begin cleansing for a low, transverse abdominal incision. Extend preparation from midthorax to knees, and down to the table at the sides.

Draping

Folded towels and a transverse sheet (cut as necessary) or individual drape sheets

Equipment

Electrosurgical unit
Suction
Fiberoptic headlight and light source (available)
Scales (for weighing specimen)

Instrumentation

Basic/Minor procedures tray
Extra Crile and Kocher (or other grasping) clamps,
    many

Supplies

Basin set
Blades (4) No. 10
Needle magnet or counter
Marking pen
Electrosurgical pencil
Suction tubing
Drainage unit (e.g., Hemovac, Jackson-Pratt)

Special notes

Weigh and record the weight of the specimen.

LIPOSUCTION

Definition

Removal of subcutaneous fat deposits employing a
high-pressure vacuum-suctioning device.

Discussion

This procedure is performed for cosmetic purposes
to reduce disproportionately large collections of fat
in a specific area such as the hips, thighs, or abdomen; it is not performed for weight reduction. Other
areas of the body for which liposuction may be employed include the chin, breasts, arms, knees, calves,
buttocks, and ankles.

Procedure

The surgeon may preinject the areas where liposuction is to be employed with a solution of local anesthesia with epinephrine, to reduce bleeding and hyaluronidase (Wydase), to minimize tissue swelling. Through a 1-cm incision a blunt suction tip is inserted and used to tunnel under the skin, separating it from the underlying subcutaneous and connective tissues. The excess subcutaneous fat is then suctioned from the pretunneled areas using a high-pressure vacuum. The incisions are closed. A compression dressing is applied.

Preparation of the patient

The patient is positioned as for any other surgery performed on that particular part of the body. When liposuction is employed for reducing the abdomen, hips, and thighs, the patient is supine with arms extended on armboards.

Skin preparation

Begin at the site of the most central incision and extend the preparation appropriate distance.

Abdomen, hips, and thighs: Prepare from the nipples to below the knees, and down to the table at the sides. Ideally, two people are needed to elevate the lower extremities, abducting and adducting them as necessary, in order to ensure that the areas around and under each thigh and hip are adequately prepared. The pubic area is prepared last.

Draping

The patient is draped appropriately for performing surgery on that particular area of the body.

Abdomen, hips, and thighs: The legs are held up and abducted as each foot is grasped in a tube (or impervious) stockinette. Each stockinette is brought up over the leg covering the knee. A sheet is draped over the end of the table. A towel (folded in thirds, lengthwise) is placed over the pubic area and may be secured with a sterile, plastic adhesive drape. Cuffed drape sheets are tucked in at the patient's sides. An additional sheet is draped under the legs and thighs. The legs are lowered onto the table. A drape sheet covers the top of the field.

Equipment

High-pressure vacuum unit (e.g., Dean medical suction unit)

Instrumentation

Limited procedure tray
Blunt suction tips or blunt cannulas

Supplies

Basin set
Marking pen
Sterile, plastic adhesive drape, optional
Tube (or impervious) stockinette (2), optional
Blade (1) No. 15
Suction tubing (flexible, noncollapsing)
Syringes (2) 30 ml
Needles (2) 22 gauge
Intravenous antibiotic (e.g., cefazolin sodium (Ancef)), optional
Local anesthetic with epinephrine
Hyaluronidase (Wydase)
Pressure girdle

Special notes

Prepare a local solution as directed by the surgeon (e.g., 250 ml saline, 75 ml lidocaine (Xylocaine) 0.5% with epinephrine, and 2 ml (300 units) Wydase).

Keep 30-ml syringes (with 22-gauge needles) filled with the local solution.

Keep an accurate record of the total amount of solution that has been injected.

A special pressure girdle that covers the abdomen, hips, thighs, and buttocks should be put on the patient immediately after the wounds are dressed. The girdle is opened on the gurney and the patient is lifted onto it. The girdle is then hooked together.

Chapter 18

OTORHINOLARYNGO-
LOGIC (ENT) SURGERY

MYRINGOTOMY

Definition

Incision into the tympanic membrane to remove fluid accumulation.

Discussion

Myringotomy is indicated in acute chronic otitis media. Myringotomy tubes of polyethylene are often implanted through the myringotomy incision to facilitate drainage of the middle ear. In children, the procedure is performed under general anesthesia.

Procedure

A speculum is inserted in the ear canal. Wax, if present, is removed. The inferior posterior portion of the drumhead is incised for acute and some chronic conditions; an incision may also be made in other positions on the drumhead for chronic otitis media. Culture may be taken. Fluid or pus is suctioned. A drainage tube may be inserted. A small amount of cotton may be placed in the ear canal.

Preparation of the patient

The patient is supine; the head is positioned at the edge of the table with the affected ear up and the other ear well padded. The arm on the affected side may be restrained at the patient's side and the other arm may be extended on an armboard. For preparation of the pediatric patient see Pediatric General Information, p. 467.

Skin preparation

The auricle and periauricular skin may be prepared; some surgeons do not require skin preparation.

Draping

Three folded towels around the ear (optional) and a drape (or split) sheet; usually gloves only are worn.

Equipment

Restraints, padded
Microscope
Suction

Instrumentation

Basic ear procedures tray
Handgrips for the microscope

Supplies

Small basin
Suction tubing
Myringotomy knife, disposable
Myringotomy tube, disposable (e.g., Pepparella, Sheppard)

Grommet (0.045 size most frequently used)
Culture tubes (aerobic and anaerobic), optional
Cotton, optional

Special notes

The table may be turned for easier access.

Check with the surgeon regarding whether the ear is to be prepared and choice of preparation solution. Do not allow preparation solution to pool in or around the ear.

Remove wax from curettes, alligator forceps, etc., with moistened saline sponge.

Guide suction tip and instruments into the speculum as necessary.

The scrub person grasps the drainage tube in alligator forceps to pass it to the surgeon.

MASTOIDECTOMY

Definition

Removal of bony partitions forming the mastoid air cells.

Discussion

This procedure eradicates infected tissue to obtain an aseptic dry ear. Until this is achieved, procedures to restore hearing, for example, tympanoplasty (see p. 389), are not likely to succeed.

Types
Simple. Removal of the air cells only.

Modified Radical. Removal of the air cells and the posterior external auditory canal wall. (The middle ear is not disturbed.)

Radical. Removal of the air cells and tympanic membrane and the malleus, incus, tensor tympani muscle, and mucoperiosteal lining.

Procedure

In *simple mastoidectomy* a postauricular incision is made and carried down to bone exposing the cortex. The mastoid cells are exenterated with a burr. A drain is placed and the incision is closed. A myringotomy may be performed.

In the *modified radical procedure,* the posterior and superior walls of the auditory canal are resected, combining the middle ear, the attic, and the mastoid cavity into a single space. Drills and burrs are employed; care is taken to avoid injury to the facial nerve and canal skin. A tympanomeatal flap is created and draped over the ossicles to partially line the mastoid cavity. A gelatin sponge may be used to pack the cavity. The incision is closed and the wound is dressed.

In the *radical procedure* the malleus, incus, tympanic membrane, tensor tympani muscle, and the mucosa of the middle ear are excised. A strip of temporalis muscle may be used to fill the cavity. The cavity may be left to heal by secondary intention. The wound is packed and dressed.

Preparation of the patient

The patient is supine; the head is positioned on a headrest, and turned to the side with the operative ear up; the other ear is well padded. The arm on the affected side may be tucked in at the patient's side, and the arm on the other side may be extended on an armboard; both arms may be secured with padded restraints. Hair is secured out of the field. Apply electrosurgical dispersive pad if the electrosurgical unit is to be used. Local anesthetic may be administered before the skin preparation; see p. 31 for circulator responsibilities regarding local anesthesia.

Skin preparation

Begin cleansing the operative ear extending from the hairline to the shoulder, and well beyond the midline of the face. Prepare well behind the ear on the operative side.

Draping

Before scrubbing, the surgeon adjusts the microscope. The scrub person drapes the microscope with a sterile cover. The patient may be draped with three or four towels placed around the ear followed by a sterile, plastic adhesive drape (optional). The head is draped with a disposable sheet placing the adhesive strip at the forehead. Two folded towels (V shape) are draped at the patient's neck. The patient's body is covered with a split (or drape) sheet.

If disposable drapes are unavailable, the patient is draped with a head drape (drape sheet and two towels under the head with the uppermost towel wrapped around the head and clipped). Three or four towels are draped around the ear followed by a sterile, plastic adhesive drape (optional). Two folded towels are draped at the patient's neck and the patient's body is covered with a drape sheet.

Equipment

Headrest (e.g., Shea)
Restraints, padded
Microscope
Suction
Power source for power drill
Electrosurgical unit, optional

Instrumentation

Limited procedure tray
Basic ear procedures tray
Drill, (e.g. micro Stryker), burrs, and cord
Suction-electrocoagulator and cord (optional)

Supplies

Basin set
Sterile, plastic adhesive drape, optional

Blades (2) No. 15
Needle magnet or counter
Suction tubing (latex preferred because of flexibility)
Gelfoam (cut 1 mm × 1 mm)
Local anesthetic (e.g. lidocaine (Xylocaine) with epinephrine)
Control syringes (2) 5 ml
Needles, e.g., 27 gauge (1½"), 25 gauge (1½")
Bulb syringe
Eye patch (available)

Special notes

The table may be turned to facilitate access.

Check with the surgeon regarding the necessity for shaving any hair around the ear.

Check with the surgeon regarding the choice of preparation solution.

Do not allow preparation solution to pool in or around eyes and ears.

Some surgeons use continuous irrigation. Equipment needed includes irrigation solution (e.g., Physiosol), suction tubing, small Y-connector, irrigation set, and straight polyethylene tubing.

TYMPANOPLASTY

Definition

Refers to a variety of reconstructive procedures of the tympanic membrane and middle ear structures.

Discussion

Tympanoplasty restores or improves hearing in patients with a conductive-type hearing loss. This procedure may be performed for chronic otitis media, adhesive otitis, tympanosclerosis, and in conjunction with mastoidectomy (see p. 386), as necessitated by the disease process. Often a flap of atrophic epithelium has retracted into the middle ear; this must be excised along with any infected or questionably infected tissue.

Tympanoplasty is classified according to the condition of the ossicles.

Types:
I   Malleus, incus, and stapes intact and mobile.
II   Malleus is eroded.
III Malleus and incus are absent; stapes intact and mobile.
IV   All ossicles absent, except a mobile stapes footplate.
V   All ossicles absent, except an immobile stapes footplate.

Procedure

An endaural approach is employed. The tympanic membrane, if not widely perforated, is incised and reflected. The pathology within is assessed; mastoidectomy (see p. 386) may be required. Diseased tissues including atrophic epithelium, fibrotic tissue, and damaged ossicles, or any portions thereof are excised. The ossicular chain is reconstructed using artificial materials, homograft, ossicular bone, or fragments of the ossicles. Myringoplasty is performed using temporalis fascia, perichondrium, vein, or periosteum. The edges of the perforation are separated and the graft is placed on the inner surface of the drum remnant. The middle ear is filled with gelatin sponge fragments combined with blood, which support and nourish the graft. Skin flaps, if employed, may be sutured. A protective dressing is applied.

Preparation of the patient, Skin preparation, and Draping

See Mastoidectomy, p. 386.

Equipment

Microscope

Suction
Power source for power drill

Instrumentation

Basic ear procedures tray
Drill (e.g., micro Stryker), burrs, and cord

Supplies

Basin set
Blades (3) No. 15
Needle magnet or counter
Suction tubing (latex preferred because of flexibility)
Gelfoam (cut 1 mm × 1 mm)
Control syringes (2) 5 ml
Local anesthetic with epinephrine
Needles 27 gauge (1½"), 25 gauge (1½")
Sterile, plastic adhesive drape, optional
Bulb syringe
Tongue blade (to smooth graft)

Special notes

The table may be turned to facilitate access.

Do not allow preparation solutions to pool in or around eyes and ears.

New blades are used on a graft.

The graft may be smoothed over a flat surface such as an overturned basin.

STAPEDECTOMY

Definition

Removal of the stapes and the establishment of a linkage between the incus and the oval window by placement of a prosthesis.

Discussion

Stapedectomy reestablishes the chain of sound transmission in otosclerosis. Part or all of the stapes footplate may be removed. The oval window can be covered with vein, mucous membrane, connective tissue, collagen, or Gelfoam. Sound transmission may be reestablished with a large variety of materials including the crus of the stapes, Teflon, stainless steel wire, platinum prosthesis, fat, and carved autogenous bone prosthesis.

Procedure

An incision is made in the posterior and superior auditory canal wall above the anulus, creating a skin flap. Bone is excised, to visualize the oval window, using burrs or curettes. The tympanic membrane is reflected. Care is taken to avoid injury to the chorda tympani nerve. The extent of the pathologic process is assessed to determine the extent of the stapes excision. The type of prosthesis to be used is based on the dimensions and the degree of sclerosis. The crus of the stapes and the footplate are transsected and removed (completely or partially). The stapedius tendon is sectioned. The remaining footplate is distracted and the oval window is sealed by connective tissue and the stapes replaced. In total stapedectomy, after the stapes is separated from the incus and removed, a wire (or other prosthesis) is attached to the incus and placed on the oval window graft. A dry field is aided by the use of epinephrine-soaked Gelfoam pledgets. The skin flap is replaced. Gelfoam is placed over the flap and cotton is placed in the canal. Antibiotic irrigation and/or systemic antibiotics may be used.

Preparation of the patient, Skin preparation, Draping, and Equipment

See Mastoidectomy, p. 386.

Instrumentation

Basic ear procedures tray
Power drill (e.g., micro Stryker), burrs, and cord
Suction-electrocoagulator and cord

Supplies

Basin set
Blade (1) No. 15
Suction tubing (latex preferred for flexibility)
Gelfoam (cut 1 mm × 1 mm)
Local anesthetic with epinephrine
Control syringe (e.g., 5 ml), and needle (e.g., 25- or
    27-gauge [1½"])
Bulb syringe
Syringe (to flush suction)
Prostheses (variety available)
Antibiotic irrigation (optional)

Special notes

Do not allow preparation solution to pool in or
around eyes and ears.

Gelfoam may be moistened with epinephrine,
e.g., 1:1000.

The prosthesis packaging is not opened until the
surgeon determines the type and size.

If a graft is needed, check with the surgeon regarding the donor site.

SUBMUCOUS RESECTION OF THE NASAL SEPTUM (SMR)

Definition

Excision of a portion of the cartilaginous or osseous
nasal septum beneath flaps of mucous membrane,
perichondrium, and/or periosteum.

Discussion

The procedure is performed to provide a clear airway by establishing an adequate partition between
the left and right nasal cavity. The procedure may
be combined with rhinoplasty (see p. 353). Numerous anatomic configurations of the intranasal structure may be responsibile for the obstructive airway.

Procedure

An incision is made anteriorly over the septum to include the mucous membrane and perichondrium, which is then reflected with elevators beyond the septal area to be resected. The septal cartilage is excised carefully, avoiding penetration of the opposite mucoperichondrium. The mucoperichondrium of the opposite side is elevated (not contiguous with the first side) to avoid later communication that may result in fistula. Retracting the flaps, the cartilage is excised. Excessive cartilage should not be removed to prevent postoperative deformity. Occasionally, a cartilage graft may be placed within the flaps. A punch, rongeur, or cutting forceps is used to excise bony fragments of the ethmoid and deviated vomer. A gouge and mallet may be used for the vomer. The intranasal incisions are sutured. A petrolatum gauze packing is inserted to join the membranes in the midline and to aid in hemostasis. An external splint may be applied. A dressing is placed under the nose.

Preparation of the patient, Preliminary nasal preparation, Skin preparation, Draping, Equipment, Instrumentation, Supplies, and Special notes

See Rhinoplasty, p. 353.

INTRANASAL ANTROSTOMY/INTRANASAL FENESTRATION OF THE NASOANTRAL WALL

Definition

An opening made into the maxillary sinus through the nasoantral wall beneath the inferior turbinate.

Discussion

The indication for this procedure is chronic purulent maxillary sinusitis.

Procedure

A mucosal incision is made over the inferior turbinate, which is then elevated superiorly with a periosteal elevator. The nasoantral wall and the inferior turbinate are fenestrated and the opening is enlarged with a rongeur. The inferior meatus of the nasal wall is removed down to the level of the floor of the nasal cavity. Polyps and diseased mucosa are excised, if present. The sinus may be irrigated with saline and suctioned. The sinus cavity is inspected by direct vision. If the disease process appears irreversible a Caldwell-Luc procedure (see p. 397) is performed. Intranasal packing is indicated only for hemostasis as necessary. A dressing is placed under the nose.

Preparation of the patient

The patient is supine; the arm on the affected side may be tucked in at the patient's side and the other arm may be extended on an armboard. Arms may be restrained by padded restraints. The procedure is usually performed under local anesthesia. The surgeon does a preliminary nasal preparation even if general anesthesia is administered. For circulator responsibilities regarding local anesthesia, see p. 31.

Preliminary nasal preparation (on a "clean" Mayo stand)

Bayonet forceps
Nasal speculum
Scissors
Atomizer
Packing of choice
Cups (2) medium
Cotton-tipped applicators
Local anesthetic (e.g., lidocaine (Xylocaine) 1% with epinephrine)
Topical anesthetic (e.g., cocaine 4% or 5%)

Skin preparation

Check with the surgeon regarding the choice of preparation solution. Begin preparing the nose extending from the hairline to the shoulders, and down to the table at the sides of the neck. The surgeon may prepare the inside of the nose and mouth.

Draping

The patient is draped with a head drape (a drape sheet and two towels under the head; the uppermost towel may be wrapped around the head, over the eyelids, and clipped). The patient's body is covered with a split (or drape) sheet.

Equipment

Restraints, padded
Fiberoptic headlight and source
Suction
Electrosurgical unit (bipolar)

Instrumentation

Nasal procedures tray
Limited procedure tray
Metal tongue depressor
Polyp forceps
Nasal snare with wires

Supplies

Basin set
Blades (2) No. 15
Needle magnet or counter
Bulb syringe
Bayonet bipolar electrocoagulating forceps
Nasal packing, e.g., ½" or iodoform gauze or petrolatum-impregnated gauze (for bleeding)

Special notes

The table may be turned to facilitate access.

Do not allow preparation solution to pool in and around the eyes.

Eyes may be protected with eye patches prior to draping.

CALDWELL-LUC PROCEDURE
(RADICAL DRAINAGE OF THE ANTRUM OF THE MAXILLARY SINUSES)

Definition

Creation of an opening into the antrum of the maxillary sinus through the canine fossa.

Discussion

This procedure permits evacuation of diseased sinus and scar tissue under direct vision when intranasal antrostomy alone is inadequate to accomplish satisfactory drainage.

Procedure

An incision is made above the canine and second molar teeth. The periosteum is elevated. The infraorbital nerve is identified and protected. The anterior wall of the sinus is fenestrated with a burr or osteotome and the opening is enlarged with a rongeur. The pathologic process is assessed. Diseased mucosa, cysts, polyps, etc. are excised. The nasoantral wall in the inferior meatus is perforated, e.g., with a trocar. The opening is enlarged under direct vision from the antral incision. The gingival incision is closed with absorbable suture. Intranasal packing is used only for hemostasis as necessary. An ice pack is applied to the cheek.

Preparation of the patient

The patient is supine; the arm on the affected side may be tucked in at the patient's side and the other arm may be extended on an armboard. Arms may be restrained by padded restraints. The procedure may be performed under local or general anesthesia. The surgeon usually does a preliminary nasal preparation.

Preliminary nasal preparation, Skin preparation, Draping, Equipment, Instrumentation, Supplies, and Special notes

See Intranasal Antrostomy, p. 394.

Additional special notes

Have ice pack ready at the conclusion of the procedure.

NASAL POLYPECTOMY

Definition

Excision of an edematous hypertrophy of the nasal mucosa resulting from a chronic edematous inflammatory process.

Discussion

Nasal polyps, usually located in the middle meatus, may occur singly or in numbers, and may be pedunculated or sessile. The antrochoanal polyp arises from the mucosa of the maxillary sinus near the posterior sinus wall; these polyps may grow large enough to obstruct the entire nasopharynx. The antrochoanal polyp may recur unless a Caldwell-Luc procedure (see p. 397) is performed.

Procedure

Each polyp is individually encircled with the wire of a nasal polyp snare, grasped with forceps, and amputated. The nasal cavity is packed with a petrolatum-impregnated gauze. The choanal polyp is removed under general anesthesia. The snare wire is passed into the nasal cavity and into the nasopharynx. The wire is looped around the polyp. The polyp is grasped by forceps introduced through the oropharynx and amputated with the snare.

Preparation of the patient, Preliminary nasal preparation, Skin preparation, Draping, and Equipment

See Rhinoplasty, p. 353.

Instrumentation

Nasal prodedures tray
Limited procedure tray
Metal tongue depressor
Polyp forceps
Nasal snare, with wires

Supplies

Basin set
Blade (1) No. 15
Cotton-tipped applicators (long)
Nasal packing (e.g., petrolatum-impregnated gauze)

Special notes

Check with the surgeon regarding the choice of preparation solution. Do not allow preparation solution to pool in or around the eyes.

The table may be turned to facilitate access.

The table may be slightly flexed for the patient's comfort.

DRAINAGE OF THE FRONTAL SINUS

Definition

Permits drainage of the infected frontal sinus by incision through its bony envelope by any of several approaches.

Discussion

This procedure is indicated for chronic infection not responsive to antibiotics and antihistamines, and for spreading acute infection. Drainage is directed externally with obliteration of the sinus cavity, or intranasally.

Procedure

An incision is made along the inferior margin of the eyebrow to the anterolateral aspect of the nasal bone. The periosteum is reflected. The lacrimal crest is identified. Ethmoidal vessels are controlled and the ethmoid sinus entered; the frontal sinus is then likewise entered after bone is rongeured, removing the floor of the sinus. Diseased mucous membrane is excised using curettes, periosteal elevators, and pituitary forceps. Care is taken to remove all involved membrane to avoid later mucocele formation and recurrent infection. Additional ethmoidal cells may be removed. A nasofrontal passage is made by removing a portion of the middle turbinate. Drains are placed to maintain the passage. The external wound is closed and dressed.

Preparation of the patient

The procedure is usually performed under general anesthesia. The patient is supine; the arm on the affected side may be tucked in at the patient's side and the other arm may be extended on an armboard. The surgeon usually does a preliminary nasal preparation. Apply electrosurgical dispersive pad.

Preliminary nasal preparation (on a "clean" Mayo stand)

Bayonet forceps
Nasal speculum
Packing of choice
Scissors
Atomizer
Cups (2) medium
Cotton-tipped applicators
Local anesthetic (e.g., lidocaine (Xylocaine) 1% with epinephrine)
Topical anesthetic (e.g., cocaine 4% or 5%)

Skin preparation

Check with the surgeon regarding the choice of preparation solution. The patient's face is cleansed beginning at the eyebrow on the affected side extending from the hairline to the shoulders, and down to the table at the sides of the neck.

Draping

See Intranasal Antrostomy, p. 394.

Equipment

Suction
Fiberoptic headlight and light source
Electrosurgical unit
Power source for saw

Instrumentation

Limited procedure tray
Nasal procedures tray
Weitlaner self-retaining retractor
Power saw (e.g., Stryker), with oscillating blade and cord

Supplies

Basin set
Suction tubing
Blades (2) No. 15
Needle magnet or counter
Bulb syringe
Drain (e.g., small Penrose)
Electrosurgical pencil
Nasal packing

Special notes

The table may be turned to facilitate access.
Do not allow preparation solution to pool in or around the eyes.
The table may be slightly flexed for the patient's comfort.
Cultures may be taken.

TONSILLECTOMY AND ADENOIDECTOMY (T & A)

Definition

Tonsillectomy is the excision of the faucial (palatine) tonsils. Adenoidectomy is the excision of the naso-pharyngeal tonsils (adenoids).

Discussion

The faucial tonsils and the nasopharyngeal tonsils are aggregates of lymphoid tissue in the posterior nasopharynx that hypertrophy secondary to infection. In children tonsillectomy is relatively simple, whereas in adults, because of long-standing fibrosis, the procedure is more difficult. The adenoids are usually atrophied by age 15.

Procedure

The mouth is retracted open with a self-retaining mouth gag. The tongue is depressed with a tongue blade. Adenoids are removed with an adenotome and/or a curette. A tonsil is grasped and the mucosa is dissected free preserving the posterior tonsil pillar. The capsule of the tonsil is separated from its bed. A forceps is passed through the loop of the snare and the tonsil is seized. The snare loop is passed over the free portion of the tonsil and the tonsil is amputated. The fossa may be packed with a tonsil sponge. Bleeding may be controlled with cautery, ties (slip knot), and/or suture. The procedure is repeated on the opposite tonsil.

Preparation of the patient

The patient is supine; arms may be extended on armboards or tucked in at the patient's side and restrained with padded restraints. A rolled towel may be placed under the shoulders to extend the neck. General anesthesia is given to all children and some adults. Apply electrosurgical dispersive pad if the suction-electrocoagulator is used.

Skin preparation

None usually required.

Draping

A sheet may be draped over the patient's body.

Equipment

Restraints, padded
Fiberoptic headlight and light source
Footrest, padded (local, adult)
Suction
Electrosurgical unit (monopolar or bipolar)

Instrumentation

Tonsillectomy and adenoidectomy tray
Suction-electrocoagulator and cord (optional)
Bayonet electrocoagulating forceps and cord (optional)

Supplies

Basin set
Suction tubing
Blade (1) No. 12
Tonsil sponges
Anesthetic with epinephrine (for local procedure);
    syringes (2) Luer-lock control, needles (2) 25-
    gauge spinal

Special notes

Have alternate suction available.

The table may be turned.

Have ties mounted on a tonsil clamp ready in advance.

Keep tonsils separate and identify specimens as right and left.

Do not dismantle suction or remove instruments until the patient leaves the room so that they are available in case of sudden bleeding.

LARYNGOSCOPY

Definition

Endoscopic examination of the larynx.

Discussion

Laryngoscopy is perfomed for diagnosis, biopsy, and/or treatment of laryngeal lesions, for aspiration of secretions, to assess laryngeal trauma, or to remove a foreign body. Use of a microscope facilitates visualization. In suspension laryngoscopy, a self-retaining laryngoscope holder gives the surgeon bimanual freedom. A carbon dioxide laser (see laser precautions in Appendix, p. 572) may be used in conjunction with microlaryngoscopy to remove benign lesions and early malignant tumors of the larynx. With the carbon dioxide laser, excision is facilitated, hemostasis is readily achieved, and there is rapid wound healing with a minimum of postoperative pain and swelling. Lesions removed by laser energy are vaporized by intense heat leaving a small crater. One disadvantage of using the laser is that tissue can be biopsied, but vaporized tissues are unavailable for histologic examination.

Procedure

The patient's head is tipped back and the laryngoscope is inserted. The oropharynx and the larynx are inspected; the scope is lifted as necessary. Care is taken not to use the teeth as a fulcrum; a bite block may be used. A self-retaining laryngoscope holder may be employed. The microscope may be used. Lesions may be biopsied, secretions may be aspirated, etc. For carbon dioxide laser microlaryngoscopy, a micromanipulator, used to direct the laser beam, is coupled to a standard microscope. Stainless steel mirrors reflect the beam to inaccessible areas. A special vocal cord retractor with suction attachments is used to clear smoke from tissue evaporation. Two suctions are employed when performing cancer surgery for rapid clearing of the plume.

Preparation of the patient

Anesthesia may be general or topical. *General anesthesia:* The patient is supine; arms may be tucked in at the patient's sides. Following intubation with a small endotracheal tube, the table is turned so that the surgeon is at the head of the table. General anesthesia is required for microlaryngoscopy.

Topical anesthesia: The patient is usually sitting up while the anesthetic is administered; the patient is supine for the procedure. To facilitate passage of the laryngoscope the patient's head is tilted backward; the neck may be supported with a roll or small sandbag.

Topical anesthesia preparation (on a "clean" Mayo stand)

Laryngeal spatulas
Laryngeal mirror
Small basin with very warm water (for mirror)
Topical anesthetic spray (e.g., Cetacaine)
Gauze sponges
Laryngeal syringe with straight and curved cannulas
Cup, medium (medication)
Topical anesthetic (e.g., cocaine 4% or 5%)
Cotton-tipped applicators
Cotton
Tissues

Skin preparation

None required.

Draping

The patient may be covered with a drape sheet. The back table is covered with a drape sheet. Folded towels are used to stabilize the laryngoscope holder. Gloves are worn.

Equipment

Small roll or sandbag
Fiberoptic headlight and light source
Fiberoptic light source (for laryngoscope)
Suction
Footstool
Microscope and 400-mm lens (microlaryngoscopy)
Carbon dioxide laser (optional); see Appendix, p. 572 for laser precautions.

Instrumentation and Supplies

Bite block
Laryngoscope and cord (e.g., Jackson)

Laryngoscope holder (e.g., Lewy)
Suction tubing
Aspirating tubes (2), e.g., Lukens
Biopsy forceps (assorted)
Suction tip
Sponge carriers (2), loaded with sponges
Telfa and needle, 25 gauge (for specimen removal)
Small basin with saline
Toluidine blue (stain to detect carcinoma)

Add for Microlaryngoscopy

Double barrel scope (e.g., Dedo, Jako) and cord (use with laryngoscope holder)

Microlaryngeal forceps (assorted), scissors, knife, hook, aspiration tube, vocal cord retractor (with suction attachments)

Special notes

Protective eye goggles should be worn.

Have sitting stool available for surgeon.

Very small amount of toluidine blue is needed (approximately 1 ml).

The scrub person works directly from the back table without the Mayo stand.

Pass biopsy forceps with tip closed.

Guide suction tip, forceps, etc. into the scope as necessary.

The biopsy specimen may be removed from forceps with a needle and placed on Telfa; do not crush the specimen.

TRACHEOSTOMY

Definition

An opening made into the trachea with the insertion of a cannula to facilitate breathing.

Discussion

The procedure may be done as an emergency, or electively, in order to maintain an airway. Several techniques are used; numerous cannulas are available including those adapted for anesthesia and/or the respirator.

Procedure

A transverse (or longitudinal) incision is made overlying the proximal trachea. The platysma and deep fascia are incised; the thyroid isthmus is retracted superiorly and the superior tracheal rings are exposed. An anterior disc of the third and fourth tracheal rings is excised (or incised). Stay sutures may be used to mark the stoma, and for retraction, in case of the need to replace the cannula. Several sutures approximate the skin. The tracheostomy tube is held in place with umbilical tapes tied into a square knot behind the neck. A gauze dressing split around the tube is applied to the wound.

Preparation of the patient

The patient is supine with a folded sheet behind the shoulders to extend the neck; arms may be tucked in at the patient's side. The procedure may be performed under local or general anesthesia.

Skin preparation

Begin cleansing the entire neck extending from the infra-auricular border to the axillae, and down to the table at the neck and shoulders.

Draping

Folded towels and a sheet with a small fenestration

Equipment

Suction
Electrosurgical unit

Instrumentation

Tracheostomy tray

Supplies

Basin set
Suction tubing
Blades (1) No. 10, (2) No. 15, and (1) No. 11
Tracheostomy tubes, silicone or Portex (preferred), adults size No. 6 to No. 8
Catheters (2) for suctioning tracheostomy tube (e.g., Robinson 14Fr or 16Fr)
Electrosurgical pencil
Umbilical tapes
10-ml syringe (to inflate cuff)
Local anesthetic, syringe (Luer-lock control), and needles, 25- or 27-gauge
Marking pen, optional

Special notes

If the procedure is performed under general anesthesia, an endotracheal tube is inserted. As the tracheostomy tube is placed, the endotracheal tube is withdrawn.

A gauze dressing split around the tube is the customary dressing.

The obturator for the tracheostomy tube must accompany the patient out of the room. It will be needed to reinsert the tube if it becomes dislodged. Tape the obturator to the top of the gurney.

Be certain that a cardiac arrest cart is nearby.

The scrub person needs to test the tube cuff for leakage.

EXCISION OF THE SUBMAXILLARY (SUBMANDIBULAR) GLAND

Definition

Excision of the submaxillary salivary gland.

Discussion

The procedure is performed most often for benign disease such as chronic inflammation (sialadenitis), stone (sialolithiasis), or ductal stricture. Tumor, including malignancy, is less often encountered.

Procedure

A transverse incision is made over the gland below the lower edge of and parallel to the mandible. Structures to be protected during dissection are the mandibular branch of the facial nerve, the lingual nerve, and the hypoglossal nerve. The anterior facial vein is divided and the fascial envelope around the gland incised. The gland is dissected free of surrounding tissues. The facial artery is ligated. Wharton's duct is identified adjacent to the lingual nerve, ligated, and divided. The wound is closed in layers. A closed suction drain is employed.

Preparation of the patient

The patient is supine with the head turned and the affected side up. A folded sheet may be placed under the shoulders to facilitate access. The procedure is usually performed under general anesthesia. Apply electrosurgical dispersive pad.

Skin preparation

Begin under the chin extending from the infraauricular border to the axilla. Prepare beyond the midline and down to the table at the neck and shoulder.

Draping

Four folded towels and a sheet with a small fenestration

Instrumentation

Basic plastic procedures tray
Extra mosquito clamps
Lacrimal duct probes available (exploration of sub-
   maxillary duct)

Supplies

Basin set
Suction tubing
Blades (2) No. 15
Needle magnet or counter
Electrosurgical pencil
Dissectors (e.g., peanut)
Drainage unit (e.g., Hemovac)
Bulb syringe
Nerve stimulator (locator), optional

Special notes

The table may be turned to facilitate access.

Do not allow preparation solution to pool in or
around the eyes and ears.

A sterile magnetic instrument pad may be
helpful.

PAROTIDECTOMY

Definition

Excision of all or a portion of the largest salivary
gland.

Discussion

The procedure is performed for inflammatory disease and benign and malignant tumors. Most significant in parotid gland surgery is the course of the
facial nerve through the gland dividing the larger
superficial portion from the deeper portion. In ma-

lignancy, if suspicious lymph nodes are encountered, a radical neck dissection (see p. 416) may be done.

Procedure

An incision is made in the preauricular region, continued inferiorly around the earlobe, and then anteriorly toward the hyoid bone. The fascia is incised. Careful exposure of the facial nerve is necessary; a nerve stimulator can be used to help in its identification. The superficial portion of the gland may be resected after blunt and sharp dissection; removal of the deeper portion may be necessary for malignancy. If a major nerve branch courses through the tumor, it must be sacrificed and a nerve graft substituted. The graft may be obtained from the great auricular nerve or superficial branches of the cervical plexus. Stenson's duct is ligated and divided. The wound is closed, often employing a drain.

Preparation of the patient

The patient is supine with the operative side of the face uppermost. A headrest may be used. The arms may be tucked in at the patient's sides. Apply electrosurgical dispersive pad.

Skin preparation

Check with the surgeon regarding choice of preparation solution. Begin with the affected cheek; cleanse the entire side of the face well beyond the midline including the ear extending from the hairline to the axilla. Some surgeons request the ear canal be dried and a cotton ball placed in the ear.

Draping

Folded towels, sterile, plastic adhesive drape (optional), and a sheet with a small fenestration

Equipment

Suction
Electrosurgical unit
Fiberoptic headlight and light source
Headrest (e.g., Richards), optional

Instrumentation

Basic/Minor procedures tray
Thyroid tray
Extra right-angle clamps
Nerve hooks

Supplies

Basin set
Blades (1) No. 10, (3) No. 15
Suction tubing
Electrosurgical pencil (needle tip available)
Dissectors (e.g., peanut)
Bulb syringe
Marking pen
Drain (e.g., ¼" Penrose, Hemovac)
Sterile, plastic adhesive drape, optional
Nerve stimulator (locator)

Special notes

The table may be turned to facilitate access.

Do not allow preparation solution to pool in or around the eyes and ears.

A sterile magnetic instrument pad may be helpful.

LARYNGECTOMY

Definition

Complete or partial removal of the larynx.

Discussion

Laryngectomy is primarily performed for malignancy. Cancers of the larynx are classified according to anatomic position.

Supraglottic: From the epiglottis to and including the false cords.

Glottic: Floor of the ventricle to below the glottis including the true cords.

Infraglottic: From below the true vocal cords to the cricoid cartilage.

Transglottic: Lesions that extend from above the ventricle to true and false cords and subglottically.

Associated with these cancers are those of the hypopharynx and pyriform sinus. Numerous presentations may occur from small unilateral lesions to extensive ones, invading widely, with cervical lymph node metastasis. Treatment modalities include radiation, surgery, laser surgery, and palliative measures and chemotherapy in advanced lesions. Hemilaryngectomy, partial or total laryngectomy, local lesion excision, laser treatment, or adjunctive radical neck dissection will be determined by the clinical extent of the malignancy and the patient's general status.

Procedure

For more extensive lesions involving both cords, transglottic lesions, or when laryngeal cartilage is involved, total laryngectomy is done. A curvilinear incision is made above the suprasternal notch. The strap muscles are divided, as is the isthmus of the thyroid gland. The trachea may be divided between rings two and three, and the endotracheal tube replaced in the distal trachea, with the infraglottic area packed to prevent secretions from filling the wound or entering the airway. Skin flaps are elevated. The larynx is sutured closed inferiorly. The superior cornua of the thyroid cartilage and hyoid bone are freed from strap and supraglottic muscles (which may also be excised). A portion of the thyroid may be excised. The constrictor muscles are divided posterolaterally. The posterior aspect of the cricoid cartilage is entered. Dissection continues to the base of the tongue. With traction on the epiglottis and the severed end of the trachea, dissection is completed. The pharynx is closed. The tracheostomy stoma is matured to the surrounding skin and a tracheostomy tube is placed. The wound flaps are approximated over a closed-suction catheter. A moderate pressure dressing is placed.

Preparation of the patient

The patient is supine; arms may be tucked in at the patient's sides. A folded sheet may be placed under the shoulders to facilitate exposure. Apply electrosurgical dispersive pad.

Skin preparation

Begin at the neck extending from the inferior auricular border to the axilla, and to the table at the sides.

Draping

Folded towels, sterile, plastic adhesive drape (optinal), and a sheet with a small fenestration

Equipment

Suction
Electrosurgical unit

Instrumentation

Basic/Minor procedures tray
Thyroid tray
Tracheostomy tray (available)
Right-angle clamps (finely pointed)
Small Yankauer suction

Supplies

Basin set
Blades (2) No. 10, (3) No. 15
Needle magnet or counter
Dissectors (e.g., peanut)
Marking pen
Suction tubing
Sterile, plastic adhesive drape, optional
Umbilical tape
Electrosurgical pencil (with needle tip)
Catheters (2) flexible, open ended for suctioning tra-
    cheostomy tube
Tracheostomy tubes (assorted types and sizes)

Special notes

Have alternate suction available.
A sterile magnetic instrument pad may be
helpful.
A cuffed tracheostomy tube is inserted in the tracheal stoma until the edema subsides (about 48
hours). It is then replaced with a laryngectomy tube.

RADICAL NECK DISSECTION

Definition

Excision of cervical lymph node bearing tissue and
adjacent muscular and vascular structures.

Discussion

The procedure is done for malignancy of the head
and neck region. It may be performed as an independent procedure or in conjunction with primary
tumor resection of local structures whose lymphatics
drain to the cervical lymph nodes, for example, thyroid, larynx, and jaw. When combined with more
extensive resections about the pharynx and larynx,

a tracheostomy (see p. 407) is performed as well. Radiation therapy may be performed in conjunction with this procedure.

Procedure

An incision (Y, double Y, T, parallel-transverse, Z) is made in the lateral neck usually from beneath the jaw to the supraclavicular region. Skin flaps are mobilized. The external jugular vein is severed, the deep cervical fascia is incised (including some cutaneous nerve branches), and the sternoclavicular origins of the sternomastoid muscle are divided. The internal jugular vein is isolated and divided. The omohyoid muscle is transsected. Fatty tissues bearing lymph nodes are dissected from underlying structures in continuity with other transsected structures. The insertion of the sternomastoid muscle is divided, as is the lower pole of the parotid gland avoiding injury to branches of the facial nerve. The facial artery and vein are divided, and the submaxillary gland and proximal end of the internal jugular vein are divided after dissecting additional fatty tissues from under the jaw. The tissue bloc is then excised. The accessory nerve may be preserved, and on the left the thoracic duct is protected. The flaps are closed over suction drains. A moderate pressure dressing is applied.

Preparation of the patient

The patient is supine; the arm on the operative side may be tucked in at the patient's side and the other arm may be extended on an armboard. Following intubation, the patient's head is turned with the face and neck on the operative side facing uppermost. Pad the lowermost ear to prevent pressure injury. A folded sheet may be placed under the shoulder to facilitate access. A Foley catheter may be inserted in the patient's bladder. Apply electrosurgical dispersive pad.

Skin preparation

Check with the surgeon regarding choice of preparation solution. Begin by cleansing the neck and face extending from the hairline to the nipples, and down to the table at the sides.

Draping

The patient may be draped with a head drape (drape sheet and two towels under the head with the uppermost towel wrapped around the head and clipped). The neck is draped with folded towels secured with a sterile, plastic adhesive drape or sutured or stapled to the skin. The field is covered with a fenestrated sheet.

Equipment

Suction
Electrosurgical unit
Scales (to weigh sponges)

Instrumentation

Basic/Minor procedures tray
Thyroid tray
Tracheostomy tray (available)
Extra mosquito clamps (24)
Extra towel clips (8)
Right-angle clamps (finely pointed)
Andrews suction

Supplies

Foley catheter and urimeter
Basin set
Marking pen
Suction tubing
Electrosurgical pencil
Blades (2) No. 10, (3) No. 15
Needle magnet or counter

Graduate
Bulb syringes (2)
Dissectors (e.g., peanut)
Umbilical tapes, vessel loops
Nerve stimulator (locator)
Suction drainage unit (e.g., Hemovac)

Special notes

A sterile magnetic instrument pad may be helpful.

Check with blood bank that blood is ready and available as ordered.

Weigh sponges.

Measure irrigation fluids accurately.

EXCISION OF LESIONS OF THE ORAL CAVITY (PARTIAL GLOSSECTOMY WITH MARGINAL RESECTION OF THE MANDIBLE)

Definition

Excision of a portion of the mandible and lymphoid-bearing tissues of the ipsilateral neck.

Discussion

Lymph channels drain the tongue and floor of the mouth into the cervical glands. Tumor cells may extend directly into the periosteum and cortex of the mandible. When the lesions of the oral cavity (i.e., tongue and floor of the mouth) are excised lymphoid-bearing tissues as well as a portion of the mandible must also be excised. If inadequate tissue remains for closure, a flap may be transposed (e.g., from the forehead or deltopectoral area) which allows some degree of mobility for the remaining tongue and cheek. The mandible may be transsected for exposure, and later repaired with stainless steel wire. Radiation therapy may be combined with surgical treatment.

Procedure

A tracheostomy (see p. 407) is performed under local anesthesia. Following induction of general anesthesia a radical neck dissection is done (see p. 416). The lower lip is transsected in the midline. The submental region is dissected excising adipose tissue and lymph nodes. The outer cortex of the mandible is exposed and transsected with a Gigli saw. The tongue is split in the midline to the posterior third and a cheek flap is mobilized behind the last molar. The inner cortex of the mandible including the alveolar ridge is transsected from the outer cortex with a power saw, preserving the latter. The outer cortex is retracted, and the intrinsic muscles of the tongue and the muscles attached to the hyoid bone are further transsected in continuity with the remainder of the specimen. The anterior and posterior bellies of the digastric muscle, submaxillary gland, and hypoglossal and lingual nerves are included in the specimen. Reconstruction is begun by stabilizing the remaining mandible with a short Kirschner wire centrally and stainless steel wires passed through drill holes and tightened. Soft tissues are approximated from the tongue to tissue above the hyoid bone and platysma, tying those sutures over the mandible. Additional coverage may be obtained from mobilization of the forehead or a deltopectoral flap. The tongue is again sutured to the platysma. The remaining exposed mandible is covered by tissues of the floor of the mouth and skin. Mucosal sutures complete the repair of the floor of the mouth. The lip is repaired in layers, snugly, to prevent excessive drooling. The neck incisions are closed over suction drains.

Preparation of the patient

The patient is supine; arms may be tucked in at the patient's sides. A folded sheet may be placed under the patient's shoulders to facilitate exposure. Apply electrosurgical dispersive pad.

Skin preparation

Check with the surgeon regarding choice of preparation solution and the area to be prepared, particularly regarding the mouth. The entire face and neck may be prepared extending from the hairline to nipples, and down to the table at the sides around the neck and shoulders. The inside of the mouth may be painted with swabs.

Draping

The patient may be draped with a head drape (drape sheet and two towels under the head with uppermost towel wrapped around the head and clipped). The neck is draped with folded towels secured with a sterile, plastic adhesive drape, staples, or sutures. The field is covered with a fenestrated sheet.

Equipment

Scales (to weigh sponges)
Suction
Electrosurgical unit
Fiberoptic headlight and light source
Power source for power saw

Instrumentation

Tracheostomy tray
Basic/Minor procedures tray
Thyroid tray
Tonsillectomy and adenoidectomy tray
Andrews suction
Right-angle clamps (4), finely pointed
Tonsil clamps (4)
Gigli saws, wire cutters, nerve hook
Power saw and cord (e.g., Stryker)

Supplies

Basin set
Marking pen

Suction tubing
Electrosurgical pencil
Blades (2) No. 10, (3) No. 15
Needle magnet or counter
Sterile, plastic adhesive drape
Graduate
Bulb syringes (2)
Umbilical tapes, vessel loops
Nerve stimulator (locator)
Dissectors (e.g., peanut)
Bone wax
Stainless steel wire
Local anesthetic, syringe (Luer-lock control), and
    needles 25- or 27-gauge
Tracheostomy tubes, silicone or Portex (preferred),
    adults sizes No. 6 to No. 8
Syringe, 10 ml (to inflate cuff)
Magnetic instrument pad, optional
Suction drainage unit (e.g., Hemovac)

Special notes

Check with blood bank that blood is available
as ordered.

Measure irrigation used for accurate assessment
of blood loss.

Weigh sponges.

Be certain a cardiac arrest cart is nearby.

Test tracheostomy cuff for leakage.

Tape the obturator to top of gurney when patient is transferred to the recovery room; it will be
needed to reinsert the tube if the tube becomes dislodged.

Chapter 19

OPHTHALMIC SURGERY

GENERAL INFORMATION

Ophthalmic surgery requires close attention to detail. A minor breach of technique could potentially lead to complete or partial loss of vision of the operated eye. Preparation and protection of the operative site and prevention of infection are of paramount importance.

In order to avoid undue repetition the following will apply to all procedures in this section unless otherwise stated.

Anesthesia

Anesthesia for ophthalmic surgery may require immobility (akinesia) of the globe and lids, anesthesia of the globe and adnexae, control of intraocular pressure, general relaxation of the patient, and prevention of retching, coughing, and blood pressure fluctuations, even after the procedure is completed. The choice of anesthetic depends on the nature of the procedure, the surgeon's (and patient's) preference, and the general status and level of anxiety of the patient.

Topical anesthesia is effected by the instillation

of the agent (e.g., tetracaine 0.5%) into the conjunctival sac. This method may suffice for superficial procedures (e.g., excision of a pterygium) or may precede administration of local anesthesia. Infiltration anesthesia is the direct injection of an agent into the surgical site (as in surgery of the lids). For more involved procedures regional block of cranial nerve branches can be employed. For procedures requiring immobilization of the globe, a retrobulbar block and an O'Brien and/or Van Lint block (or their modifications) are performed to provide akinesia of the lids and extraocular muscles. In retrobulbar block the anesthetic agent is injected into the muscle cone (behind the globe) blocking cranial nerves III, IV, and VI to immobilize the extraocular muscles and to produce anesthesia of the conjunctiva, cornea, and uvea by blocking the ciliary nerve branches. The O'Brien block deposits the anesthetic by the branches of the facial nerve (over the condyle of the mandible, inferior to the posterior zygomatic process) to paralyze the orbicularis oculi muscle. The Van Lint block similarly produces paralysis of the orbicularis muscle, anesthetizing facial nerve branches over the periosteum just lateral to the orbital rim. Combining these blocks ensures complete akinesia. General anesthesia or heavy sedation may be preferred and/or combined with conduction anesthesia.

Skin preparation

Unilateral: Prepare the affected eye extending from the hairline to the inferior border of the mandible (the preparation may extend only to the superior border at some hospitals), and at the sides from the anterior auricular border to well beyond the midline. Begin by cleansing the eyelid, eyelashes, eyebrow, and skin around the operative eye. Do not allow preparation solution to pool in the eye. Using applicator sticks, carefully cleanse the lid margins. Irrigate the eye from inner to outer canthus using a bulb syringe containing normal saline.

Bilateral: Prepare the eyes extending from the hairline to the inferior border of the mandible. Cleanse both eyes in the manner employed for a unilateral preparation, as just described.

Draping

In an attempt to eliminate lint on the field, most ophthalmic surgeons use disposable drapes. *Unilateral:* The adhesive-backed strip of a sheet is placed on the forehead. A split sheet is then draped so that the operative eye and the surrounding area fit into the split ("V") of the drape; the adhesive-backed tails of the split sheet are secured at the top of the head, and the remainder of the split sheet is draped over the patient's body. A sterile, plastic adhesive drape is placed over the operative eye and the surrounding field.

Bilateral: The adhesive-backed strip of a sheet is placed on the forehead. A split sheet is then draped so that the bridge of the nose fits into the split ("V") of the drape; the adhesive-backed tails of the split sheet are secured at the top of the head and the remainder of the split sheet is draped over the patient's body. A sterile, plastic adhesive drape is placed over both eyes and the surrounding field.

Special notes

Keep talking and movement in the room to a minimum. Remember the patient is often awake. Distractions can interfere with the surgeon's concentration and performance.

For procedures in which local anesthesia is used without the presence of an anesthetist, see circulator responsibilities, p. 31.

Local anesthesia (infiltration or block) may be administered prior to final skin preparation and draping.

Hyaluronidase (Wydase) may be added to the local anesthetic solution to enhance absorption and dispersion of the agent.

Eyelashes are not routinely clipped; if lashes are trimmed it is done prior to the skin preparation. Coat the lashes with a thin layer of petrolatum so that the severed lashes adhere to the scissors (rather than fall into the eye).

Eyes are *always* irrigated from inner to outer canthus.

Powder is meticulously removed from gloves to prevent corneal irritation.

The scrub person may be required to irrigate the eye frequently during the procedure.

Extreme care is taken to protect instruments, especially microsurgical instruments, from damage, particularly the tips and cutting surfaces.

Precautions are taken to keep lint off the instruments and the surgical field.

Ophthalmic drops are instilled into the conjunctival sac.

EXCISION OF A CHALAZION

Definition

Incision and curettage of a granulomatous swelling of the Meibomian gland(s).

Discussion

A chalazion can be a single swelling or multiple swellings, either noninfected or infected, which may sometimes subside spontaneously, but otherwise is excised through a conjunctival or skin approach.

Procedure

A *conjunctival approach* is employed when the chalazion is pointing through the conjunctiva. The chalazion is centered in a chalazion clamp and the lid is everted. The chalazion is incised at right angles to the lid margin and its contents are evacuated with a curette. The clamp is slowly removed when hemostasis has been effected.

For the *skin approach* the chalazion is centered in a chalazion clamp. An incision is made parallel to the lid. The orbicularis oculi muscle is cut exposing the Meibomian gland. The gland is incised and its contents thoroughly curetted. The wound is approximated. Antibiotic ophthalmic ointment may be instilled and an eye pad is applied.

Preparation of the patient

The patient is supine. One arm may be extended on an armboard; the other arm may be tucked in at the patient's side. The head may be supported by a headrest with the head turned (affected side up). The procedure is usually performed under local anesthesia. Topical anesthetic eyedrops may be instilled. See p. 31 for circulator responsibilities regarding local anesthesia.

Skin preparation and Draping

See Ophthalmic Surgery, General Information, p. 423.

Equipment

Headrest (e.g., horseshoe), optional
Sitting stools

Instrumentation

Basic eye procedures tray
Eyelid and conjunctival procedures tray

Supplies

Basin set
Sterile, plastic adhesive drape
Cotton-tipped applicators or cellulose sponges
Blade (1) No. 15 or (1) No. 11
Cautery (wet field or disposable)
Balanced Salt Solution (BSS), tear substitute
Topical anesthetic eyedrops, e.g., tetracaine (optional)

Local anesthetic (e.g., lidocaine (Xylocaine) 2% with
   epinephrine)
Dye (e.g., methylene blue), optional
Antibiotic ophthalmic ointment (optional)

CANTHOTOMY

Definition

Incision of the canthus.

Discussion

The procedure is indicated when there is an adhe-
sion of the eyelids or when exposure to the globe is
inadequate. Canthotomy may be performed prior to
cataract extraction or in conjunction with other procedures.

Procedure

A straight mosquito hemostat is clamped over
the outer canthus for at least 60 seconds to effect hemostasis. The skin and conjunctiva are incised. Antibiotic ophthalmic ointment may be instilled and an
eye patch applied.

Preparation of the patient, Skin preparation, and Draping

See Excision of a Chalazion, p. 426.

Instrumentation

Basic eye procedures tray

Equipment

Headrest (e.g., horseshoe), optional
Sitting stools

Supplies

Basin set
Sterile, plastic adhesive drape
Cotton-tipped applicators or cellulose sponges
Blade (1) No. 15
Cautery (wet field or disposable)
Balanced Salt Solution (BSS), tear substitute
Anesthetic drops (e.g., tetracaine), optional
Local anesthetic (e.g., lidocaine (Xylocaine) 2% with
    epinephrine)
Antibiotic ophthalmic ointment (optional)

CORRECTION OF ECTROPION

Definition

Correction of an eversion and drooping of the lower
eyelid.

Discussion

The method of correction employed depends on the
type and severity of the deformity. Ectropion usually
occurs bilaterally.

Types:

Involutional, most common type, caused by a
relaxation of the orbicular muscle, may occur as a
result of aging.

Congenital, associated with Down's syndrome, is
the result of an elongation of the lower lid.

Paralytic, in which the orbicularis oculi has lost
its tone caused by cranial nerve VII paralysis.

The Byron-Smith procedure, a modification of
the Kuhrt-Szymanowski procedure, is employed for
involutional ectropion.

Procedure

Byron-Smith Procedure

A skin incision is made below the lid margin extending from the punctum to just beyond the lateral

canthus. A second incision (an extension of the first) is made in the direction of the earlobe. A skin-muscle flap is developed and elevated across the lower lid. A vertical incision is made through the tarsus (in the lateral third of the eyelid) and angled into the inferior cul-de-sac. The two free edges of the lid are overlapped until tight, and the redundant portion excised. The two lid edges are approximated. The orbicularis oculi muscle is approximated. The skin is pulled laterally; redundant skin is resected. The skin is approximated. In younger patients, if the punctum is still everted, a tarsal-conjunctival resection may be necessary. Antibiotic ophthalmic ointment may be instilled and an eye pad placed.

Preparation of the patient

The patient is supine; the arm on the side of the operative eye may be tucked in at the patient's side, and the other arm may be extended on an armboard. A headrest may be used. The procedure may be performed under local or general anesthesia. See circulator responsibilities regarding local anesthesia, p. 31. Tetracaine drops may be instilled.

Skin preparation and Draping

See Ophthalmic Surgery, General Information, p. 31.

Equipment

Headrest (e.g., horseshoe), optional
Sitting stools

Instrumentation

Basic eye procedures tray
Eyelid and conjunctival procedures tray

Supplies

Basin set
Sterile, plastic adhesive drape
Cotton-tipped applicators or cellulose sponges
Blade (1) No. 15 or (1) No. 11
Cautery (wet field or disposable)
Balanced Salt Solution (BSS), tear substitute
Topical anesthetic drops (e.g., tetracaine), optional
Local anesthesia (e.g., lidocaine (Xylocaine) 2% with epinephrine)
Marking pen
Antibiotic ophthalmic ointment (optional)

CORRECTION OF ENTROPION

Definition

Correction of an inversion of the lid margins and eyelashes.

Discussion

Entropion usually affects the lower lid. The condition may be corrected by various procedures.

Types:

Congenital is due to hypertrophy of the marginal and pretarsal orbicularis oculi muscle, which causes the eyelid margin to be pushed up and against the globe.

Involutional (most common) occurs when canthal tendons retain their rigidity but the apposition of the lid to the globe is changed (e.g., from senile atrophy of orbital fat) resulting in the inversion of the eyelid, or it may occur as the result of weakness of the retractor muscles of the lower lid.

Procedure

Internal Tarsal-Orbicularis Resection. The lower lid is everted with a chalazion clamp. The line of incision may be marked inside the eyelid. A base-down triangle of skin, orbicularis oculi muscle, and tarsus is excised. The edges are sutured together and the "dog-ear" edge of remaining tissue is excised. In an alternate method (skin-tarsal fixation), the orbicular muscle is divided and sutured to the lower border of the tarsus.

Preparation of the patient, Skin preparation, Draping, Equipment, Instrumentation, and Supplies

See Correction of Ectropion, p. 429.

BLEPHAROPTOSIS REPAIR

Definition

Correction of a drooping upper eyelid.

Discussion

The condition may be unilateral or bilateral. Any one of a number of techniques may be employed depending on the type and severity of the deformity.

Types:
Congenital: Mild to severe (eyelid droops 1.5 mm to 4 mm or more)
Acquired: May be neurogenic or caused by myogenic and aponeurosis defects
Traumatic: Also as a result of ocular surgery
Mechanical: Blepharochalasis or enophthalmos may be the cause
External levator resection is indicated in patients with moderate to severe ptosis and fair to poor levator function.

Procedure

External Levator Resection. A traction suture is placed in the lid to permit downward traction. An incision is made from canthus to canthus and carried through the orbicularis oculi to the superior border of the tarsus. The upper half of the tarsus is exposed. The upper skin edge is grasped and the orbicularis is separated from the orbital septum. The fat is retracted posteriorly, and the levator aponeurosis is excised. The eyelid is everted and the conjunctiva is incised. The aponeurosis is buttonholed at its medial and lateral border, a straight hemostat is placed across it and Müller's muscle and the tissues are transsected. The conjunctiva is reapproximated. Müller's muscle and the levator are sutured to the tarsus. The excess levator is excised. Lid crease skin sutures are placed. The lower lid is pulled up over the globe by sutures placed in the lower lid through a silicone peg or bolster, which are taped to the forehead. These sutures are removed the next day.

Preparation of the patient, Skin preparation, Draping, Equipment, Instrumentation, and Supplies

See Correction of Ectropion, p. 429.

LACRIMAL DUCT PROBING

Definition

Opening of the nasolacrimal duct.

Discussion

The procedure is done to prevent acute infection of the lacrimal drainage system. If conservative management of a lacrimal duct obstruction is unsuccessful, probing is indicated. When repeated probings are technically successful but have otherwise failed, an indwelling silicone tube is inserted.

Procedure

The upper canaliculus is dilated with a lacrimal dilator. A lacrimal probe (e.g., size 000) is inserted and passed through the imperforate opening into the nose. The procedure may be repeated with the next larger size lacrimal probe, and so on. A lacrimal cannula is used to irrigate through the upper canaliculus into the nose. Antibiotic ophthalmic drops may be instilled.

Preparation of the patient

In infants (up to 6 months), the procedure may be performed using a topical anesthetic. The patient is positioned in a mummylike wrap. The procedure is usually performed under general anesthesia for the child over 6 months. The child is supine. The head and foot of the table may be dropped to provide closer access to the patient. Extremities are restrained using padded restraints. For preparation of the pediatric patient see Pediatric General Information, p. 467.

Skin preparation

See Ophthalmic Surgery, General Information, p. 423.

Draping

The patient is usually draped very simply with folded towels around the eye; a body sheet may be used.

Equipment

Sitting stools, optional
Restraints, padded or mummy wrap (optional)

Instrumentation

Basic eye procedures tray
Lacrimal dilators (e.g., Bowman)
Lacrimal probes
Lacrimal cannula
Safety pins

Supplies

Small basin
Balanced Salt Solution (BSS), tear substitute
Cotton-tipped applicators or cellulose sponges
Antibiotic ophthalmic drops (optional)

Special notes

Gloves only may be worn.
Fluorescein dye may be requested to test the patency of the duct.

DACRYOCYSTORHINOSTOMY

Definition

Reestablishment of a passageway between the lacrimal duct and the nasal cavity.

Discussion

This procedure is indicated in patients with chronic dacryocystitis who have not responded to probing, irrigation, and silicone intubation.

Procedure

An incision is made along the side of the nose 1 cm from the canthus to just above the level of the alar cartilages. Traction is placed on the skin so that the deeper incision does not lie directly under the skin incision, avoiding a direct cutaneous-osseous scar. The periosteum is incised and separated from the bone with a periosteal elevator. The sac is separated from the fossa and the superior punctum probed to identify its location. An H-incision is made in the sac, which is retracted laterally as a power drill is used to remove the lacrimal crest. The nasal packing (from the preliminary nasal preparation) is removed. The nasal mucosa is exposed and a Kerrison rongeur is employed to enlarge the opening.

Care is taken to protect the corneas. An H-incision is made in the nasal mucosa. The flaps of the lacrimal sac and the flaps of the nasal mucosa are reapproximated. Hemostasis is achieved. The nose is packed with thrombin-soaked Gelfoam pledgets or gauze packing (e.g., Aaptic, iodoform, or petrolatum-impregnated gauze). The subcutaneous and skin layers are closed. A catheter may be passed through the nasolacrimal duct for postoperative irrigation. A folded eye pad may be placed over the incision only.

Preparation of the patient

The patient is supine; the arm on the side of the operative eye is tucked in at the patient's side, and the other arm may be extended on an armboard. The table is placed in reverse Trendelenburg position; a padded footboard is used. The procedure is performed under general anesthesia; however, the surgeon does a preliminary nasal preparation prior to the skin preparation, and local anesthesia with epinephrine may be administered during the procedure.

Preliminary nasal preparation (on a "clean" Mayo stand)

Topical anesthetic (e.g., cocaine 4% or 5% or phenylephrine (Neo-Synephrine) 0.25% or 0.5%)
Bayonet forceps
Nasal speculum
Packing material
Medicine cup

Skin preparation

See Ophthalmic Surgery, General Information, p. 423; prepare for a bilateral eye procedure.

Draping

See Ophthalmic Surgery, General Information, p. 423. Drape as for a unilateral eye procedure. In addition to the eye, the entire nose is draped into the field.

Equipment

Footboard, padded
Suction
Power source for power drill
Sitting stools

Instrumentation

Limited procedure tray
Basic eye procedures tray
Dacrocystorhinostomy tray
Kerrison rongeurs
Power drill (e.g., Stryker), burrs, and cord

Supplies

Basin set
Balanced Salt Solution (BSS), tear substitute
Cotton-tipped applicators or cellulose sponges
Blades (1) No. 15, (1) No. 11
Needle magnet or counter
Suction tubing
Local anesthetic (e.g., lidocaine (Xylocaine) 1% with epinephrine)
Bulb syringe
Topical anesthetic (e.g., cocaine 4% or 5% or phenylephrine (Neo-Synephrine) 0.25% or 0.5%)
Catheter (e.g., 10Fr Robinson) or infant feeding tube (optional)
Packing (e.g., ½" gauze and Adaptic)
Cautery, disposable
Thrombin (e.g., 5000 units)
Gelfoam (cut into pledgets 2 cm × 1 cm)

Special notes

Local anesthesia with epinephrine may be administered during the procedure to aid in hemostasis.

Protective goggles may be worn.

The area being drilled is lightly irrigated with saline to minimize friction and buildup of heat; saline and bone fragments are suctioned.

CORRECTION OF STRABISMUS

Definition

Alignment of the visual axes of the eyes.

Discussion

When medical treatment (glasses, patching, and fusion exercises) fails to align the axes of the eyes, surgical treatment is indicated. Complete restoration to normal alignment cannot always be achieved.

Types:

Lateral rectus resection is the shortening of this extraocular muscle by removing a portion of it and the reanastomosis of the cut ends.

Medial rectus recession is the lengthening of this extraocular muscle by detaching it from its original insertion and reattaching it more posteriorly on the sclera.

Procedure

Lateral Rectus Resection. An eye speculum is inserted. An incision is made in the conjunctiva at the limbus to expose the lateral rectus muscle. The eye is rotated medially as far as possible. Two traction sutures are placed in the conjunctiva. The conjunctiva is freed from underlying tissue. A muscle hook is passed under the muscle insertion. The amount of muscle to be resected is measured with a caliper (previously adjusted). A muscle clamp is clamped over the muscle and the measured portion (specimen) is excised. The end of the muscle is reattached to the original point of insertion. Hemostasis is achieved. The conjunctiva is closed. Antibiotic ophthalmic ointment may be instilled and an eye pad is applied.

Medial Rectus Recession. An eye speculum is inserted. An incision is made in the conjunctiva at the limbus; the conjunctiva is undermined. The distance from the original point of insertion to the new one is measured with a caliper (previously adjusted). The new point of insertion may be marked. Two absorbable sutures are placed in the end of the muscle (and left untied with the needles attached). A straight mosquito hemostat is clamped across the muscle (between the sutures and the insertion) in order to compress small blood vessels and discourage oozing. The clamp is removed and a muscle hook is passed under the muscle. The muscle is incised and the cautery is employed as necessary to achieve hemostasis. The muscle is reattached at the new point of insertion further back on the globe with the previously placed sutures. The conjunctiva is closed. Antibiotic ophthalmic ointment is instilled and an eye pad is applied.

Preparation of the patient

The procedure is usually performed under general anesthesia. A retrobulbar injection may be administered prior to the skin preparation. The patient is supine; the arm on the side of the affected eye may be tucked in at the patient's side, and the other arm may be extended on an armboard.

Skin preparation and Draping

See Ophthalmic Surgery, General Information, p. 423.

Equipment

Headrest
Loupes (optional)
Sitting stools

Instrumentation

Basic eye procedures tray
Basic eye muscle procedures tray

Supplies

Basin set
Cotton-tipped applicators or cellulose sponges
Cautery, disposable
Balanced Salt Solution (BSS), tear substitute
Needle magnet or counter
Antibiotic ophthalmic ointment
Marking pen, optional

EVISCERATION OF THE EYE

Definition

Removal of the entire contents of the eye within the scleral shell.

Discussion

The sclera and muscles attached to the sclera remain intact to accommodate a prosthesis. Indication for evisceration is a hopelessly traumatized eye in a young person with no history of previous eye disease. The cosmetic result is superior to the result of enucleation because the extraocular muscles still attached to the scleral shell result in a moveable implant.

Procedure

A peritomy is made superiorly from the 3 o'clock to 9 o'clock position. An incision (same length) is made in the exposed sclera through to the uvea. The entire uvea is separated from the sclera by an evisceration spoon and is completely removed. The remaining uvea may be removed with a gauze sponge on a hemostat rotated within the scleral shell or with a chalazion curette. The wound is irrigated. Hemostasis is achieved. Scleral edges are held open by tagged sutures while the implant is inserted by a sphere introducer. The posterior surface of the cornea is removed to reduce its sensitivity. The sclera is closed with interrupted sutures. The conjunctiva is approximated with interrupted sutures. A conformer is placed in the cul-de-sac. Antibiotic ophthalmic ointment is instilled and an eye patch is applied.

Preparation of the patient

The patient is supine; the arm on the side of the operative eye may be tucked in at the patient's side, and the other arm may be extended on an armboard.

Skin preparation and Draping

See Ophthalmic Surgery, General Information, p. 423.

Equipment

Suction
Sitting stools

Instrumentation

Basic eye procedures tray
Globe and orbit procedures tray
Curettes
Sphere prosthesis and conformer

Supplies

Basin set
Balanced Salt Solution (BSS), tear substitute
Cautery (wet field or disposable)
Cotton-tipped applicators or cellulose sponges
Blade (1) No. 11
Suction tubing
Antibiotic ophthalmic ointment

Special notes

Have prosthesis ready to implant.

Follow hospital policy for recording the insertion of a prosthesis.

Complete manufacturer's forms.

ENUCLEATION OF THE GLOBE

Definition

Removal of an eye (without rupture of the globe).

Discussion

The procedure is indicated in certain instances of severe trauma, intraocular malignancy, intolerable pain, and unsightly appearance. A plastic or silicone sphere is placed within Tenon's capsule. A conformer is placed over the sphere. The conformer is replaced with an artificial eye 8 weeks postoperatively.

Procedure

A peritomy is made at the limbus circumferentially separating the conjunctiva and Tenon's capsule from the globe. The superior oblique tendon is grasped with a muscle hook and divided. The inferior oblique muscle is double-clamped with hemostats for hemostasis; the muscle is cut. Hemostats are released after several minutes. All attachments to the globe are separated, permitting the globe to move freely. The eye is held steady by the medial rectus insertion. The location of the optic nerve is identified. The optic nerve is transsected, the globe delivered, and the remaining attachments are separated. Hemostasis is achieved. A sphere implant is sutured into Tenon's capsule. The conjunctiva is approximated. A conformer is placed over the sphere in the cul-de-sac. An intermarginal suture is placed to produce a mild pressure effect. Antibiotic ointment may be instilled, an eye pad is placed, and a pressure dressing is applied.

Preparation of the patient

The patient is supine; the arm on the side of the operative eye may be tucked in at the patient's side, and the other arm may be extended on an armboard.

Skin preparation and Draping

See Ophthalmic Surgery, General Information, p. 423.

Equipment

Suction
Sitting stools

Instrumentation

Basic eye procedures tray
Globe and orbit procedures tray
Sphere prosthesis and conformer

Supplies

Basin set
Balanced Salt Solution (BSS), tear substitute
Cautery (wet field or disposable)
Cotton-tipped applicators or cellulose sponges
Suction tubing
Antibiotic ophthalmic ointment

Special notes

Have prosthesis ready to implant.
Follow hospital policy for recording the insertion of a prosthesis.

ORBITAL EXENTERATION

Definition

Removal of the eye and a significant portion of the orbital tissues.

Discussion

The amount of tissues removed beyond the globe depends on the origin and extent of the disease process. Exenteration is usually performed for neoplasms, but may also be performed for benign disease such as phycomycosis.

Classification
1. *Subtotal:* Eye and epibulbar tissues excised
2. *Total* (with or without eyelid skin): Removal of all tissues within the bony orbit, including the periorbita
3. *Radical:* Removal of one or more bony orbital walls in addition to soft tissues and periosteum

The subtotal procedure is used to remove tumors involving the anterior portion of the eye and the conjunctiva. The total procedure is indicated when an intraocular tumor (e.g., melanoma) extends into the orbit. Malignant tumors not involving bone that do not respond to radiation may require total exenteration. Radical exenteration is indicated when a malignant sinus tumor invades the orbit or when a malignant skin tumor involves the orbital bones. After the wound has healed the cavity may be covered with a black patch or a cosmetic plastic prosthesis.

Procedure

For *total exenteration,* with preservation of eyelid skin, an incision is made circumferentially around the palpebral fissure. The skin is dissected to the orbital rim. Orbicularis muscle may be incised with the cutting blade of an electrosurgical pencil. The periosteum is separated from the orbital rim and walls; care is taken to avoid the perforation of bony walls. The eye and soft tissues within the orbit are removed. The skin is undermined and closed over the lateral orbital rim. A split-thickness skin graft may be used to cover denuded orbital walls. The orbital cavity is packed with gauze impregnated with antibiotic ointment, and a moderate pressure dressing is applied. Alternatively, the bone surfaces may be permitted to heal by spontaneous epithelialization.

Preparation of the patient

The patient is supine; the arm on the side of the operative eye may be extended on an armboard, and the other arm may be tucked in at the patient's side. Apply electrosurgical dispersive pad.

Skin preparation and Draping

See Ophthalmic Surgery, General Information, p. 423.

Equipment

Suction
Electrosurgical unit
Sitting stools
Power unit for dermatome (optional)

Instrumentation

Limited procedure tray
Basic eye procedures tray
Globe and orbit procedures tray
Dermatome (e.g., Brown), optional

Supplies

Basin set
Balanced Salt Solution (BSS), tear substitute

Electrosurgical pencil
Cotton-tipped applicators or cellulose sponges
Needle magnet or counter
Bone wax
Suction tubing
Packing (e.g., ¼" gauze)
Antibiotic ophthalmic ointment
Mineral oil (if dermatome is used)

Special notes

Determine if a skin graft is to be obtained and prepare the donor site.

CORNEAL TRANSPLANT/KERATOPLASTY

Definition

The grafting of corneal tissue from the eye of one person to another.

Discussion

The indications for corneal transplant are corneal injury or disease resulting in opacification of the cornea. The procedure is performed to improve vision; the retina and optic nerve must be functioning properly.

Types:
Lamellar: Replacement of a partial thickness of the cornea
Penetrating: Replacement of a full thickness of the cornea
Total: Replacement of the entire corneal area (limbus to limbus)
Lamellar and total keratoplasty are rarely performed. Penetrating keratoplasty is often performed as an emergency procedure.

Procedure

Penetrating Keratoplasty. The trephine size is chosen and the donor button is prepared. If the donor button has been prepared by the excision of a cornea with a scleral rim, this is placed into a Teflon block, and the button punched from behind (on the endothelial surface). The trephine used for the donor button is 0.5 mm larger than the host trephine. A single nonabsorbable suture is placed through the cut edge of the button. When the whole eye is used as the donor, the button can be trephined from the anterior surface with a trephine the same size or 0.5 mm larger than the one used for the recipient. The depth of the trephine blade is set at 1.5 mm, placed against the anterior surface of the cornea, and the button may be removed in toto. If the anterior chamber is entered (aqueous escapes), the trephine is removed and the excision is completed with scissors. A single suture is placed through the excised button. The excised button is placed epithelial-side down on a moistened (with saline or McCarey-Kaufman medium) gauze pad, and fluid is placed on the endothelial surface to prevent drying. The host cornea is now removed by trephining the cornea 0.4 mm deep. The anterior chamber is entered with a sharp knife and the excision is completed with scissors. Care is taken to remove any adventitious tissue from the host site. Lens extraction, vitrectomy, or any other necessary procedures are performed. The donor button is placed into the host and the previously placed suture is tied at 12 o'clock. The graft is fixed at the 6 o'clock, 3 o'clock, and 9 o'clock positions. The graft is secured with additional sutures. Before the last suture is tied, the anterior chamber is reformed to normal depth with balanced salt solution. Any leaks are repaired. Steroids, as well as antibiotics, may be applied topically.

Preparation of the patient

The patient is supine; the arm on the side of the

operative eye may be tucked in at the patient's side, and the other arm may be extended on an armboard. Tetracaine drops may be instilled. Eyelashes may be clipped. The procedure is performed under general anesthesia. A retrobulbar injection may be administered prior to the skin preparation.

Skin preparation and draping

See Ophthalmic Surgery, General Information, p. 423. A drape is needed to cover the microscope.

Equipment

Headrest
Microscope
Sitting stools

Instrumentation

Basic eye procedures tray
Corneal procedures tray

Supplies

Basin set
Cautery (wet field or disposable)
Balanced Salt Solution (BSS), tear substitute
Cotton-tipped applicators and cellulose sponges
Culture dishes (to store donor corneal button)
Blades (1) No. 15, (1) No. 64 Beaver, (1) superblade
     30°
Fluorescein strip (topical stain that temporarily stains
     denuded corneal epithelium)
Antibiotic solution (to wash transplant)
Anti-inflammatory agent (e.g., betamethasone [Cele-
     stone Soluspan])

Special notes

Confirm that the donor cornea is available.
When a portable floor-model microscope is

used, it is brought over the patient on the side opposite the operative eye.

A separate sterile table may be requested to cut
out the donor transplant.

CATARACT EXTRACTION

Definition

Removal of an opaque ocular lens.

Discussion

The ocular lens becomes opacified for a number of
reasons including trauma, and congenital, drug,
and metabolic effects, but is primarily due to aging.
At an appropriate time in the maturation of the cataract, and with sufficient loss of vision, surgery is indicated.

Types:

Intracapsular method: Removal of the opaque
lens within its capsule. A cryoprobe is usually applied to the cataract and the lens, and they are removed by gentle pressure.

Extracapsular method: Removal of an opaque
lens by irrigation and expression, leaving the posterior capsule in situ.

Phacoemulsification: A variation of the irriga-
tion/aspiration technique; the contents of the lens
capsule is fragmented with ultrasonic energy as the
lens material is simultaneously irrigated and aspirated.

An artificial lens is commonly implanted after
the cataract has been removed. The surgeon will se-
lect a lens prosthesis prior to surgery.

Procedure

Intracapsular. A lid speculum is placed. Traction sutures are placed in the sclera. The conjunctiva

is reflected from the corneal superior hemicircumference. Bleeders are cauterized. The anterior chamber is entered. An iridotomy is performed as the cornea is retracted by suture traction. Alpha-chymotrypsin (Zolyse) is instilled into the anterior chamber (to dissolve the zonules suspending the lens). After 3 minutes a cryoextractor is applied to the lens, which adheres to it and the lens is withdrawn from the eye. The corneal incision is closed. Traction sutures are removed and the conjunctival flap is approximated. Ophthalmic ointment may be instilled and an eye pad is applied.

An intraocular lens implant may be inserted following the extraction of the lens. Several varieties of intraocular lens prostheses are used. The prosthesis is either sutured to the iris or simply held in place (by virtue of its shape) by the iris. The wound closure then proceeds as above.

Extracapsular. This procedure is similar to the intracapsular procedure, except that the lens capsule is incised, and the lens is expressed or irrigated out leaving the posterior capsule, which remains as a barrier to the vitreous humor. When *phacoemulsification* is employed the anterior lens capsule is excised, the lens nucleus is prolapsed into the anterior chamber, and the ultrasonic probe (with capabilities of irrigation and aspiration, as well as delivery of ultrasonic energy) is inserted into the capsule. Alternately, the probe is set to irrigate; irrigate and aspirate; and irrigate, aspirate, and fragment the remaining lens substance (cortex). The posterior capsule is "polished" with a moist cellulose sponge (removal of any lens fragments) or partially excised. Phacoemulsification permits a smaller (more cosmetic) wound and iridotomy incision. After phacoemulsification is complete, the wound is closed as above. An intraocular lens may be placed, as described earlier.

Preparation of the patient

The patient is supine; the arm on the side of the affected eye may be tucked in at the patient's side, and the other arm may be extended on an arm-board. The head may be supported by a headrest. Prior to the skin preparation tetracaine drops may be instilled in both eyes followed by the application of a Honan intraocular pressure reducer cuff for 10 to 15 minutes. Lashes may be trimmed (infrequently).

Skin preparation and Draping

See Ophthalmic Surgery, General Information, p. 423.

Equipment

Honan intraocular pressure reducer cuff
Lift sheet for operating table
Headrest (e.g., horseshoe) optional
Sitting stools
Microscope
　　Intracapsular: Cryoextractor (e.g., Frigitonics)
　　Phacoemulsification: Irrigation/Aspiration (I/A)
unit (e.g., Cavitron)

Instrumentation

Basic eye procedures tray
Cataract extraction and lens procedure tray
Phacoemulsification tray, as indicated by the brand
　　of the I/A unit (e.g., Cavitron Phaco Emulsifier
　　unit with AVIT handpiece, I/A handpiece, ultra-
　　sonic handpiece, and irrigation cystotome)
Handgrips (or drape) for microscope
Intraocular lens implant (IOL)

Supplies

Basin set
Sterile, plastic adhesive drape
Balanced Salt Solution (BSS) 500 ml
I/A pack (for phacoemulsification)
Cellulose sponges
Cautery (wet field or disposable)

Beaver blade No. 69
Super blade 30°
Millipore filter (for acetylcholine (Miochol))
Medications (available)
Anesthetic for retrobulbar block (e.g., lidocaine (Xylocaine) 2% with epinephrine or bupivacaine (Marcaine) 0.5% with epinephrine)
Corticosteroid, an anti-inflammatory agent (e.g., betamethasone (Celestone) drops)
Enzyme to increase absorption and dispersion of other drugs (e.g., hyaluronidase (Wydase))
Miotic agent to irrigate and rapidly constrict the pupil (e.g., acetylcholine (Miochol))
Viscoelastic agent acts as a tamponade and a vitreous substitute (e.g., sodium hyaluronate (Healon))

Special notes

A lift sheet placed on the table will be helpful in transferring the patient to the gurney postoperatively.

A portable (floor model) microscope, when used, is brought over the patient on the side opposite the affected eye.

Be thoroughly familiar with equipment (i.e., Frigitonics and Cavitron).

Thoroughly check the functioning of the Cavitron unit preoperatively.

When using the Cavitron unit inform the surgeon as different positions are entered, that is, *one* (on irrigation alone), *two* (on irrigation and aspiration), and *three* (on irrigation, aspiration, and ultrasound). The surgeon is advised by the numbers (e.g., "one, two, three, two, three").

Follow hospital policy for recording the insertion of a lens.

Complete lens manufacturer's forms.

IRIDECTOMY

Definition

Excision of a section of the iris.

Discussion

The prodedure provides a new channel for aqueous humor to flow from the posterior to anterior chamber. Chief indications for iridectomy are treatment of primary angle-closure glaucoma, secondary angle-closure glaucoma, and occludable angle glaucoma. The new communication relieves pupillary block and reestablishes the flow of aqueous through Schlemm's canal.

Procedure

A 2-mm peritomy is made at the superior limbus. Epithelium is scraped away from the corneoscleral junction. Preplaced sutures are placed in the cornea. Prolapse of the iris is facilitated by gentle traction on the sutures. The iris is grasped (lifted slightly superiorly) and excision is performed. Balanced Salt Solution is used to flush away remaining pigment epithelium. The preplaced sutures are tied. Additional sutures may be necessary. Topical corticosteroids and antibiotic ointment may be instilled; an eye pad is applied.

Preparation of the patient

The patient is supine; the arm on the side of the affected eye may be tucked in at the patient's side and the other arm extended on an armboard. A headrest may be used. Tetracaine drops are instilled. A facial nerve block may be administered prior to the skin preparation. Retrobulbar anesthesia is avoided (it causes increased intraocular pressure and dilation of the pupil). Lashes may be trimmed (infrequently).

Skin preparation and Draping

See Ophthalmic Surgery, General Information, p. 423.

Equipment

Headrest (optional)
Sitting stools
Microscope or loupes (optional)

Instrumentation

Basic eye procedures tray
Glaucoma procedures tray
Handgrips (or drape) for microscope, if used

Supplies

Basin set
Sterile, plastic adhesive drape
Cotton-tipped applicators or cellulose sponges
Blade (e.g., Beaver No. 69 or No. 67)
Millipore filter (for acetylcholine [Miochol])
Cautery (wet field or disposable)
Local anesthetic
Balanced Salt Solution (BSS)
Antibiotic ophthalmic ointment
Miochol, to irrigate anterior chamber and rapidly
    constrict pupil
Topical corticosteroid (e.g., prednisolone acetate
    1%)

TRABECULECTOMY

Definition

Drainage of the anterior chamber employing a
partial-thickness limbal-based scleral flap.

Discussion

Trabeculectomy is the procedure of choice for primary glaucomas when iridectomy is considered inadequate. Trabeculectomy may also be performed to treat infantile glaucoma and several types of secondary glaucoma.

Procedure

Intraocular pressure is checked; if it is excessively high, measures are taken to bring it into the satisfactory range. A superior rectus bridle suture is placed. A limbal-based conjunctival flap is developed; episcleral tissue is cleaned anteriorly up to and including the corneoscleral sulcus. A caliper is used to measure the width of the flap on the globe. The sclera is cauterized lightly in the shape of the flap to be developed. The sclera is incised to a depth of two thirds its thickness with the cautery. Atropine eyedrops may be administered to dilate the pupil. The edge of the flap is developed with a Beaver blade; care is taken not to penetrate the base of the flap. The flap is continued to the anterior junction of the conjunctiva and the cornea. A paracentesis track is placed with a sharp-tipped knife into the cornea 1 mm anterior to the limbus. An incision is made through the sclera, through which the iris will prolapse. An iridotomy is performed. The sclera is incised radially. The block of scleral wall is excised. Iridectomy is performed. The scleral flap is sutured in place; after two sutures are placed the anterior chamber is filled with Balanced Salt Solution through the paracentesis track, as the intraocular pressure is monitored. When filtration is desired postoperatively, a filtering bleb develops as the anterior chamber is shaped. Antibiotic drops or ointment may be instilled and an eye patch is placed.

Preparation of the patient

The patient is supine; the arm on the side of the operative eye may be tucked in at the patient's side, and the other arm may be extended on an armboard. A headrest may be used. Tetracaine eyedrops may be instilled. Facial and retrobulbar blocks may be administered. Lashes may be trimmed.

Skin preparation and Draping

See Ophthalmic Surgery, General Information, p. 423.

Equipment

Headrest (optional)
Sitting stools
Microscope

Instrumentation

Basic eye procedures tray
Glaucoma procedures tray
Handgrips (or drape) for microscope

Supplies

Basin set
Sterile, plastic adhesive drape
Cotton-tipped applicators or cellulose sponges
Blades (e.g., No. 57 Beaver and 15° super blade)
Balanced Salt Solution (BSS), tear substitute
Cautery (wet field or disposable)
Local and retrobulbar anesthetic (e.g., bupivacaine
    (Marcaine) 0.5%)
Antibiotic ophthalmic drops or ointment

EXCISION OF A PTERYGIUM

Definition

Removal of a growth of fibrovascular tissue that extends from the conjunctiva onto the cornea.

Discussion

True pterygia are located in the interpalpebral zone, particularly on the medial aspect of the globe; pterygia often occur bilaterally. All pterygia need not be excised. Indications for removal include an inflamed eye that does not respond to topical medication, growth of a pterygium so that it interferes or is expected to interfere with vision, a change in corneal astigmatism associated with growth of the pterygium, or cosmetic reasons. Several different techniques are advocated.

Procedure

A speculum is inserted. The head of the pterygium may be dissected from the cornea and undermined toward the sclera by superficial stripping (or from sclera to cornea). Alternatively, an incision may be made above or below the pterygium, a suture passed under the body of the pterygium, and with a sawing motion of the suture the pterygium is stripped from the cornea as the suture is pulled medially. The corneoscleral limbus is made smooth with a Beaver or No. 15 blade. Hemostasis is achieved with the cautery. With recurrent or large pterygia, every effort is made to carefully excise this tissue to prevent recurrence.

Preparation of the patient

The patient is supine; the arm on the side of the affected eye may be tucked in at the patient's side, and the other arm may be extended on an armboard. A headrest may be used. The procedure may be performed with a topical anesthetic of cocaine 10%, subconjunctival injection of lidocaine, retrobulbar injection of lidocaine, or a similar agent. See circulator responsibilities regarding local anesthesia, p. 31.

Skin preparation and Draping

See Ophthalmic Surgery, General Information, p. 423.

Equipment

Headrest (optional)
Sitting stools
Microscope (optional)

Instrumentation

Basic eye procedures tray
Basic eye procedures microscope tray
Handgrips (or drape) for microscope, if used

Supplies

Basin set
Balanced Salt Solution (BSS), tear substitute
Sterile, plastic adhesive drape
Blades (1) No. 15, and Beaver (1) No. 57 or No. 64
Anesthetic agent
Cotton-tipped applicators or cellulose sponges
Cautery (wet field or disposable)
Anti-inflammatory agent (e.g., hydrocortisone ophthalmic ointment), optional

REPAIR OF RETINAL DETACHMENT/SCLERAL BUCKLING

Definition

The sealing of a localized retinal defect by inciting an inflammatory reaction near the defect or by compressing the globe buckling the sclera to seal a linear defect in the retina.

Discussion

When the neural retinal layer becomes detached from its underlying pigmented layer either because of a defect in the retina or because of accumulation of fluid behind the retina, serious visual disturbance results. The inciting events include tumor of the choroid, trauma, and degeneration. Vitreous humor, blood, or tissue may accumulate between the retinal layers and the choroid. Treatment consists of sealing the retinal defect and drainage of the subretinal fluid. Several modalities are employed to effect closure of the defects. Diathermy coagulation to the sclera overlying the retinal defect creates an inflammatory reaction that seals the defect. Similarly, laser surgery (see Appendix, p. 570) or cryosurgery may be used. To achieve reattachment of the retina, the globe is encircled by suturing a band of silicone to maintain the buckle of the sclera, which decreases the potential space in which unwanted fluids can accumulate.

Procedure

A discrete retinal defect, not surrounded by a detachment, can be sealed by photocoagulation or laser (performed in an "eye laboratory" rather than the operating room). To effect adhesions with a diathermy or cryoprobe, the preoperatively mapped out section of the globe overlying the defect is exposed. The conjunctiva and Tenon's capsule are incised. The diathermy is applied to create adhesions to seal the defect. This maneuver can be controlled by the surgeon viewing through the microscope as the assistant depresses the sclera with the diathermy probe against the defect. An incision can also be made into the subretinal fluid accumulations to evacuate them. The buckling is achieved by incising a groove around the equator of the globe, undermining the edges. A Silastic band is placed in the groove, secured by multiple mattress sutures, which also closes the groove. The Silastic band is then tightened around the globe to effect the buckling and maintenance of the retinal layers in apposition. A silicone sponge may be used under the band to exert additional pressure and assure the proper degree of buckling. On occasion, one of the extraocular muscles must be retracted (transiently detached) to provide adequate exposure. The conjunctiva is closed. Antibiotic ophthalmic drops and/or ointment may be instilled.

Preparation of the patient

The patient is supine; the arm on the side of the operative eye may be tucked in at the patient's side, and the other arm may be extended on an armboard. A headrest may be used. General anesthesia is employed.

Skin preparation and Draping

See Ophthalmic Surgery, General Information, p. 423. Additional drapes may be needed to cover the cryosurgical unit and the microscope.

Equipment

Headrest (optional)
Sitting stools
Diathermy unit
Indirect ophthalmoscope
Cryosurgical unit
Microscope
Laser, optional

Instrumentation

Basic eye procedures tray
Retinal procedures tray
Tonometer and weights
Cryosurgical retinal probes (curved and straight with rubber covering) and cords
Diathermy cords and probes
Implant

Supplies

Basin set
Sterile, plastic adhesive drape

Balanced Salt Solution (BSS), tear substitute
Cotton-tipped applicators and cellulose sponges
Cautery (wet field or disposable)
Beaver blade No. 69 or No. 59
Antibiotic ophthalmic drops and/or ointment, op-
tional

Special notes

The surgeon chooses the Silastic band and scleral sponge prior to the procedure.

Soak ophthalmoscope lens in aqueous glutaraldehyde (e.g., Cidex).

Have cryosurgical unit and diathermy machine
ready.

Implants may be soaked in antibiotic solution
after being flash-autoclaved.

Acetazolamide (Diamox) may be requested (to
reduce intraocular pressure).

The ophthalmoscope may be handled using a
sterile plastic covering for it.

Sterile back vests may be helpful in maintaining
the sterility of the field.

If laser is used, see precautions in Appendix,
p. 572.

A culture may be taken prior to closure.

VITRECTOMY

Definition

Removal of vitreous humor (vitreous body).

Discussion

The vitreous body may opacify secondary to retinal
hemorrhage (as in diabetes), endophthalmitis, foreign bodies and trauma, and preretinal membranes. The vitreous may also opacify as a result of
the formation of bands following anterior chamber
surgery (e.g., cataract extraction). Surgery can re-

move or lyse the bands, restore contour to the globe, and remove organized hemorrhagic areas or foreign matter in order to restore a clear visual pathway to the retina. The argon or the neodymium: yttrium aluminum garnet (Nd:YAG) laser may be used to lyse the bands noninvasively, when applicable. See Appendix, p. 572 for laser precautions.

Procedure

The vitreous is approached by an incision in the pars plana (the anterior attachment of the retina) or by a paralimbal incision. The lens, if not already absent, may be removed. Vitreous, if displaced into the anterior chamber during prior cataract extraction, is removed. A vitrector (e.g., Ocutome), which is a fine, blunt-tipped suction, cutting cannula with the capacity for irrigation (console controlled), is inserted. An additional incision through the pars plana permits endoillumination. The vitreous and its opacities are removed using a combination of diathermy, cryosurgery, irrigation, and suction. If a retinal tear is present, it is treated by cryoprobe, photocoagulation, or a scleral buckle (see p. 458). During the procedure Balanced Salt Solution or sodium hyaluronate (Healon) is infused by catheter to replace vitreous loss and give tonicity to the globe. The incisions are closed. Antibiotics and steroids are instilled or injected subconjunctivally, and an eye patch is applied.

Preparation of the patient

The patient is supine; the arm on the side of the operative eye may be tucked in at the patient's side, and the other arm may be extended on an armboard. The procedure is usually performed under general anesthesia. The table is placed in slight reverse Trendelenburg position, the neck is extended, and the head is stabilized with a headrest. Antiembolic hose or elastic bandages may be used. Pressure points are well padded.

Skin preparation and Draping

See Ophthalmic Surgery, General Information, p. 423. The microscope is draped.

Equipment

Headrest (e.g., doughnut)
Microscope with x-y coupling (allows surgeon to move microscope head over the field)
Endoilluminator light source
Endocoagulator (bipolar, wet field)
Frigitonics unit
Vitrector (e.g., Ocutome II)
Sitting stools

Instrumentation

Basic eye procedures tray
Retinal procedures tray
Forceps (e.g., Lister, curved and straight Pierse-Hoskins, and curved and straight McPherson tying)
Cryoprobe and cord
Endocoagulator handpiece with cord
Endoilluminator handpiece with cord
Vitrectomy instrumentation, vitrectomy handpiece (AVIT) and tubing, scleral plugs (19- or 20-gauge), scleral plug forceps, hand-held lens (with irrigator), caliper, special knife and blade, infusion cannula, vitreous scissors, membrane pick, flute needle, foreign body forceps

Supplies

Basin set
Sterile, plastic adhesive drape
Balanced Salt Solution (BSS), tear substitute
Sodium hyaluronate (Healon), vitreous substitute
Cotton-tipped applicators and cellulose sponges
Acetylcholine (Miochol) and filter to constrict the pupil

Antibiotic and/or steroid ophthalmic drops or injection

Special notes

Check equipment before beginning the procedure.

The vitrectomy handpiece is attached to sterile tubing, which is connected to the Ocutome unit.

Test suction vacuum and assess the cutting function of the vitrector.

Prime the infusion cannula with solution (surgeon's choice) and remove air bubbles.

Vitrector unit rates are set (infusion, cutting, and aspiration).

Cultures may be taken (from vitreous washings).

REFRACTIVE KERATOPLASTY

Definition

Reshaping of the cornea in order to alter its refractive power.

Discussion

Refractive keratoplasty refers to a variety of procedures including those performed to correct or improve myopia, astigmatism, hyperopia, aphakia, and keratoconus. In radial keratoplasty, multiple radial incisions are made in the peripheral and paracentral cornea through as much as 90% of its depth so that the uncut central cornea may be flattened to correct myopia. For other conditions, such as aphakia, a button of cornea from either the patient (keratomileusis) or a donor (keratophakia) is cryolathed by means of a computer-controlled instrument, (re)-inserted, and sutured to the cornea. Sophisticated measurements of the corneal shape, thickness, and refractive parameters are performed preoperatively. Following one of these procedures, the patient may see well enough to eliminate the need for glasses.

Procedure

Radial keratotomy requires the patient's cooperation as he or she focuses his or her gaze while being observed through the operating microscope. Employing a micrometer, controlled radial incisions are made in the cornea using a sapphire, diamond, or steel knife, according to preoperative measurements regarding number, depth, and position. Antibiotic ointment and an eye patch may be applied.

Preparation of the patient

The patient is supine; the arm on the side of the operative eye may be tucked in at the patient's side, and the other arm may be extended on an armboard. A headrest may be employed. The procedure is performed with topical and local anesthesia.

Skin preparation and Draping

See Ophthalmic Surgery, General Information, p. 423.

Equipment

Headrest (e.g., doughnut)
Microscope (with fixation device attached to the objective lens)
Sitting stools

Instrumentation

Basic eye procedures tray
Cataract extraction and lens procedure tray

Supplies

Basin set
Sterile, plastic adhesive drape

Balanced Salt Solution (BSS), tear substitute
Cotton-tipped applicators and cellulose sponges
Cautery, disposable
Antibiotic ophthalmic ointment (optional)

Special notes

Surgery is usually performed as an outpatient procedure.

Chapter 20

PEDIATRIC PROCEDURES

PEDIATRIC GENERAL INFORMATION

The surgical care of the infant and small child mandates attention to numerous considerations not ordinarily required for older children or adult surgical patients. The need for appropriately sized smaller instruments, equipment, drapes, supplies, and so on is obvious. Other important factors must be heeded regarding the pediatric patient. It is in this context that the propriety of the phrase "the pediatric patient is not a small adult" is particularly evident. Special precautions for preoperative medication, administration of anesthesia, maintenance of body temperature, accurate fluid balance, etc., are essential. In addition to the age of the patient, size and weight, nutritional status, degree of hydration, and general medical condition influence the care of these children. The operating room is to be prepared prior to transporting the pediatric patient into the room so that specific measures may be instituted immediately on arrival.

Specific requirements follow.

**Maintenance of body temperature and/or
prevention of heat loss considerations**

Neonates and small infants are transported in a
heated isolette
Room temperature regulated by adjusting the ther-
mostat
26° to 27°C (80° to 85°F) infants under 11 kg (25
pounds)
23° to 24°C (75° to 80°F) older children
Radiant heat lamps (newborns)
Warming mattress temperature approximately
37.7°C (100°F)
Head covering (e.g., stockinette cap)
Covering for extremities (e.g., with Webril and plas-
tic wrap or tube stockinette)
Warmed intravenous fluids, blood, etc., to body tem-
perature
Warmed skin preparation solutions
Not allowing preparation solution to pool under the
patient
Avoidance of excessive draping
Warmed irrigation fluids to body temperature
Warmed blankets to cover patient postoperatively

Anesthesia measures

Assorted intravenous catheters
Assorted endotracheal tubes
2.5 to 3 mm (8 to 9Fr) newborn
3.5 to 4.5 mm (10 to 14Fr) infant
5 mm (15Fr) small child
Pediatric anesthesia circuit
Pediatric rebreathing bag
Small suction catheters
Humidifier (available)
Temperature probe, telethermometer with digital
display, e.g., axillary, esophageal, rectal (avoid
perforation)
Pediatric electrodes for ECG

Restraints

Mummylike wrap (newborn, small infants, or for older children when procedure is performed under local anesthesia)
Soft, padded, nonconstricting extremity restraints

Skin care precautions

Avoid pooling of preparation solutions to prevent skin maceration and/or chemical irritation
Avoid use of direct application of adhesive tape whenever possible
Use hypoallergenic tape (e.g., Durapore, Transpore, Micropore, Microfoam)
Pad pressure points when positioning patient (e.g., sacrum, elbows, heels, and knees) to avoid skin breakdown and nerve injuries, especially in lengthy surgeries

Positioning considerations

Avoid hyperextension and hyperflexion to prevent nerve traction injuries (e.g., brachial plexus)
Pad bony prominences to avoid nerve and skin damage, especially in lengthy procedures
Drop the foot and/or head of the table to facilitate access to the pediatric patient

Fluid balance monitoring

Irrigation solutions accurately measured
Sponges weighed (when significant blood loss anticipated; immediate weighing of sponges reduces evaporation factor)

The surgeon and/or anesthetist may request additional supportive measures. Preferably they will be reviewed prior to transporting the patient into the room.

PEDIATRIC TRACHEOSTOMY

Definition

An opening made into the trachea with the insertion of a cannula to facilitate breathing.

Discussion

The procedure is usually performed under general anesthesia. In infants the trachea is relatively shorter and the cartilaginous structures are soft and more difficult to palpate than in adults. The thyroid may be situated lower than in the adult, and a pretracheal fat pad may contain substantial blood vessels. In acute respiratory emergencies the cricothyroid membrane may be incised and a trocar and any available hollow tube inserted.

Procedure

The procedure is similar to the procedure for the adult patient (see p. 407), except that segments of the tracheal rings are not excised.

Preparation of the patient

See Pediatric General Information, p. 467. The patient is supine with the neck extended; a small roll is placed under the shoulders. Small sandbags may be placed at the sides of the head. The extremities are covered and restrained using padded restraints. Apply pediatric electrosurgical dispersive pad.

Skin preparation

Using warm preparation solutions only, begin cleansing the entire neck extending from the level of the infra-auricular border to the axillae, and down to the table around the shoulders.

Draping

Folded towels and a sheet with a small fenestration

Equipment

Body heat maintenance equipment (e.g., heat lamps, warming mattress)
Small roll and 2 or 3 small sandbags
Covering for extremities
Electrosurgical unit
Suction

Instrumentation

Tracheostomy tray
Pediatric minor procedures tray

Supplies

Basin set
Blades (2) No. 15, (1) No. 11
Needle magnet or counter
Suction tubing
Tracheostomy tubes, assorted pediatric 2.5 to 5 mm
Umbilical tape
Electrosurgical pencil (with needle tip)

Special notes

The tracheostomy tube will be held in place with umbilical tapes tied behind the neck.

A gauze dressing split around the tube is applied after the tube is connected to the ventilation equipment.

Tape the obturator to the top of the isolette or crib so that it does not become misplaced while transporting the patient. It will be needed to reinsert the tube if it becomes dislodged.

BRANCHIAL CLEFT SINUSECTOMY

Definition

Excision of a tract resulting from the nonclosure of a branchial cleft.

Discussion

These congenital anomalies are most often noted in later childhood, but can be treated in infants. Remnants of the first and second branchial clefts are the most common.

The first branchial cleft sinus extends from the auditory canal to just below the midpoint of the mandible.

The second branchial cleft sinus extends from the tonsillar fossae to the lower anterior border of the sternocleidomastoid muscle. The lesion presents as an abscess or a chronically draining sinus.

Procedure

Sinusectomy of first branchial cleft: A transverse elliptical incision is made around the external sinus opening (usually in the submandibular or upper neck region). The tract is dissected and the incision is extended posteriorly toward the angle of the mandible and lower portion of the auditory canal. Care is taken to avoid injury to the mandibular (and other) branches of the facial nerve. The tract is divided at the external auditory canal and ligated. The wound is closed in layers, usually over a small drain secured with a stitch or safety pin.

Preparation of the patient

See Pediatric General Information, p. 467; the head and extremities are covered prior to positioning. The patient is supine with the head turned to the side (the affected side is uppermost). A folded sheet may be placed under the shoulders to extend the neck. The extremities are restrained using padded restraints. Apply pediatric electrosurgical dispersive pad.

Skin preparation

Using warm preparation solutions only, begin by cleansing the entire neck extending from the infraauricular border to the nipples, and down to the table at the sides of the neck and shoulders.

Draping

Folded towels and a sheet with a small fenestration

Equipment

Body heat maintenance equipment (e.g., heat lamps, warming mattress)
Covering for head and extremities
Restraints, padded
Suction
Electrosurgical unit

Instrumentation

Pediatric major procedures tray
Weitlaner retractor

Supplies

Basin set
Blades (2) No. 15
Electrosurgical pencil (with needle point)
Suction tubing
Dissectors (e.g., peanut)
Nerve stimulator (locator), optional
Drain (e.g., rubber band, ¼″ Penrose)

REPAIR OF CONGENITAL DIAPHRAGMATIC HERNIA

Definition

Repair of an opening in the diaphragm through which the abdominal viscera protrude into the thoracic cavity.

Discussion

Several types of diaphragmatic hernias are seen in the newborn. These hernias require prompt repair to prevent life-threatening cardiorespiratory and obstructive phenomena. The most common of these hernias is through the pleuroperitoneal canal (Bochdalek's hernia). A sac is usually not present; the abdominal viscera enter the pleural space. Hernias through the anterior diaphragm at the sternocostal junction (foramen of Morgagni) are usually small, have a true sac, and are closed by a thoracic or abdominal approach. Eventration of the diaphragm (an attenuation, not a true hernia) is treated by plication of the diaphragm transthoracically. Esophageal hiatal hernia is repaired by a transthoracic approach and is less urgent, the diagnosis often not being suspected in the newborn. Congenital absence of a portion of the diaphragm is rarely encountered; it is repaired by mobilizing the remaining portions or by employing prosthetic sheeting (e.g., Silastic). In all of these patients additional congenital abnormalities may be present.

Procedure

The approach may be abdominal or transthoracic. The abdominal approach is most often employed for Bochdalek hernia repair. A paramedian or subcostal incision is made on the side of the hernia. Air is introduced intrapleurally to assist with the delivery of the viscera out of the pleural space. The hernia is repaired with interrupted sutures. Prior to tying the final sutures air is aspirated from the pleural space as the compressed lung is inflated. If the lung is hypoplastic, an indwelling thoracotomy tube is left in place. Before the abdomen is closed the viscera are inspected for other abnormalities, especially malrotation, adhesive bands, and intestinal atresia. If the abdomen accommodates the viscera poorly, only skin is closed over the incision in order to avoid respiratory embarrassment because of too tight a closure. Two weeks later as the abdominal wall stretches, peritoneal and fascial closure may be effected.

Preparation of the patient

See Pediatric General Information, p. 467; the head and extremities are covered prior to positioning. The patient is supine. The extremities are restrained using padded restraints. Apply pediatric electrosurgical dispersive pad.

Skin preparation

Using warm preparation solution only, begin cleansing the abdomen for a paramedian or subcostal incision (same side as the hernia), extending from the suprasternal notch to the pubic symphysis, and down to the table at the sides.

Draping

Folded towels and a pediatric laparotomy sheet

Equipment

Body heat maintenance equipment (e.g., heat lamps, warming mattress)
Covering for head and extremities
Restraints, padded
Suction (with a specimen trap for accurate blood loss measurement)
Electrosurgical unit

Instrumentation

Pediatric major procedures tray
Hemoclip appliers (short, medium)

Supplies

Basin set
Blades (2) No. 15
Needle magnet or counter
Electrosurgical pencil with needle tip
Syringe, 60 ml (for accurate irrigation measurement)
Vessel loops or umbilical tapes, ¼"
Infant chest drainage unit (e.g., Pleurevac), optional
Small chest tube (e.g., 10Fr Argyle), optional
Hemoclips (small, medium)
Gastrostomy tube, optional
Silastic sheeting (for defect repair), optional

Special notes

See Repair of Congenital Atresia of the Esophagus, p. 482.

OMPHALOCELE REPAIR

Definition

Correction of a defect of the umbilicus through which the abdominal viscera protrude outside of the abdominal cavity.

Discussion

This congenital defect is evident at birth. The size and extent of an omphalocele is variable, from one containing the greater portion of the intra-abdominal viscera including the spleen and liver, to one containing a small loop of intestine. There is no skin covering the defect, but rather amnion or peri-

toneum that may rupture at birth, exposing the patient to increased risk of infection. The viscera involved have not undergone the usual rotation and posterior fixation; the blood supply may be under tension and torsion leading to edema and/or circulatory compromise. Additional congenital abnormalities are present in approximately half of these newborns. These considerations and the ability of the abdominal cavity to safely contain the contents of the omphalocele will determine whether a single or a staged repair will be necessary. Hyperalimentation may be required to assure adequate nutrition.

Procedure

Single-Stage Repair. The omphalocele is covered with warm-saline-moistened laparotomy pads. An incision is made separating the skin from the borders of the sac. The umbilical vessels are ligated. The sac and the rim of the defect are excised. A gastrostomy (see Pediatric Gastrostomy, p. 490) may be performed. The viscera are reduced within the abdomen. The abdomen is closed in layers.

Multiple-Stage Repair. In the larger omphalocele when the defect cannot be closed and/or the abdominal cavity is too limited to contain the contents of the sac, an attempt is made to mobilize surrounding skin to cover the protruding viscera. When this, too, is not possible, a synthetic material such as Silastic or silicone mesh or cone is sutured around the periphery over the viscera. As growth permits, in 6 to 24 months complete repair of the defect may be achieved in one or more additional procedures.

Preparation of the patient

See Pediatric General Information, p. 467; the head and extremities are covered prior to positioning. The patient is supine. Extremities are restrained using padded restraints. Apply pediatric electrosurgical dispersive pad. A nasogastric tube is passed.

Skin preparation

The surgeon usually prefers to do skin preparation. If the circulator performs skin preparation, full instructions must be obtained regarding treatment of the omphalocele. Using warm preparation solutions only cleanse the omphalocele according to directions; cleanse the rest of the abdomen extending from the axillae to midthighs, and down to the table at the sides.

Draping

Folded towels and a pediatric laparotomy sheet

Equipment

Body heat maintenance equipment (e.g., heating lamps, warming mattress)
Covering for head and extremities
Padded restraints
Electrosurgical unit
Suction (with specimen trap for accurate blood loss measurement)
Scale (to weigh sponges)

Instrumentation

Pediatric major procedures tray
Hemoclip appliers (short, medium)

Supplies

Basin set
Blades (2) No. 15
Needle magnet or counter
Electrosurgical pencil (with needle tip)
Syringe, 60 ml (for accurate irrigation measurement), optional
Hemoclips (small, medium)
Silastic or silicone mesh or cone (for defect repair), available

Special notes

Do not begin the skin preparation without instructions from the surgeon.

Determine if an intravenous cutdown and/or hyperalimentation line are to be done first.

Accurately measure irrigation fluids.

Weigh sponges immediately to reduce evaporation factor.

Check with blood bank that blood is available as ordered.

PEDIATRIC UMBILICAL HERNIORRHAPHY

Definition

Repair of an abdominal wall defect at the umbilicus through which viscera protrude.

Discussion

Umbilical hernia is the incomplete closure of the umbilical ring at the fascial level. Skin coverage is intact. Although noted at birth or early infancy, a significant number of these defects close in time. Unless there is a large defect, or symptoms present, surgery may be delayed for 18 months or longer. The umbilicus is preserved rather than excised to maintain body image.

Procedure

Usually an infraumbilical hemicircumferential incision is made. The sac is dissected free and the fascial rim of the defect exposed. The dome of the sac is transsected and can be left attached to the undersurface of the umbilical skin. The sac is closed (excess sac is excised) and replaced intra-abdominally. The fascial anterior rectus sheath defect is closed by any of several simple or overlapping layer techniques. The umbilical skin or retained dome of the sac is sutured to the fascia to recreate the umbilical identation. The skin incision is closed; fine catgut sutures may be used.

Preparation of the patient

See Pediatric General Information, p. 467. The patient is supine. Extremities are covered and restrained with padded restraints. Apply pediatric electrosurgical dispersive pad.

Skin preparation

Using warm preparation solutions only, begin by cleansing the abdomen at the umbilicus extending from the axillae to the upper thighs, and down to the table at the sides.

Draping

Folded towels and a pediatric laparotomy sheet

Equipment

Body heat maintenance equipment (e.g., heating
    lamps, warming mattress)
Covering for head and extremities
Restraints, padded
Electrosurgical unit

Instrumentation

Pediatric minor procedures tray

Supplies

Basin set
Electrosurgical pencil (with needle tip)
Blades (2) No. 15
Needle magnet or counter
Dissectors (e.g., peanut)

PEDIATRIC INGUINAL HERNIORRHAPHY

Definition

Ligation of the patent processus vaginalis through which intra-abdominal viscera have passed into the inguinal canal.

Discussion

Most pediatric inguinal hernias are indirect; correction is accomplished by high ligation of the patent processus vaginalis (sac) without repair of the inguinal floor. In the male, care is taken to avoid injury to the spermatic cord structures. A hydrocele or undescended testis may be associated with the hernia and is corrected at the same time. In females, ovary and fallopian tubes may be encountered within the hernial sac. These hernias are repaired when the diagnosis is made (as an emergency if incarceration occurs). Some surgeons explore the opposite side even if no evidence of contralateral hernia is present preoperatively.

Procedure

A transverse incision is made. The external oblique aponeurosis is exposed and incised. The ilioinguinal nerve is avoided. The contents of the inguinal canal are explored and the sac identified. High ligation is performed; the sac is transsected. If a hydrocele is present, the sac is delivered into the wound and opened to the testis; a portion may be excised. The external oblique aponeurosis is closed, and the skin is closed using a subcuticular suture. In the female, if a sliding component is present (i.e., part of the sac wall is broad ligament or mesentery), the sac is transsected and ligated including the round ligament, as close to the sliding portion as possible. Transversalis fascia is closed over the defect prior to closure of the external oblique aponeurosis. The skin is closed.

Preparation of the patient

See Pediatric General Information, p. 467. The patient is supine. The extremities are covered and restrained using padded restraints. Apply pediatric electrosurgical dispersive pad.

Skin preparation

Using warm preparation solutions only, begin cleansing the inguinal area on the affected side extending from nipples to midthighs, and down to the table at the sides.

Draping

Folded towels and a pediatric transverse sheet or sheet with a small fenestration

Equipment, Instrumentation, Supplies, and Special notes

See Pediatric Umbilical Herniorrhaphy, p. 479.

REPAIR OF CONGENITAL ATRESIA OF THE ESOPHAGUS

Definition

The restoration of esophageal continuity and the repair of the often associated tracheoesophageal fistula.

Discussion

Several types of these anomalies are found. In all there is lack of a patent esophagus in continuity with the stomach. The stomach either may or may not contain air by virtue of the connection with the trachea. In the most common type the upper esophagus ends blindly, and the lower esophagus communicates with the trachea. The upper and lower esophagus may exhibit muscular continuity, but without luminal continuity. Air distends the stomach. The upper esophagus may end blindly, with the lower esophagus extending above the diaphragm for a variable distance, but not communicating with the trachea. Here the stomach is empty. Diagnosis is made by the newborn's inability to take oral fluids without regurgitation and aspiration; it is confirmed by x-ray studies. Antibiotics are given and dehydration is corrected. Additional anomalies including those of the cardiovascular and gastrointestinal systems may be encountered.

When air is not present in the stomach a gastrostomy (see Pediatric Gastrostomy, p. 490) is performed and tube feedings are begun. Cervical esophagostomy for drainage of secretions and definitive reconstruction is performed in stages. Final restoration may be delayed (even for as long as 2 years). A colonic segment interposition is employed to restore esophageal continuity. If the air-filled stomach compromises respiration and there is reflux of gastric contents into the trachea, gastrostomy is performed immediately and the definitive surgery is delayed. When the stomach is only moderately distended, definitive single-stage correction may be done employing a transpleural or extrapleural approach.

Procedure

A transpleural approach may be used. A right posterolateral incision is made over the fifth rib. The pleura is entered in the fourth intercostal space; the azygous vein is divided. The mediastinal pleura is incised and the lower esophagus is exposed and mobilized. The tracheoesophageal fistula is transsected and closed. The integrity of the tracheal closure is tested for air leaks by filling the chest with saline. Esophageal continuity is established by any of several one- or two-layer techniques depending on the diameter and muscular wall thickness of the upper and lower segments. A small-gauge feeding tube may be passed transnasally into the esophagus across the anastomotic site into the stomach for postoperative feeding. The connective tissues about the divided azygous vein may be used to reinforce the anastomosis, as may the mediastinal pleura. A chest tube is placed and the chest is closed.

Preparation of the patient

See Pediatric General Information, p. 467; the head and the extremities are covered prior to positioning. Following endotracheal intubation the patient is placed in a left lateral position (right side up). A small pillow is placed between the legs. The left leg is straight. The left arm is extended; a small roll may be required just below the axilla to decrease pressure on the brachial plexus. The right arm is positioned on a pillow. The extremities may be restrained with padded restraints. The feet are padded, positioned, and supported as necessary to maintain good body alignment. Apply pediatric electrosurgical dispersive pad.

Skin preparation

Using warm preparation solutions only, begin cleansing the chest at the level of the fifth rib extending from the neck to the iliac crest, and down to the table anteriorly and posteriorly.

Draping

Four folded towels, sterile, plastic adhesive drape (optional), and pediatric laparotomy sheet

Equipment

Body heat maintenance equipment (e.g., heat lamps, warming mattress)
Covering for head and extremities

Restraints, padded
Small pillow, small roll
Suction (with specimen trap for accurate blood loss
    measurement)
Electrosurgical unit
Scale (to weigh sponges)

Instrumentation

Pediatric major procedures tray
Pediatric thoracotomy tray
Bone cutter, small
Hemoclip appliers (short, medium)
Beaver knife handle, optional

Supplies

Basin set
Sterile, plastic adhesive drape, optional
Blades (2) No. 15
Beaver blade, optional
Suction tubing
Needle magnet or counter
Electrosurgical pencil (with needle tip)
60-ml syringe with cone tip (for accurate irrigation
    measurement), optional
Vessel loops or ¼" umbilical tape
Infant chest drainage unit (e.g., Pleurevac)
Chest tube (e.g., No. 10 Argyle)
Double cone connector
Hemoclips (small, medium)
Bone wax

Special notes

Determine if an intravenous cutdown and/or
hyperalimentation line are to be done first.
Check with blood bank that blood is ready and
available as ordered.
Weigh used sponges immediately to reduce
evaporation factor.
Measure irrigation fluids accurately.

When transferring patient keep the closed drainage system below body level.

INSERTION OF A CENTRAL VENOUS CATHETER (PEDIATRIC)

Definition

Introduction of Silastic tubing into the subclavian, internal jugular, cephalic, or facial vein in order to administer parenteral nutrition or chemotherapy, or to monitor hemodynamics and to replace fluids and blood.

Discussion

A central venous pressure catheter may be inserted on an acute basis for hemodynamic monitoring and for rapid replacement of fluids and blood, or for ongoing access for purposes of parenteral nutrition or administration of chemotherapy or any other drug. The main advantage of this technique is to spare the patient frequent venipunctures and to decrease the likelihood of inducing phlebitis if more peripheral veins are used. Several types of Silastic catheters are available.

Procedure

A small incision is made over the external jugular vein in the lateral neck. The catheter is passed into the incised vein (confirmed by the aspiration of blood) to a predetermined length in order to be in the superior vena cava. A subcutaneous tunnel is made from the incision, employing a blunt tunneling instrument, to the anterior chest lateral to the sternum. The catheter exits through the tunnel and is sutured to the skin. The position of the catheter is confirmed by x-ray or fluoroscopy. The catheter is immediately connected by a heparin lock or a three-way stopcock to an appropriate intravenous solution. The venotomy and initial incision are closed.

Preparation of the patient

See Pediatric General Information, p. 467; the head and extremities may be covered prior to positioning. The patient is supine with the head and neck turned to the left (right side up); a small roll may be used to extend the neck. Cover the extremities and restrain them using padded restraints. The procedure may be done under local anesthesia with anesthesia standby on newborns and cooperative children; otherwise, general anesthesia is administered. Apply pediatric electrosurgical dispersive pad.

Skin preparation

Using warm preparation solution only begin cleansing the supraclavicular area, extending from the infra-auricular border to the umbilicus (including the right shoulder) if the catheter is to exit the anterior thorax. If the catheter is to exit from the epigastrium, extend the preparation to the pubic symphysis. Prepare the skin to the table on the right side and well beyond the midline on the left side.

Draping

Folded towels and a pediatric laparotomy sheet

Equipment

Body heat maintenance equipment (e.g., heating lamps or warming mattress)
Covering for head and extremities
Image intensifier or portable x-ray machine with cassettes
Restraints, padded
Small roll
Electrosurgical unit

Instrumentation

Pediatric major procedures tray
Bulldog clamps (assorted small)
Tunneling instrument

Supplies

Basin set
Blades (1) No. 15, (1) No. 11
Needle magnet or counter
Electrosurgical pencil (with needle tip)
Graduate and syringe for heparin solution (optional)
Local anesthetic, e.g., lidocaine (Xylocaine) 1%, with syringe and needle (local)
Silastic catheter and introducer (e.g., Broviac)
Radiopaque dye (e.g., Hypaque), optional
Intravenous tubing
Heparin lock or three-way stopcock
Intravenous solution (e.g., 10% dextrose)

Special notes

Determine if image intensifier or portable x-ray is to be used and prepare the table accordingly. Notify x-ray department.

Some warming mattresses interfere with fluoroscopy.

Observe x-ray precautions, see p. 20.

PYLOROMYOTOMY FOR CONGENITAL HYPERTROPHIC PYLORIC STENOSIS

Definition

Incision of the hypertrophied muscles of the pylorus in order to relieve pyloric obstruction.

Discussion

This congenital condition usually becomes evident a few weeks after birth with progressive episodes of vomiting caused by pyloric muscular hypertrophy creating a mechanical obstruction. The muscle mass ("olive") can often be palpated transabdominally. A thin solution of barium contrast medium may be necessary to confirm the diagnosis. A Ramsted-Fredet pyloromyotomy, the procedure of choice, divides the pyloric muscle leaving the mucosa (and submucosa) intact and relieving the condition.

Procedure

A high right rectus splitting incision is made over the liver; a transverse or oblique incision can also be used. The peritoneum is incised and the pylorus delivered into the wound. The pylorus is incised longitudinally anteriorly from the pyloric vein and pyloroduodenal junction proximally over the extent of the hypertrophic muscle. Using a pyloric spreading forceps all remaining circular muscle fibers are separated to the level of the submucosa. Any laceration of the gastric or duodenal mucosa is immediately repaired. After hemostasis is obtained the wound is closed.

Preparation of the patient

See Pediatric General Information, p. 467; the head and extremities are covered prior to positioning. The patient is supine. Extremities are restrained using padded restraints. Apply pediatric electrosurgical dispersive pad.

Skin preparation

Using warm preparation solutions only begin cleansing over the right upper abdomen extending from the axillae to the pubic symphysis, and down to the table at the sides.

Draping

Folded towels and a pediatric laparotomy sheet

Equipment

Body heat maintenance equipment (e.g., heating lamps, warming mattress)
Restraints, padded
Electrosurgical unit
Suction (available)

Instrumentation

Pediatric major procedures tray
Pyloric spreader

Supplies

Basin set
Electrosurgical pencil (with needle tip)
Blades (2) No. 15
Needle magnet or counter
Dissectors (e.g., peanut)

PEDIATRIC GASTROSTOMY

Definition

Establishment of an artificial opening into the stomach exiting onto the skin of the abdominal wall.

Discussion

Gastrostomy is most frequently performed to permit liquid feedings; it may also be done to permit gastric drainage or retrograde dilation of an esophageal stricture. Gastrostomy can be an independent procedure or performed in conjunction with other abdominal surgeries.

Procedure

As an independent procedure: A short left-upper-quadrant transverse or vertical incision is made. The greater curvature of the stomach is identified. Two pursestring sutures are placed in the stomach; a stab wound is made in the center of the pursestrings, and a gastrostomy catheter is inserted. The pursestring sutures are then tightened and tied to secure the tube. The tube is brought out through a stab wound lateral to the incision. The stomach is sutured to the peritoneum about the stab wound. The tube is sutured to the skin. The wound is closed.

Preparation of the patient, Skin preparation, Draping, and Equipment

See Pediatric Umbilical Herniorrhaphy, p. 479.

Instrumentation

Pediatric major procedures tray

Supplies

Basin set
Electrosurgical pencil (with needle tip)
Needle magnet
Blades (2) No. 15, (1) No. 11
Gastrostomy catheter (e.g., Pezzer, Malecot, or Foley)

Special notes

Check with the surgeon regarding the type and size of gastrostomy catheter.
Keep soiled instruments isolated in a basin.

RELIEF OF INTESTINAL OBSTRUCTION (PEDIATRIC)

Definition

Refers to the reestablishment of intestinal patency in any number of conditions that present with blockage of the intestinal tract.

Discussion

Intestinal obstruction in the newborn becomes apparent shortly after birth with symptoms of emesis, abdominal distention, and failure to pass flatus and meconium. Urgent treatment is often mandatory. The conditions responsible for obstruction are numerous including intussusception, esophageal atresia, atresia and stenosis of the duodenum, small bowel, and colon, annular pancreas, hypertrophic pyloric stenosis, imperforate anus, congenital malrotation, volvulus, congenital bands, infarction, meconium ileus, aganglionic megacolon, internal hernias, strangulated hernias, and infection. Treatment depends on the diagnosis; during the course of surgery the search is made for additional abnormalities. Intestinal obstructive symptoms may also be seen in otherwise unrelated conditions such as cerebral injury with persistent emesis and in pulmonary infections.

Procedure

For duodenal atresia a paramedian or transverse incision is made in the upper abdomen. The abdomen is explored, and the site of obstruction and other conditions are identified. Bypass rather than resection of the obstructed duodenal segment (usually second portion) is performed. An antecolic duodenojejunostomy is usually the procedure of choice. A loop of proximal jejunum is brought anterior to the transverse colon to the side of the distended proximal duodenum. A side-to-side anastomosis is fashioned in one or two layers according to the surgeon's preference and size of the small jejunal lumen. The abdomen is closed in layers.

Preparation of the patient, Skin preparation, and Draping

See Pyloromyotomy for Congenital Hypertophic Pyloric Stenosis, p. 488.

Equipment

Body heat maintenance equipment (e.g., heating
    lamps, warming mattress)
Restraints, padded
Electrosurgical unit
Suction

Instrumentation

Pediatric major procedures tray
Pediatric gastrointestinal tray
Automatic stapling device (optional)

Supplies

Basin set
Electrosurgical pencil (with needle tip)
Blades (2) No. 15
Needle magnet or counter
Dissectors (e.g., peanut)
Staples, optional

Special notes

Keep all soiled instruments isolated in a basin.

REDUCTION OF PEDIATRIC INTUSSUSCEPTION

Definition

Reduction of intussusception (in the child) is the correction of a condition in which there is an invagination of a segment of the intestine into an adjacent segment.

Discussion

This entity, typically seen in the older male infant, is characterized by sudden episodes of severe abdominal pain, emesis, and subsequent passage of bloody mucus. The infant seems to feel well shortly thereafter. Additional bouts follow until intestinal obstruction becomes evident. The most common site of intussusception is about the ileocecal valve, in which the terminal ileum (intussusceptum) becomes invaginated into the cecum (intussuscipiens). If not reduced, either spontaneously or by the hydrostatic pressure of a barium enema examination, gangrene will ultimately ensue.

Procedure

A low midline incision is employed. The intussusception is manually reduced. If there is resistance to reduction or compromised bowel is encountered, a resection is done with primary anastomosis or the ends of the bowel are brought out as stomas through separate incisions. Anastomosis is performed as a secondary procedure. The abdomen is closed.

Preparation of the patient

See Pediatric General Information, p. 467; the head and extremities are covered prior to positioning the patient. The patient is supine. Extremities are restrained using padded restraints. Apply pediatric electrosurgical dispersive pad.

Skin preparation

Using warm preparation solutions only, begin cleansing for a low midline incision extending from the nipples to the upper thighs, and down to the table at the sides.

Draping

Folded towels and a pediatric laparotomy sheet

Equipment

Body heat maintenance equipment (e.g., warming mattress, heating lamps)
Restraints, padded
Electrosurgical unit
Suction

Instrumentation

Pediatric major procedures tray
Pediatric gastrointestinal procedures tray
Automatic stapling device (optional)

Supplies

Blades (3) No. 15
Needle magnet or counter
Electrosurgical pencil (with needle tip)
Suction tubing
Vessel loops or umbilical tape, ¼"
Staples, optional

Special notes

If a bowel resection is performed, isolate soiled instruments in a basin.

PEDIATRIC COLOSTOMY

Definition

Formation of an opening into the colon, which is exteriorized onto the anterior abdominal wall as a stoma.

Discssion

Colostomy is performed to bypass an obstructed colonic segment distally or for diversion of the fecal stream to minimize contamination because of perforation or infection and to "protect" a distal anastomosis by eliminating passage of the fecal stream across it. Several types of colostomy may be created; transverse and sigmoid are the most common. Most pediatric colostomies are temporary, but may be permanent when the rectum is congenitally absent, or unable to be reconstructed, or in cases of neurologic and neoplastic processes. Colostomy may be performed as an independent procedure or in conjunction with other abdominal surgery. X-ray studies help to determine the appropriate site. Colostomy may be done as an emergency procedure.

Procedure

For an obstructive process or congenital absence of the distal sigmoid colon or rectum, a sigmoid or descending colon colostomy is made. An oblique incision is made in the left lower abdomen, and the muscles are either separated (as in gridiron incision) or divided. The abdomen is explored to identify any associated abnormalities or obstructive bands. The colon may be brought out as a loop over a rod or bridge to prevent retraction, or it can be divided, the distal end closed, and the proximal end brought out through the incision, or through an adjacent limited incision as an end-colostomy. In either situation, the colon and mesentery are sutured to ensuing layers of abdominal wall to prevent prolapse or herniation. The stoma wall is matured by suturing the full thickness of the stoma of the skin. Tension is avoided in order to prevent retraction or circulatory compromise, and to allow for increasing thickness of the abdominal wall, with growth and improved postoperative nutrition. The main incision is closed; additional draping is used to avoid undue contamination. The sequence of closure of the wound and final preparation of the stoma varies with the surgeon. At the completion of the procedure a colostomy pouch is applied to the stoma.

Preparation of the patient

See Pediatric General Information, p. 467; the head and extremities are covered prior to positioning. The patient is supine. Extremities are restrained using padded restraints. Apply pediatric electrosurgical dispersive pad.

Skin preparation

Using warm preparation solutions only, begin cleansing the left lower abdomen extending from the nipples to the upper thighs, and down to the table at the sides.

Draping

Folded towels and a pediatric laparotomy sheet

Equipment

Body heat maintenance equipment (e.g., heating lamps, warming mattress)
Restraints, padded
Electrosurgical unit
Suction (available)

Instrumentation

Pediatric major procedures tray
Pediatric gastrointestinal procedures tray

Supplies

Basin set
Blades (1) No. 10, (2) No. 15
Electrosurgical pencil (with needle tip)
Vessel loops or umbilical tape ¼"
Dissectors (e.g., peanut)
Suction tubing, optional
Glass rod and tubing with colostomy pouch (e.g.,
    Karaya Seal or plastic bridge) and loop colos-
    tomy set (e.g., Hollister)

Special notes

Keep soiled instruments isolated in a basin.

PEDIATRIC COLORECTAL RESECTION FOR AGANGLIONIC MEGACOLON/HIRSCHSPRUNG'S DISEASE

Definition

Removal of the aganglionic portion of the colon and
rectum with the anastomosis of the proximal normal
colon to the distal rectum or anus.

Discussion

The section of colon removed, which can include a
short segment of rectum and/or colon, or less often
the entire colon, represents a functional obstruction
caused by a lack of ganglion cells in the muscular
layer (myenteric plexus) and the inability of this distal segment to relax permitting passage of feces. The
problem may be recognized soon after birth or in
later infancy (or if the absence of ganglion cells is
partial, diagnosis may be delayed until adulthood).
Constipation with abdominal distention, growth failure, anemia, and episodes of paradoxical diarrhea
occur. Necrotizing enterocolitis can develop in the
neonate and is often fatal if not treated promptly.

Barium enema examination and rectal muscle biopsy to demonstrate absence of ganglion cells are diagnostic. Colostomy (see Pediatric Colostomy, p. 496) is indicated in newborns and children who are either ill or not responsive to measures to alleviate constipation and abdominal distention. The site of the colostomy must be proximal to the aganglionic segment, as confirmed by histologic examination. When the infant has regained good health and weight of 13.5 kg (30 pounds), or even until late childhood, surgical correction is undertaken. The aganglionic segment is resected and the proximal colon anastomosed to the distal rectum or anus.

The Swenson "pull-through" procedure is most often employed. The Duhamel procedure, in which the distal rectum is not excised, but allowed to form a common lumen with a segment of normal proximal colon brought anterior to the rectum by crushing the adjacent bowel walls with clamps, has its advocates. In the Soave procedure the distal rectum is preserved, but denuded of mucosa, forming a sleeve through which a normal colonic segment is passed to the anus with local anastomosis. These latter procedures avoid dissection in the pelvis sparing possible injury to genital nerves, but do not necessarily give better results than the Swenson procedure or its several modifications.

Procedure

A left paramedian incision is made. The colostomy, if present, is excised. The sigmoid colon is mobilized and superior hemorrhoidal vessels are divided, taking care not to injure the ureters. Frozen section of colon muscle biopsies may be done at the level of the division of the bowel to make certain of the presence of ganglia. The pelvis is entered, the lateral rectal ligaments are cut, and the rectum is further mobilized, staying close to the bowel to avoid injury to the autonomic nerves. A ring clamp or long Babcock forceps is inserted transanally and a segment of dissected colon is seized from within; with counterpressure from the pelvis the colon is everted and "pulled through" the anus. The coats of the everted bowel are circumferentially incised, suturing the rim of the retained portion of colon to the anal canal in a single or double layer. The specimen is thereby amputated and the anastomosis completed. The anastomotic ring is then inverted, replacing it within the anal canal. The abdominal incision is closed.

Preparation of the patient

See Pediatric General Information, p. 467; the head and extremities are covered prior to positioning. Following the induction of anesthesia, the patient is positioned in modified lithotomy or supine position with the knees bent in a modified frog-leg position. A folded towel is placed under the buttocks. The legs may be held in position using abdominal dressing pads and adhesive tape. Padded restraints are used on the upper extremities. Apply pediatric electrosurgical dispersive pad. Check with the surgeon regarding insertion of a Foley catheter and irrigation of the rectum with warm saline.

Skin preparation

Use warm preparation solutions only. For a *combined approach:* Begin cleansing for a left paramedian incision extending from the nipples to the knees, and down to the table at the sides. Cleanse inner thighs, genitalia, exposed buttocks, perineum, and anus (discarding each sponge after preparing anus).

For *separate approaches: (Perineal):* Begin at the pubic symphysis, cleanse inner thighs, genitalia, exposed buttocks, perineum, and anus (discarding each sponge after preparing anus). *(Abdominal):* Begin cleansing for a left paramedian incision extending from the nipples to the midthighs, and down to the table at the sides.

Draping

The patient may be draped all at once for both the abdominal and perineal approaches, or the patient may be reprepared and redraped for the perineal approach.

Combined approach: Tuck a drape sheet under the patient's buttocks. Drape the abdomen and perineal area with folded towels. Towels may be secured by a sterile, plastic adhesive drape, staples, or with sutures. A pediatric laparotomy sheet covers the field.

For the *perineal approach* the abdominal wound is covered and a hole is cut in the laparotomy sheet in the perineal area. If the patient is to be reprepared and redraped: tuck a drape sheet under the patient's buttocks; drape the perineum with folded towels and a pediatric laparotomy sheet.

For the *abdominal approach* gowns and gloves are changed, the patient is reprepared, redraped, and the instruments are changed. The patient is draped with folded towels on the abdomen and a pediatric laparotomy sheet.

Equipment

Body heat maintenance equipment (e.g., heating lamps, warming mattress)
Covering for the head and extremities
Pediatric stirrups (modified lithotomy)
Suction (with specimen trap for accurate blood loss measurement)
Electrosurgical unit
Scale (to weigh sponges)
Mayo stand (additional) and/or back table for perineal approach

Instrumentation

Abdominal Approach
Pediatric major procedures tray

Pediatric Balfour retractors
Brain/Ribbon/Malleable retractor (small)
Hemoclip appliers (short, medium)
Hegar dilators, small
Automatic stapling device (optional)

Perineal approach
Pediatric major procedures tray
Ruler

Supplies

Basin set
Electrosurgical pencil (with needle tip)
Bulb syringe
Hemoclips (small, medium)
Suction tubing
Sterile, plastic adhesive drape, optional
Needle magnet or counter
Blades (1) No. 10, (4) No. 15
Foley catheter (e.g., No. 8) for bladder
Dissectors (e.g., peanut)
Staples, optional

Special notes

In positioning the patient do not allow adhesive tape to come in direct contact with the skin. Protect skin with tincture of benzoin.

Check with blood bank to determine that blood is available as ordered.

Weigh used sponges immediately to reduce evaporation factor.

Measure irrigation fluids accurately.

Be prepared for multiple bowel tissue biopsies.

REPAIR OF IMPERFORATE ANUS

Definition

Establishment of colorectal continuity where there is an absence of an anal opening.

Discussion

There are four classes of imperforate anus.

Types

   I Stenosis at the anus or distal rectum
  II Membranous barrier at the anus
 III Rectum ends in a blind pouch above the perineum
 IV Anal canal canal and distal rectum end in a blind pouch proximally, and the more proximal rectum ends in a blind pouch above the distal segment

Type I may be treated by dilation; ultimately if stricture persists a plastic procedure will be necessary.

In *Type II* a simple anal membrane needs only to be incised and dilated. The mucosa can be sutured to the skin.

Type III is often associated with various fistulas (rectovesical, rectourethral, rectovaginal, rectoperineal) that may allow the passage of the fecal stream by way of the genitourinary tract. Correction of these conditions depends on the presentation.

Type IV, which is rare, is treated by preliminary colostomy with definitive repair several months later by direct anastomosis or "pull-through" procedure. Type III with its variety of fistulas is initially treated by colostomy, especially if other abnormalities are present and the infant is in otherwise ill health or premature. Definitive repair can be performed after 3 months of age.

Procedure

In the male type III procedure without fistula, the procedure is done by the *perineal approach* only if x-ray confirms the blind pouch is less than 1.5 cm from the anal dimple. A catheter (8Fr or 10Fr) is passed into the bladder. The location of the anal sphincter is determined by a nerve stimulator. A small vertical incision is made within the anal dimple. The rectal pouch is dissected free from surrounding stricture so that it can be brought to skin level without tension. The bowel is opened and meconium aspirated. The full thickness of the rectal wall is sutured to the skin.

When the rectal pouch is greater than 1.5 cm above the sphincter, a *combined abdominoperineal approach* is used. The bladder is catheterized with the patient in modified lithotomy position. (This gives simultaneous access to abdomen and perineum.) An incision is made within the anal dimple as above and the sphincter is dilated. A left lower oblique or a left paramedial abdominal incision is made. The sigmoid colon and rectum are mobilized taking care not to injure the ureters. Meconium is aspirated from the distal portion of the colon with a large-bore needle and the puncture site sutured closed. Dissection continues until the rectum can reach the perineal floor without tension. Care is taken to preserve vascular arcades. The end of the bowel is passed through a tunnel within the levator muscles, made via the perineal incision. The pelvic peritoneum is closed. The abdominal wound is closed. The full thickness of the rectum is sutured to the skin overlying the sphincter as above.

Preparation of the patient

See Pediatric General Information, p. 467; the head and extremities are covered prior to positioning. Following the induction of anesthesia the patient is positioned in modified lithotomy or supine position with the knees bent in a modified frog-leg position. A folded towel is placed under the buttocks. The legs may be held in position using abdominal dressing pads and adhesive tape. Padded restraints are used on the upper extremities. Apply pediatric electrosurgical dispersive pad. Check with the surgeon regarding the insertion of a Foley catheter.

Skin preparation

Use warm preparation solutions only. See Pediatric Colorectal Resection, p. 498. For an extensive procedure, follow the preparation for a combined approach; for a limited procedure, follow the preparation for a perineal approach.

Draping

See Pediatric Colorectal Resection, p. 498. For an extensive procedure, drape as for a combined approach; for a limited procedure, drape as for a perineal approach.

Equipment

Covering for head and extremities
Body heat maintenance equipment (e.g., heat lamp, warming mattress)
Electrosurgical unit
Suction (with specimen trap for accurate blood loss measurement)
Scale (to weigh sponges for an extensive procedure)

Instrumentation

Pediatric major procedures tray
Hegar dilators, probes
For extensive procedures: See Pediatric Colorectal Resection, p. 498

Supplies

Basin set
Blades (2) No. 15
Needle magnet or counter
Suction tubing
Bulb syringe
Electrosurgical pencil (with needle tip)
Nerve stimulator (locator)

For extensive procedures: See Pediatric Colorectal
Resection, p. 498

Special notes

In positioning the patient do not allow adhesive
tape to come into direct contact with the skin. Protect
the skin with tincture of benzoin.

For extensive procedures: See Pediatric Colorectal Resection, p. 498.

Isolate soiled instruments in a basin.

Part IV

INSTRUMENT TRAYS

The chapters on instrument trays complement the instrumentation section of each procedure. The instruments included are meant to be representative of particular types used for specific functions. Substitutions for instruments that can be similarly used can be made according to the preference of the surgeons at each institution.

Today there is an ever-increasing number and variety of surgical instruments. Many traditionally used instruments have been discarded or modified. Some instruments are known by more than one name or by various colloquial names even within the same institution. The composition of the trays appearing in this guide, therefore, will be familiar to most readers, although perhaps not precisely what might be encountered at their own surgical facility.

These trays are based on anatomic regions or frequently performed specific procedures. To simplify the listings of the tray components certain liberties have been taken to avoid excessive terminology and subsections. Therefore, the category of forceps refers only to "thumb" forceps; the category of clamps includes hemostatic forceps, grasping forceps, towel clips, and needle holders. The miscellaneous subheading is an all-inclusive category for all instruments that do not fit under any of the main categories.

Chapter 21

GENERAL SURGERY TRAYS

MAJOR PROCEDURES TRAY

Retractors

2 Ribbon/Malleable (1) 1½", (1) 2½"
3 Richardson (1) small, (1) medium, (1) large
2 Goulet
2 Army-Navy
3 Deaver (1) narrow, (1) medium, (1) wide

Forceps

2 Tissue without teeth (1) 5½", (1) 10"
3 Tissue with teeth (1) 5½", (1) 8", (1) 10"
2 Russian (1) 7", (1) 10"
6 DeBakey (2) 6", (2) 7¾", (2) 9"
2 Adson with teeth

Scissors

2 Straight Mayo 6¼"
1 Curved Mayo 6¼"
1 Metzenbaum 7"
1 Wire cutter

Clamps

10 Towel clip 5½"
18 Curved Crile 5½"
 6 Straight Crile 5½"
 6 Straight Kocher 6¼"
 6 Allis 6"
 4 Babcock 6"
12 Curved Pean (6) 6¼", (6) 8"
 4 Tonsil (Schnidt) 7½"
 2 Right-angle 8"
 6 Needle holder (2) 6", (2) 7", (2) 8"
 4 Sponge forceps 10"
 2 Carmalt 8"

Suction tubes or tips

1 Poole
1 Yankauer 10⅜"

Miscellaneous

3 Knife handles (2) No. 3, (1) No. 7
1 Probe, malleable
1 Grooved director

BASIC/MINOR PROCEDURES TRAY

Retractors

2 Goulet
2 Army-Navy
1 Weitlaner, sharp 6½"
1 Ribbon/Malleable 1"
1 Deaver, narrow
1 Richardson, small
2 Senn, sharp

Forceps

2 Tissue without teeth 5½"

2 Tissue with teeth 5½"
1 Adson without teeth
2 Adson with teeth
1 Russian 7"
4 DeBakey (2) 6", (2) 7¾"

Scissors

1 Curved Mayo 6¼"
2 Straight Mayo 6¼"
3 Metzenbaum (1) 5¼", (1) 6", (1) 7"
1 Stevens tenotomy
1 Straight iris
1 Curved iris

Clamps

10 Towel clip (6) 3½", (4) 5½"
12 Curved mosquito 5¼"
2 Straight mosquito 5¼"
12 Curved Crile 5½"
2 Babcock 6"
4 Allis 6"
4 Straight Kocher 6¼"
2 Webster needle holder
4 Needle holder (2) 6", (2) 7"
2 Sponge forceps 7"

Suction tubes or tips

1 Yankauer 10⅜"
1 Poole
1 Frazier No. 10

Miscellaneous

3 Knife handles (2) No. 3, (1) No. 7
1 Probe, malleable
1 Grooved director
2 Medicine cups

LIMITED PROCEDURE TRAY

Retractors

2 Joseph skin hook
2 Senn, sharp

Forceps

1 Tissue with teeth 5½"
2 Adson with teeth
1 Adson without teeth
1 Adson-Brown

Scissors

1 Straight Mayo 6¼"
2 Metzenbaum (1) 5¼", (1) 6"
1 Stevens tenotomy
1 Curved iris
1 Straight iris

Clamps

4 Curved Crile 5½"
2 Straight Crile 5½"
4 Curved mosquito 5¼"
2 Needle holder 6"
8 Towel clip (4) 3½", (4) 5½"

Suction tubes or tips

1 Frazier No. 10

Miscellaneous

2 Knife handles No. 3
2 Medicine cups

THYROID TRAY

Retractors

2 Senn, sharp
1 Mahorner
2 Greene
2 Cushing vein
2 Gelpi
1 Weitlaner, sharp 5½"
2 Lahey

Forceps

2 Tissue without teeth 5½"
2 Tissue with teeth 5½"
2 Adson with teeth
2 DeBakey 6"

Scissors

2 Straight Mayo (1) 5¼", (1) 6¼"
2 Metzenbaum (1) 5¼", (1) 6"
1 Straight Metzenbaum 5¼"

Clamps

12 Curved mosquito 5¼"
 6 Curved Crile 5½"
 2 Curved Pean 6¼"
 6 Allis 6"
 2 Right-angle, fine
 2 Right-angle 6¼"
 2 Straight Kocher 6"
 2 Lahey
 2 Needle holder 6"
12 Towel clip 3½"

Suction tubes or tips

1 Frazier No. 8
1 Andrews 9½"

Miscellaneous

2 Knife handles No. 3

LONG INSTRUMENTS TRAY

Forceps

1 Tissue without teeth 10″
1 Tissue with teeth 10″

Scissors

1 Metzenbaum 9″

Clamps

4 Collier 10½″
3 Right-angle 11″
6 Pean 10″
4 Allis 10″
2 Babcock 10″
2 Needle holder 10″

Miscellaneous

1 Knife handle No. 3L, 8″

BILIARY TRACT PROCEDURES TRAY

Forceps

4 Randall stone (¼ curved length through 1 full
   curved length)

Scissors

1 Metzenbaum 9″

Scoops

3 Ferguson gallstone scoops (1) small, (1) medium, (1) large

Miscellaneous

9 Bakes common duct dilators (sizes 3 to 11)
1 Knife handle No. 3L
1 Spoon
1 Medicine cup
1 Probe, malleable
1 Alcock conical catheter adaptor
1 Ochsner gallbladder trocar

CHOLEDOCHOSCOPY TRAY

1 Choledochoscope
1 Light adaptor (for scope)
1 Fiberoptic cord
1 Biopsy forceps, flexible
1 Biopsy forceps, rigid
1 Foreign body forceps, flexible
1 Instrument guide
1 Stone crusher
1 Stopcock
1 Rubber washer
2 Rubber caps

BASIC RIGID SIGMOIDOSCOPY TRAY

1 Sigmoidoscope with obturator (steel) or 1 disposable sigmoidoscope with obturator
1 Illuminator head unit (for disposable scope only)
1 Sigmoidoscopy light cord
1 Insufflation bulb
1 Anoscope (e.g., Hirschmann, medium)

Special notes

Standard sigmoidoscope is 25 cm × 1.9 cm.

Disposable sigmoidoscopes are preferred over metal ones.

GASTROINTESTINAL PROCEDURES TRAY

Clamps

12 Pean (8) 6¼", (4) 10"
 4 Babcock 10"
 4 Kocher (Ochsner) 9"
 2 Straight Doyen intestinal 9¼"
 2 Curved Doyen intestinal 9¼"
Assorted variety, additional pairs of noncrushing
    bowel clamps, straight or right angle such as:
        Glassman intestinal
        DeBakey vascular
        Bainbridge intestinal
        Wertheim

Miscellaneous

8 Latex tubing pieces 6" × 3/16" (for Doyen)

RECTAL PROCEDURES TRAY

Retractors

1 Parks or 1 Pratt rectal speculum (with set screw)
3 Sawyer (1) small, (1) medium, (1) large

Forceps

1 Tissue without teeth 5½"
1 Tissue with teeth 5½"
1 Adson-Brown

Scissors

1 Straight Mayo 6¼"
1 Curved Mayo 6¼"
1 Metzenbaum 7"

Clamps

6 Curved Crile 5½"
6 Allis 6"
4 Towel clip 5½"
4 Pennington 5½"
2 Needle holder 6"

Suction tubes or tips

1 Yankauer 10⅜"

Miscellaneous

2 Knife handles No. 3
1 Probe, malleable
1 Grooved director
1 Crypt hook

Chapter 22

GYNECOLOGIC AND OBSTETRIC TRAYS

DILATATION & CURETTAGE (D & C) TRAY

Retractors

1 Auvard vaginal speculum, weighted

Forceps

1 Tissue without teeth 10"
1 Tissue with teeth 10"

Scissors

1 Straight Mayo 6¼"

Clamps

1 Straight Crile 5½"
2 Towel clip 5½"
1 Needle holder 8"

Tenaculums

1 Schroeder single-toothed
1 Jacobs

Dilators

8 Hegar (Nos. 3 to 4 through Nos. 17 to 18)
1 Goodell

Curettes

3 Sims sharp (1) small, (1) medium, (1) large
1 Thomas blunt, medium
1 Heaney endometrial

Miscellaneous

1 Biopsy punch
1 Randall stone forceps ¼ curved length
1 Bozeman packing forceps
1 Sponge forceps 10″
1 Uterine sound

CERVICAL CONE TRAY

Retractors

2 Heaney

Forceps

1 Tissue without teeth 10″
2 Tissue with teeth (1) 5½″, (1) 10″

Scissors

1 Straight Mayo 6¼″
1 Curved Mayo 6¼″
1 Metzenbaum 7″

Clamps

6 Curved Crile 5½″
2 Straight Kocher 6¼″
6 Allis 6″

2 Towel clip 5½"
1 Needle holder 7"

Miscellaneous

2 Knife handles (1) No. 3, (1) No. 7

VAGINAL HYSTERECTOMY TRAY

Retractors

1 Auvard vaginal speculum, weighted
1 Glennor, weighted
1 Deaver, narrow
2 Jackson, short
2 Heaney

Forceps

3 Tissue without teeth (1) 5½", (1) 8½", (1) 10"
3 Tissue with teeth (1) 5½", (1) 8½", (1) 10"
1 Russian 7"

Scissors

1 Curved Mayo 6¼"
2 Straight Mayo 6¼"
1 Metzenbaum 7"

Clamps

8 Straight Crile 5½"
8 Curved Crile 5½"
8 Allis 6"
4 Curved Pean 6¼"
12 Straight Kocher (Ochsner) (8) 6¼", (4) 8"
4 Curved Kocher (Ochsner) 8"
4 Heaney 8¼"
2 Babcock 10"
4 Sponge forceps 10"
4 Needle holder (2) 6", (2) 7"

2 Heaney needle holder
6 Towel clip 5½"

Suctions

1 Yankauer 10⅜"
1 Poole

Tenaculums

1 Jacobs
1 Schroeder single-toothed
1 Schroeder double-toothed

Miscellaneous

1 Bozeman packing forceps
1 Uterine sound
3 Knife handles (1) No. 3, (1) No. 3L 10", (1) No. 7

LAPAROSCOPY TRAY

Forceps

2 Adson with teeth

Scissors

1 Straight Mayo 6¼"

Clamps

3 Straight Crile 5½"
1 Needle holder 6"
4 Towel clip 5½"

Miscellaneous

1 Knife handle No. 3
1 Verres needle (2 parts)
1 Silastic tubing with connector

1 Trocar 7 mm (and trocar sleeve with valve)
1 Trocar 5 mm (and trocar sleeve)
Fiberoptic laparoscope(s):
  1 Fiberoptic light cord
  1 Electrosurgical biopsy forceps
  1 Electrosurgical cord
  1 Probe, calibrated
  1 Tissue grasping forceps
  1 Aspirating tube

ABDOMINAL HYSTERECTOMY TRAY

Forceps

1 Tissue with teeth 10"

Scissors

1 Curve Mayo 6¼"

Clamps

2 Lahey
5 Heany 8¼"
6 Straight Kocher (Ochsner) 8"
6 Curved Kocher (Ochsner) 8"
6 Curved Phaneuf 8¼"
6 Long Allis 10"

Tenaculums

1 Jacobs
1 Schroeder single-toothed
1 Schroeder double-toothed

CESAREAN SECTION TRAY

Retractors

2 Richardson (1) small, (1) medium

1 Deaver, extra wide 3"
2 Goulet
1 DeLee universal

Forceps

2 Tissue with teeth 5½"
2 Adson with teeth
1 Russian 7"

Scissors

2 Straight Mayo 6¼"
1 Curved Mayo 6¼"
1 Metzenbaum 7"
1 Umbilical
1 Lister bandage

Clamps

 4 Towel clip 5½"
12 Curved Crile 5½"
 4 Straight Crile 5½"
 2 Babcock 6"
 6 Allis 6"
 6 Straight Kocher 6¼"
 6 Pean 6¼"
 4 Sponge forceps 7"
 4 Pennington
 4 Needle holder (2) 7", (2) 8"

Suction tubes or tips

1 Poole
1 Yankauer 10⅜"

Miscellaneous

3 Knife handles (2) No. 3, (1) No. 4
5 Laparotomy rings, optional

Chapter 23

GENITOURINARY TRAYS

VASECTOMY TRAY

Retractors

2 Joseph skin hook
2 Senn, sharp

Forceps

1 Tissue without teeth 5½"
1 Tissue with teeth 5½"
1 Adson with teeth

Scissors

1 Metzenbaum 5¼"
1 Straight Mayo 6¼"

Clamps

2 Curved Crile 5½"
2 Curved mosquito 5¼"
2 Allis 6"

2 Towel clip 5½"
1 Needle holder 6"

Miscellaneous

1 Knife handle No. 3

OPEN PROSTATECTOMY TRAY

Rectractors

1 Judd-Mason

Clamps

6 Allis 10"
6 Babcock 10"
4 Lahey
1 Stratte needle holder 9"

Scissors

1 Metzenbaum 9"
1 Jorgenson 9"

KIDNEY TRAY

Forceps

4 Randall Stone (¼ curved length through 1 full
curved length)

Scissors

1 Metzenbaum 9"

Clamps

4 Babcock 9"
2 Herrick kidney pedicle 9½"
1 Pean vessel 10"

Chapter 24

THORACIC TRAYS

MEDIASTINOSCOPY TRAY

Retractors

2 Senn, sharp
2 Army-Navy
2 Carlen introducer
1 Weitlaner, blunt 5½"

Forceps

1 Tissue with teeth 5½"
1 Adson with teeth
1 DeBakey 6"

Scissors

1 Straight Mayo 6¼"
1 Metzenbaum 7"

Clamps

1 Straight Crile 5½"
4 Curved Crile 5½"
4 Towel clip 5½"
2 Needle holder, fine 6"

Suctions

1 Frazier No. 10
2 Suction-electrocoagulators and cords

Miscellaneous

1 Fiberoptic mediastinoscope
1 Fiberoptic light cord
3 Biopsy forceps, assorted
1 Circular biopsy
2 Staimey needles
1 Knife handle No. 3
1 Aspirating tube
1 Syringe, Luer lock, 5 ml

THORACOTOMY TRAY

Retractors

1 Finochietto rib (with 4 blades) adult size, total opening 10"
1 Finochietto rib (with 4 blades) child size, total opening 6"

Forceps

1 Russian 10"

Scissors

1 Metzenbaum 11"
1 Nelson 8"

Clamps

2 Duval-Crile lung
2 Mixter 9"
2 Right-angle 11"
4 Babcock 10"
1 Needle holder, fine 10½"

Rib elevators

2 Doyen elevator and raspatory, (1) left, (1) right
1 Matson stripper and elevator
1 Alexander costal periosteotome
1 Langenbeck periosteal elevator
1 Alexander rib raspatory

Rib shears

1 Bethune
2 Gluck (1) narrow, (1) wide
1 Sauerbruch double-action rongeur
1 Stille

Miscellaneous

2 Bailey rib contractors

PACEMAKER TRAY

Retractors

2 Senn, blunt
2 Weitlaner (1) 5½", (1) 7½"
2 Rake, blunt (4 prong)
2 Army-Navy

Forceps

1 Tissue without teeth 5½"
1 Tissue with teeth 5½"
1 Adson without teeth
2 Adson with teeth
1 DeBakey 6"

Scissors

1 Metzenbaum 7"
1 Straight Mayo 6¼"
1 Stevens tenotomy

1 Curved iris
1 Straight iris
1 Potts

Clamps

2 Right-angle 8″
2 Tonsil (Schnidt)
8 Curved Crile 5½″
6 Curved mosquito 5¼″
2 DeBakey, multipurpose 6″ (1) 30°, (1) 60°
1 Needle holder 6″
1 Ryder needle holder 6″
4 Towel clip 5½″
2 Sponge forceps 10″

Suction tubes or tips

1 Frazier No. 10
1 Andrews 9½″

Miscellaneous

2 Knife handles No. 3
1 Medicine cup
1 Bozeman packing forceps

Chapter 25

CARDIOVASCULAR TRAYS

VASCULAR PROCEDURES TRAY

Forceps

6 DeBakey (2) 6", (2) 8", (2) 9½"

Scissors

1 Potts

Clamps

2 DeBakey multipurpose (1) 9¾", (1) 12"
1 DeBakey curved aorta aneurysm 11¼"
5 DeBakey tangential occlusion 7½", 9¾", 10", 10¼", 10⅝"
1 Hufnagel ascending aorta
2 Angled DeBakey 90°, 10"
1 DeBakey aorta 10½"
1 Medium curved Crawfoord auricle 9¼"
1 Glover coarctation, straight 8¾"
1 Glover coarctation, angled 8¾"
1 Glover patent ductus, straight 8"

1 Glover patent ductus, angled 8"
1 Straight Glover 6¾"
2 Curved Glover (1) 6¾", (1) 8¼"
1 Cooley multipurpose, angled 6¼"
2 Cooley multipurpose, straight 7"
1 Curved Cooley 6¾"
6 Cardiovascular needle holder (2) 7", (2) 8", (2) 9"

VASCULAR SHUNT TRAY

Retractors

2 Army-Navy
2 Goulet
2 Senn, blunt
2 Rake, blunt (4 prong)
2 Cushing vein
2 Straight Weitlaner, blunt 6½"
1 Curved Weitlaner, blunt 6½"
2 Alm, blunt

Forceps

1 Tissue without teeth 5½"
1 Tissue with teeth 5½"
1 Russian 6"
2 Adson without teeth
1 Adson with teeth
1 Adson-Brown
2 DeBakey 6"

Scissors

2 Straight Mayo 6¼"
3 Metzenbaum (1) 5", (1) 5¾", (1) 7"
1 Straight Metzenbaum 5"
1 Stevens tenotomy
1 Straight iris
1 Curved iris

Clamps

- 6 Straight Crile 5½"
- 6 Curved Crile 5½"
- 3 Straight mosquito 5¼"
- 3 Curved mosquito 5¼"
- 3 Curved Pean 6¼"
- 3 Tonsil (Schnidt) 7½"
- 5 Right-angle (2) 5¼", (3) 7"
- 12 Towel clip 3½"
- 2 Sponge forceps 7"
- 2 Shunt
- 1 Needle holder, fine 6"
- 4 Ryder needle holder (2) 6", (2) 7"
- 1 Castroviejo needle holder

Suction tubes or tips

1 Andrews 9½"

Miscellaneous

1 Probe (malleable)
2 Knife handles No. 3
8 Rubber tubing pieces 2"
Various vascular clamps (e.g., DeBakey peripheral, DeBakey multipurpose, patent ductus and coarctation)

CARDIAC PROCEDURES TRAY*

Retractors

1 Richardson, small
3 Army-Navy

---

*A wide variety of instruments have been developed for cardiovascular surgery. Similar instruments with minor modifications are available. The selection and nomenclature of similar clamps varies among institutions and sections of the country.

2 Cushing vein
2 Senn, sharp
2 Rake, (3 prong) sharp
2 Adson self-retaining, straight
2 Himmelstein sternal (with hinged arms)
2 Lamina spreader (1) small, (1) large

Forceps

 4 Tissue with teeth 5½"
 3 Adson with teeth
 2 Russian 10"
10 DeBakey (1) 7¾", (8) 9½", (1) 12"

Scissors

4 Straight Mayo 6¼"
1 Curved Mayo 6¼"
5 Metzenbaum 7"
3 Potts (1) 25°, (1) 45°, (1) 60°
2 Wire cutter

Clamps

 6 Curved mosquito 5¼"
18 Curved Crile 5½"
 2 Curved Pean 6¼"
 2 Herrick kidney 9½"
 2 Straight Kocher (Ochsner) 8"
 2 Right-angle 8"
 2 Tonsil (Schnidt) 7½"
 6 Tube occluding
 3 Derra (1) small, (1) medium, (1) large
 2 DeBakey coarctation (1) 8½", (1) 8⅜"
 2 Crafoord aortic aneurysm 9½"
 2 DeBakey tangential occlusion (1) 9¾", (1) 10"
 2 Satinsky 9½"
 1 DeBakey patent ductus, straight 7½"
 1 DeBakey patent ductus, angular 7½"
12 Needle holder (6) 6", (6) 8"
16 Vascular needle holder, variety
 4 Sternal needle holder

2 Sponge forceps 10"
26 Towel clip 5½"

Suction tubes or tips

2 Yankauer 10⅜"

Miscellaneous

4 Knife handles (1) No. 3, (2) No. 7 (1) No. 3L
2 Beaver knife handles
1 Lebsche sternal knife
1 Aortic punch
2 Awls
1 Ruler
2 Aortic dilators
10 Vessel dilators
1 Toomey adaptor
3 Heparin needles
3 Olive-tipped heparin needles
1 Mallet
1 Pliers, needlenose
2 DeBakey bulldog clamps, curved
4 DeBakey bulldog clamps, straight
1 Pituitary rongeur, straight

For valves add

4 Allis clamps (2) 6", (2) 10"
4 Babcock clamps 10"
4 Richardson retractors (2) 9½" with ¾" × 1" blade,
    (2) 9½" with 1" × 1¼" blade
Valve retractor
1 atrial retractor
1 Valve dilator
1 Smithwick hook

Chapter 26

ORTHOPEDIC TRAYS

BASIC ORTHOPEDIC PROCEDURES TRAY

Retractors

2 Rake (4 prong) sharp
2 Rake (6 prong) sharp
1 Weitlaner, sharp
2 Army-Navy

Forceps

2 Tissue with teeth 5½"
2 Adson with teeth

Scissors

2 Straight Mayo 6¼"
1 Curved Mayo 6¼"
2 Metzenbaum (1) 6", (1) 7"
1 Bandage 8"
1 Wire cutter
1 Pin cutter

Clamps

2 Curved Pean 6¼"
2 Kocher-Lovelace

5 Curved Crile 5½"
2 Needle holder 7"
8 Towel clip 5½"
1 Sponge forceps

Suction tubes or tips

1 Yankauer 10⅜"

Miscellaneous

3 Knife handles (2) No. 3, (1) No. 7
2 Pliers (1) regular (1) needlenose
2 Screwdrivers (1) Phillips (1) blade
1 Mallet
1 Ruler
1 Depth gauge
3 Guidewires
1 Drill bit ⁷⁄₆₄"
1 Rasp
1 Hand drill with chuck
3 Bone cutters
1 Langenbeck elevator
1 Joker
1 Freer dissector
6 Currettes Nos. 0 to 5
1 Lewin bone holding forceps
1 Duckbill rongeur
1 Straight double-action rongeur
1 Rongeur (Stille-Luer)
1 Blunt nerve hook
1 Gigli saw with 2 handles
5 Osteotomes, various sizes

MINOR ORTHOPEDIC PROCEDURES TRAY

Retractors

2 Weitlaner, sharp 5½"
2 Senn (sharp)

2 Joseph skin hook
2 Volkmann rake, 2 prong

Forceps

1 Tissue without teeth 5½"
1 Tissue with teeth 5½"
1 Adson without teeth
2 Adson with teeth
1 Adson-Brown

Scissors

2 Straight Mayo 6¼"
3 Metzenbaum (1) 5¼", (1) 6", (1) 7"
1 Stevens tenotomy
1 Curved iris
1 Straight iris
1 Wire cutter

Clamps

4 Curved Crile 5½"
2 Straight Crile 5½"
4 Curved mosquito 5¼"
2 Straight mosquito 5¼"
2 Allis 6"
6 Kocher (Ochsner) (4) 6", (2) 10"
1 Needle holder 6"
1 Scissors needle holder
1 Webster needle holder 5"
8 Towel clip (4) 3½", (4) 5½"

Suction tips

1 Frazier No. 10

Miscellaneous

2 Knife handles No. 3
1 Langenbeck elevator
1 Small rasp

1 Small double-action rongeur (Ruskin)
1 Small bone cutter (Ruskin-Lister)
1 Small mallet
1 Small chisel
1 Freer elevator dissector
1 Short blunt nerve hook
1 Straight Key elevator ½"
1 Curved Key elevator ¼"
3 Curettes Nos. 000 to 0
1 Ruler
5 Osteotomes

BONE HOLDING INSTRUMENTS TRAY

2 Lane retractors
2 Lowman clamps
5 Verbrugge forceps (1) large, (1) medium, (1) small, (2) very small
2 Lewin bone clamps
2 Bishop clamps

HIP RETRACTORS TRAY

2 Bennett
2 Hibbs
3 Israel
2 Meyerding
3 Cobra
4 Hohmann

KNEE ARTHROTOMY TRAY

Retractors

6 Grey
1 Blount
1 Doane

Scissors

1 Cartilage

Clamps

1 Cartilage (modified Martin)
2 Lahey

Miscellaneous

1 Semilunar cartilage knife
3 Smillie cartilage knives (1) right, (1) left, (1) neutral
1 Meniscotome
1 Beaver knife handle
1 O'Donahue suture passer
1 Adson blunt hook

KNEE OR ANKLE ARTHROSCOPY TRAY

Forceps

1 Adson with teeth

Scissors

1 Straight Mayo 6¼"
1 Curved Mayo 6¼"

Clamps

2 Curved Crile 5½"
4 Straight Crile 5½"
4 Allis 6"
2 Curved Pean 6¼"
4 Towel clip 5½"
1 Needle holder 6"

Miscellaneous

1 Knife handle No. 3
Arthroscope(s) and bridge

1 Fiberoptic light cord
1 Sheath
1 Sharp obturator
1 Blunt obturator
1 Trocar
1 Sharp stylet
1 Blunt stylet
1 Connector
1 Verres needle
1 Straight probe
1 Stopcock
1 Right-angle hook and retractor
1 Knife (Smillie)
1 Hook knife
1 Retrograde knife
1 Alligator hook scissors
1 Alligator forceps
1 Alligator cutting forceps

Chapter 27

NEUROLOGIC PROCEDURES TRAYS

CRANIOTOMY TRAY

Retractors

1 Mastoid
2 Weitlaner (1) 5½", (1) 6½"
1 Curved Weitlaner 6½"
1 Adson cerebellar
2 Brain spoons
8 Malleable brain spatulas, double-ended (Davis) (¼" to 1½")
2 Nerve hooks (1) sharp, (1) blunt
2 Nerve root
2 Hoen dura separators (1) 45°, (1) 90°
2 Dura hooks

Forceps

2 Adson with teeth
2 Adson cup
4 Cushing with teeth (2) 7", (2) 8"
2 Cushing without teeth 8"
2 Bayonet 8"

Scissors

2 Straight Mayo 6¼"
1 Curved Mayo 6¼"
2 Metzenbaum (1) 6", (1) 7"
1 Wire cutter

Clamps

2 Curved Pean 6¼"
10 Curved Crile 5½"
6 Curved Mosquito 5¼"
36 Hemostatic scalp (Dandy)
2 Allis 6"
2 Tonsil (Schnidt) 7½"
2 Needle holder, fine 6"
2 Needle holder, heavy 7¼"
12 Towel clip (4) 3½", (8) 5½"

Suction tubes or tips

4 Frazier (1) No. 7, (1) No. 9, (1) No. 10, (1) No. 12

Miscellaneous

3 Knife handles (2) No. 3, (1) No. 7
1 Langenbeck periosteal elevator
1 Freer
5 Penfield dissectors Nos. 1 to 5
2 Short Kerrison rongeur, (1) 40°. (1) 90° up
1 Flat Kerrison rongeur
1 Kerrison rongeur 30° up
1 Leksell double-action rongeur
1 Small double-action rongeur
1 Straight pituitary forceps
1 Angled pituitary forceps, up
3 Blunt ventricular needles, (1) No. 11, (1) No. 14,
   (1) No. 16
1 Sharp ventricular needle
4 Stylets
4 Syringes, Luer-lock control 10 ml
3 Pituitary spoons (1) small, (1) medium, (1) large
1 Perforator (Raney, Hudson)

2 Scalp clip appliers (Raney, Michel)
4 Hemoclip appliers (2) small, (2) medium
1 Hand drill with key
1 Set drill bits
2 Gigli saws with (2) handles
1 Saw guide (Bailey)
1 Hudson brace
1 Basin (tiny)
4 Medicine cups
10 Rubber bands
1 Bayonet bipolar electrocoagulating forceps and cord
1 Neurosurgical sponge tray (pattie plate)
Prongs for skull clamp (e.g., Yasargil, Gardner, Mayfield)

LAMINECTOMY TRAY

Retractors

1 Downing (with 6 blades) (2) small, (2) medium, (2) large
4 Taylor (2) small, (2) large
2 Beckman (sharp)
2 Gelpi
2 Straight Weitlaner, blunt
2 Curved Weitlaner, sharp
2 Angled nerve root
2 Goulet
2 Army-Navy
1 Lamina spreader
4 Love root (2) 45°, (2) 90°
2 Straight Love root

Forceps

2 Tissue with teeth 5½"
1 Adson with teeth
2 Cushing without teeth
3 Bayonet without teeth

Scissors

1 Straight Mayo 6¼"
1 Curved Mayo 6¼"
1 Metzenbaum 7"

Clamps

18 Curved Crile 5½"
 6 Curved mosquito 5¼"
 2 Curved Pean 6¼"
 2 Short Kocher (Ochsner) 6¼"
 2 Kocher-Lovelace
 4 Needle holder (2) 6", (2) 7"

Suction tips

1 Frazier No. 10

Miscellaneous

4 Knife handles (2) No. 3, (2) No. 7
1 Long Beaver knife handle
1 Probe, malleable
1 Grooved director
1 Blunt nerve hook (Hoen)
1 Ruler
2 Jokers
2 Freer dissectors
1 Freer chisel
1 Langenbeck periosteal elevator ¹¹⁄₁₆"
2 Penfield dissectors
2 Medicine cups
4 Long curettes No. 0 to 3
2 Ring curettes (1) small, (1) medium
3 Cobb elevators (1) small, (1) medium, (1) large
2 Key elevators (1) ¾", (1) 1"
1 Leksell double-action rongeur
1 Stille-Luer double-action rongeur (gooseneck)
1 Neurosurgical sponge tray (pattie plate)

KERRISON RONGEURS AND PITUITARY FORCEPS TRAY

Pituitary Forceps

2 Straight (1) 2 mm × 10 mm, (1) 4 mm × 10 mm
2 Angled, up (1) 2 mm × 10 mm, (1) 4 mm × 10 mm
2 Angled, down (1) 2 mm × 10 mm, (1) 4 mm × 10 mm

Clamps

1 Ligamenta flava forceps

Kerrison Rongeurs

2 Straight (1) 3 mm, (1) 5 mm
2 Angled, up (1) 3 mm, (1) 5 mm
2 Angled, down (1) 3 mm, (1) 5 mm

Chapter 28

PLASTIC PROCEDURES TRAY

BASIC PLASTIC PROCEDURES TRAY

Retractors

- 2 Joseph skin hook, single
- 2 Joseph skin hook, double
- 2 Army-Navy
- 2 Senn, blunt
- 2 Cushing vein
- 2 Rake, blunt (four prong)
- 2 S-shaped
- 5 Malleable brain (1) ⅜", (1) ½", (1) ⅝", (1) ¾", (1) 1"

Forceps

- 1 Tissue without teeth 5½"
- 1 Tissue with teeth 5½"
- 1 Adson-Brown
- 1 Adson without teeth
- 2 Adson with teeth
- 2 Bayonet

Scissors

1 Straight Mayo 6¼"
3 Metzenbaum (1) 5¼", (1) 6", (1) 7"
1 Straight Metzenbaum 5¼"
1 Straight iris
1 Curved iris
1 Stevens tenotomy

Clamps

10 Towel clip 3½"
 4 Curved Crile 5½"
 2 Straight Crile 5½"
12 Curved mosquito 5¼"
 4 Straight mosquito 5¼"
 2 Allis 6"
 2 Kocher 6"
 2 Needle holder 6"
 2 Brown needle holder
 2 Webster needle holder

Suction tubes or tips

3 Frazier (with stylets) (1) No. 7, (1) No. 9, (1) No. 11
1 Andrews 9½"

Miscellaneous

3 Knife handles (2) No. 3, (1) No. 7
1 Probe, malleable
1 Ruler
1 Freer septal elevator
1 Caliper

Chapter 29

OTORHINOLARYNGO-LOGIC (ENT) TRAYS

BASIC EAR PROCEDURES TRAY

Retractors

2 Joseph skin hook
2 Senn, sharp
2 Army-Navy
1 Richardson, small
2 Wullstein-Weitlaner
2 Mastoid
1 Shea speculum holder (with 4 specula)
6 Ear specula sizes 1 to 6

Forceps

2 Adson with teeth
1 Adson-Brown
1 Bayonet, short (Jansen)

Scissors

1 Straight Mayo
2 Metzenbaum (1) 5¼", (1) 7"

548

1 Strabismus
3 House-Bellucci alligator (1) straight, (1) left, (1) right

Clamps

  4 Straight mosquito 5¼"
  6 Curved mosquito 5¼"
  2 Curved Crile 5½"
  2 Curved Pean 6¼"
  2 Allis 6"
  2 Webster needle holder 5"
10 Towel clip (6) 3½", (4) 5½"

Suction tubes or tips

2 Frazier with stylets (1) No. 5, (1) No. 7
4 Baron (2) No. 5, (2) No. 7
2 House
4 Rosen

Miscellaneous

1 Knife handle No. 3
1 Ruler
1 House elevator
1 Endaural speculum
1 Malleus nipper
1 House-Dieter malleus nipper
3 Cup forceps (1) small, (1) medium, (1) large
2 Alligator forceps (1) small, (1) large
1 Hartman forceps
2 Mastoid gouges (1) 2 mm, (1) 4 mm
2 House curettes (double-ended)
3 Mastoid curettes (1) size 000, (1) size 00, (1) size 0
1 House Gelfoam pressure forceps

Middle Ear Sharp Instruments (Usually in Protective Rack)
  1 Duckbill knife-elevator
  1 Right-angle elevator
  1 Oval curette

1 Excavator
1 Heavy needle
2 Picks (1) 45°, (1) 90°
1 Rosen needle
1 Attic dissector
1 Strut caliper
1 Straight chisel
1 Canal knife
1 Sickle knife (House)
1 Drum scraper
1 Oval window rasp
1 Incal stapedial knife
1 Hough hoe
2 Footplate hooks
1 House alligator crimper forceps

NASAL PROCEDURES TRAY

Retractors

2 Nasal specula (Killian) (1) 3″, (1) 2″
1 Nasal speculum, short
2 Aufricht nasal (1) long, (1) short

Forceps

1 Jansen bayonet without teeth
1 Cottle columella

Scissors

1 Fomon forsal angular
1 Fomon lower lateral
1 Cottle bulldog
1 Knight nasal

Clamps

1 Bayonet needle holder (Jacobson)

Suction tubes or tips

1 Antrum

Miscellaneous

- 1 Asch septal forceps
- 1 Mallet, small
- 2 Long metal applicators
- 1 Cartilage knife
- 2 Joseph knives (1) sharp (1) blunt
- 1 Joseph button-end knife
- 1 McKenty knife
- 1 Ballenger swivel knife
- 1 Freer septum knife
- 1 Freer septum elevator
- 1 Joseph periosteal elevator
- 1 Takahashi nasal forceps
- 1 Ferris-Smith fragment forceps
- 3 Knight polyp forceps (1) small, (1) medium, (1) large
- 1 Septal cutting forceps
- 1 Kazanjian nasal hump forceps
- 1 Double-action nasal rongeur
- 3 Kerrison rongeurs (1) 2 mm, (1) 4 mm, (1) 6 mm
- 1 Nerve hook
- 1 Reamer
- 1 Antrum trocar and stylet
- 3 Nasal rasps, assorted
- 2 Nasal saws, (1) right, (1) left
- 2 Chisels, curved, guarded (1) right, (1) left
- 2 Gouges (1) 2 mm, (1) 4 mm
- 2 Osteotomes (1) 2 mm, (1) 4 mm
- 6 Nasal curettes, angled (Coakley) assorted

MYRINGOTOMY TRAY

Retractors

- 3 Aural specula, plastic (1) small, (1) medium, (1) large
- 4 Aural specula, metal (assorted)

Forceps

- 1 Bayonet 5½"

Scissors

1 Straight iris

Suction tubes or tips

3 Frazier (with stylets), (1) No. 5, (1) No. 7, (1) No. 9

Miscellaneous

1 Smooth alligator
2 Curettes (1) small, (1) medium
1 Folding myringotomy Deaver knife
1 Medicine cup

TONSILLECTOMY AND ADENOIDECTOMY TRAY

Retractors

1 Fulton mouth gag
3 Jennings mouth gags (1) 4", (1) 4½", (1) 6"
1 Love uvula
1 Hurd dissector and pillar retractor
2 Tongue blades (1) large, (1) small

Scissors

1 Metzenbaum 7"
1 Straight Mayo 6¼"

Clamps

2 Tonsil (Schmidt) 7½"
2 Allis 6"
1 Curved Allis 10"
1 Straight sponge forceps 10"
2 Curved sponge forceps 7"
2 Towel clip 3½"
1 Needle holder 7"

Suction tubes or tips

1 Yankauer 10⅜"

Miscellaneous

1 Knife handle No. 7
1 Beck-Schenck tonsil snare with wire (and 2 extra wires)
1 Adenoid punch
1 Fisher tonsil knife
3 Barnhill adenoid curettes (1) No. 1, (1) No. 2, (1) No. 3
3 La Force adenotomes (1) small, (1) medium, (1) large
2 Medicine cups

TRACHEOSTOMY TRAY

Retractors

2 Army-Navy
2 Senn, blunt

Forceps

1 Tissue with teeth 5½"
1 Adson with teeth

Scissors

1 Metzenbaum 7"
1 Curved Mayo 6¼"
1 Straight Mayo 6¼"

Clamps

4 Curved Crile 5½"
4 Curved mosquito 5¼"
2 Allis 6"
1 Needle holder 6"
4 Towel clip 3½"

Miscellaneous

  2 Knife handles No. 3
  2 Knife blades (1) No,. 11, (1) No. 15
  1 Syringe 5 ml, Luer-lock control
  2 Needles (1) 20-gauge 1" and (1) 25-gauge 1"
  1 Tracheostomy dilator
  1 Tracheostomy hook
10 Sponges 4" × 4"
  1 Preparation cup

Chapter 30

OPHTHALMIC TRAYS

BASIC EYE PROCEDURES TRAY

Scissors

1 Blunt (Stevens)
1 Curved iris
1 Stevens tenotomy
1 Suture

Clamps

2 Halsted straight mosquito 5¼″
1 Halsted curved mosquito 5¼″
4 Towel clip 3½″

Miscellaneous

1 Irrigating tip No. 21
1 Knife handle No. 9
6 Medicine cups
Needles:
    (1) 23-gauge 1″, (1) 25-gauge ⅝″
    (2) 23-gauge retrobulbar
    (2) 25-gauge retrobulbar
Syringes:

(2) 5 ml Luer lock
(5) 2 ml Luer lock
1 Eye pad
2 Eye shields (1) metal, (1) plastic
2 Serrefine clamps

Special notes

Labeling syringes and medicine cups avoids confusion.

Leave eye pads in the wrapper when sterilizing the tray.

EYELID AND CONJUNCTIVAL PROCEDURES TRAY

Retractors

1 Eye speculum (Barraquer, Lancaster)
1 Lacrimal sac
1 Chalazion clamp (Des Marres)
2 Senn
2 Skin hook
2 Skin hook, double-prong
5 Des Marres (2) No. 1, (1) No. 2, (2) No. 3
2 von Graefe muscle hook (1) No. 1, (1) No. 3

Forceps

2 Fixation (e.g., Lester)
2 Bishop-Harmon suturing
1 Castroviejo suturing
1 Conjunctival, with teeth
1 Conjunctival, serrated
1 Dressing
1 Tying (e.g., Castroviejo)
1 Lid (Green)
1 Chalazion
1 Entropion (Snellen)

Scissors

1 Wescott tenotomy
1 Vannas iridocapsulotomy

Clamps

1 Kalt needle holder
1 Castroviejo needle holder

Miscellaneous

1 Corneal knife (Gill)
1 Beaver knife handle
1 Castroviejo caliper
3 Chalazion curettes

BASIC EYE MUSCLE PROCEDURES TRAY

Retractors

1 Eye speculum (Lancaster, Barraquer)
1 Lacrimal sac (self-retaining)
2 Muscle hook (Stevens)
4 Muscle hook (von Graefe) (2) No. 1, (2) No. 3

Forceps

1 Fixation (Lester)
1 Recession
2 Suturing (Bishop-Harmon) (1) heavy, (1) fine
2 Suturing (Castroviejo 0.5 mm)
2 Muscle (Jameson, Berens)

Scissors

1 Straight Wescott tenotomy
1 Curved Wescott tenotomy
1 Suture (Troutman)

Clamps

2 Needle holder (Kalt, Barraquer)

Miscellaneous

1 Caliper (Castroviejo)

DACRYOCYSTORHINOSTOMY TRAY

Retractors

2 Lacrimal sac, 4 prong (Knapp)
1 Lacrimal sac, self-retaining (Agricola)
2 Nasal specula (1) short, (1) medium

Forceps

2 Bayonet

Clamps

2 Webster needle holder

Suction tubes or tips

2 Frazier with stylets (1) No. 5, (1) No.7

Miscellaneous

1 Lacrimal irrigating cannula
1 Lacrimal trephine (Arruga)
3 Lacrimal dilators
2 Lacrimal cannulas (1) straight, (1) bulbous tip
2 Lid everters (Berens)
6 Lacrimal probes (sizes 0000–000 to sizes 7–8)
1 Worst pigtail probe
2 Lacrimal chisels (1) 2 mm, (1) 4 mm
2 Lacrimal gouges (1) 2 mm, (1) 4 mm
2 Lacrimal osteotomes (1) 2 mm, (1) 4 mm
1 Small mallet

2 Kerrison rongeurs (1) 2 mm, (1) 4 mm
1 Takahashi straight nasal forceps
1 Lempert rongeur, delicate curved
1 Freer elevator
1 Joseph periosteal elevator

GLOBE AND ORBIT PROCEDURES TRAY

Retractors

1 Eye speculum (Guyton-Park, Lancaster)
1 Lacrimal sac (Fink)
4 von Graefe muscle hook (2) No. 1, (2) No. 3
1 Arruga orbital/elevator
1 Schepens orbital
1 Converse alar retractor, double-ended

Forceps

2 Tissue (Bishop-Harmon)
2 Fixation (Lester, von Graefe)
2 Suturing (Castroviejo)
1 Recession (Jameson)

Scissors

1 Suture (Stevens)
2 Wescott (1) left, (1) right
1 Straight tenotomy (Stevens)
1 Curved tenotomy (Stevens)
1 Enucleation

Clamps

1 Curved mosquito 5¼"
4 Straight mosquito 5¼"
1 Straight Crile 5½"
1 Right-angle (Mixter)
2 Tonsil (Schnidt)
2 Needle holder (Barraquer, Alabama-Green)

Miscellaneous

2 Kerrison mastoid rongeurs (1) up, (1) down
1 Lacrimal sac chisel
1 Freer periosteal elevator
1 Cottle septum elevator
1 Enucleation snare
1 Evisceration spoon
1 Enucleation spoon
1 Sphere introducer
1 Small mallet
1 Bone cutter
1 Rongeur, single-action (Lempert)
1 Blade breaker and holder

CORNEAL PROCEDURES TRAY

Retractors

1 Eye speculum (Lancaster, Barraquer)
2 Muscle hook (Green, O'Connor, Jameson, von Graefe)

Forceps

2 Tissue (Bishop-Harmon)
1 Corneal (Colibri 0.12 mm)
2 Suturing (Castroviejo)
1 Corneal-scleral
1 Straight tying (McPherson)
1 Curved tying (McPherson)

Scissors

1 Curved suture
2 Troutman-Castroviejo (1) right, (1) left
1 Straight Castroviejo
1 Straight iris (Barraquer-DeWecker)

Clamps

2 Straight micro needle holder (Castroviejo, Barraquer)

Miscellaneous

1 Iris spatula
1 Paton spatula
1 Castroviejo spatula
1 Corneal knife (Gill)
1 Corneal dissector (Troutman)
1 Air cannula, 27 gauge
1 Castroviejo caliper
2 Corneal markers
2 Trephine handles (Weck)
3 Trephine blades (1) 7.5 mm, (1) 8.0 mm, (1) 8.5 mm
1 Teflon block
1 Corneal punch (Troutman), 2 parts
1 Base plate with corneal block

CATARACT EXTRACTION AND LENS PROCEDURE TRAY

Retractors

1 Eye speculum (Barraquer, child size)
1 Muscle hook (von Graefe) No. 1
1 Muscle hook (Green)

Forceps

1 Curved iris (von Graefe)
1 Capsulotomy (Arruga)
1 Corneal (Colibri 0.12 mm)
1 Straight tying (McPherson)
1 Curved tying (McPherson)
2 Suturing (Castroviejo (1) 0.12 mm, (1) 0.5 mm)
1 Lens holding forceps (Shepard)
1 Bonn forceps 0.12 mm

Scissors

1 Tenotomy (Wescott)
1 Straight iris (Barraquer-DeWecker)
1 Capsulotomy (Vannas)
1 Iridotocapsulotomy

2 Corneal (Troutman) (1) left, (1) right
1 Barraquer-DeWecker

Clamps

1 Castroviejo needle holder
1 Barraquer needle holder

Miscellaneous

1 Beaver knife handle
1 Lens loop (Knapp)
1 Olive tip irrigator
1 Iris spatula (Wheeler)
1 Castroviejo cyclodialysis spatula
1 Irrigating vectis loop
1 Corneal knife (Gill)
1 Air or Healon cannula
1 Lacrimal irrigator
1 Blade breaker
1 Castroviejo caliper
Irrigation and aspiration set
1 Micro lens hook (Sinsky)
1 Lens manipulator (Kugler)
1 Iris hook (Bonn)
1 Lens hook (Fenzl)

GLAUCOMA PROCEDURES TRAY

Retractors

1 Eye speculum (Barraquer, Lancaster)

Forceps

1 Corneal (Colibri 0.12 mm)
1 Suturing (Castroviejo 0.12 mm)
1 Bonn forceps 0.1 mm
2 Tissue (Bishop-Harmon)

Scissors

1 Wescott (blunt tipped)
1 Suture (Troutman)
1 Iris (Barraquer-DeWecker)
1 Strabismus scissors (Knapp)
1 Iridocapsulotomy (Vannas)
1 Tenotomy (Wescott)

Clamps

1 Kalt needle holder
1 Barraquer needle holder (curved, nonlocking)

Miscellaneous

1 Tonometer (Schiotz)
1 Irrigating tip No. 27
1 Corneal dissector (Troutman)
1 Castroviejo caliper
1 Castroviejo cyclodialysis spatula
1 Iris spatula (Wheeler)
1 Blade breaker (Castroviejo, Barraquer)
1 Beaver knife handle
1 Corneal knife (Gill)
1 Iris hook (Bonn)
1 Air cannula
1 Scleral punch (Holth)

BASIC EYE PROCEDURES MICROSCOPE TRAY

Retractors

1 Eye speculum (Barraquer, Lancaster)
5 Lid retractors (Des Marres) (2) No. 1, (1) No. 2, (2) No. 3
2 Muscle hook retractors

Forceps

2 Castroviejo suturing (0.12 mm, 0.5 mm)

1 Bishop-Harmon suturing
1 Fixation (Lester, von Graefe)
1 Corneal (Colibri 0.12 mm)
1 Curved tying (McPherson)
1 Straight tying (McPherson)
2 Straight suture tying (Castroviejo)

Scissors

2 Corneal (Castroviejo) (1) left, (1) right
1 Suture (Troutman)
1 Suture iris (Barraquer-DeWecker)
1 Iridocapsulotomy (Vannas)

Clamps

1 Nonlocking needle holder (Barraquer)
2 Needle holder (Kalt, Troutman-Barraquer)

Miscellaneous

1 Knife handle No. 9
1 Beaver knife handle
1 Iris spatula (Barraquer)
1 Corneal knife (Gill)

RETINAL PROCEDURES TRAY

Retractors

1 Eye speculum (Lancaster, Guyton-Park)
1 Muscle hook (von Graefe) No. 1
1 Muscle hook (Jameson)
1 Retinal detachment hook (Gass)
1 Des Marres lid No. 2
1 Arruga
1 Schepens

Forceps

1 Castroviejo suturing (0.12 mm)
2 Suturing (Bishop-Harmon) (1) heavy, (1) fine

2 Tying (McCollough, Alabama)
1 Fixation (Lester, von Graefe, Elshnig)
1 Recession (Jameson)

Scissors

1 Tenotomy (Wescott)
1 Suture
1 Straight Stevens
1 Curved Stevens
1 Iris

Clamps

1 Curved Castroviejo needle holder
1 Barraquer needle holder
1 Kalt needle holder

Miscellaneous

2 Beaver knife handles
1 Corneal knife (Gill)
1 Castroviejo caliper
2 Air cannulas (1) 27 gauge (1) 30 gauge
1 Tonometer (Schiotz)
1 Scleral depressor (Schepens)
3 Diathermy tips
1 Straight retinal probe
1 Curved retinal probe
1 Retinal probe sleeve

Chapter 31

PEDIATRIC TRAYS

PEDIATRIC MAJOR PROCEDURES TRAY

Retractors

2 Senn, blunt
4 Gans (2) No. 1, (2) No. 2
5 Malleable brain (spatulas) (1) ⅜″, (1) ½″, (1) ⅝″, (1) ¾″, (1) 1″
1 Small Balfour (total opening 3¾″)
1 Heiss self-retaining
2 Richardson (1) ¾″ × 1″, (1) 1″ × 1″

Forceps

1 Tissue with teeth 5½″
2 Adson without teeth
2 Adson with teeth
1 Cushing without teeth 7″
1 Cushing with teeth 7″
4 DeBakey (fine) (2) 6″, (2) 7¾″

Scissors

2 Straight Mayo 6¼″
1 Curved Mayo 5½″
3 Metzenbaum (1) 5¼″, (1) 6″, (1) 7″

1 Straight Metzenbaum 6"
1 Potts
1 Stevens tenotomy
1 Curved iris
1 Straight iris

Clamps

4 Straight Crile 5½"
6 Curved Crile 5½"
4 Straight mosquito 5¼"
10 Curved mosquito 5¼"
6 Curved Pean 5½"
4 Curved Kocher 5½"
6 Straight Kocher 5½"
2 Kocher-Lovelace
4 Babcock 5¾"
4 Allis 6"
6 Allis, fine 5¾"
6 Right-angle (2) 5½", (2) 7", (2) 7½"
2 Tonsil (Schnidt) 7½"
2 Needle holder 6"
2 Needle holder, fine 7½"
6 Towel clip 3½"
4 Sponge forceps 7"

Suction tubes or tips

1 Poole 9¼"
1 Andrews 9½"
1 Frazier No. 7

Miscellaneous

4 Knife handles (2) No. 3, (1) No. 7, (1) No. 9
1 Ballinger elevator
1 Elevator dissector
1 Elevator probe

PEDIATRIC MINOR PROCEDURES TRAY

Retractors

2 Gans No. 1
2 Senn, blunt

Forceps

2 Tissue without teeth
2 Adson without teeth
2 Adson with teeth
2 DeBakey 6"

Scissors

1 Straight Mayo 6¼"
2 Metzenbaum (1) 5½", (1) 6"
1 Straight Metzenbaum 5¼"
1 Stevens tenotomy
1 Curved iris
1 Straight iris

Clamps

2 Curved Crile 5½"
2 Straight mosquito 5¼"
6 Curved mosquito 5¼"
2 Babcock 5¾"
2 Needle holder 6"
4 Towel clip 3½"

Miscellaneous

2 Knife handles No. 3
1 Medicine cup

PEDIATRIC GASTROINTESTINAL PROCEDURES TRAY

Clamps

2 Curved pediatric Doyen 7½"
2 Straight pediatric Doyen 7½"
2 Curved pediatric Bainbridge 7½"
2 Straight pediatric Bainbridge 7½"

Miscellaneous

8 Robinson catheter 18 Fr, pieces 2"

PEDIATRIC THORACOTOMY TRAY

Retractors

1 Finochietto rib (4 blades) child size, total opening 6"
2 Finochietto rib, infant size, total opening (1) 2½", (1) 3½"

Miscellaneous

2 Langenbeck periosteal elevators (1) ¼", (1) $^{11}/_{16}$"
1 Beyer double-action rongeur 7"
1 Bailey rib contractor 6¾"

APPENDIX: LASER TECHNOLOGY

Definition

The laser (an acronym for light amplification by stimulated emission of radiation) is an energy source derived from light.

Discussion

The laser emits light energy produced by stimulating the electrons of various media (solid, liquid, tunable dye, or gas) with electricity (or xenon flash lamp or another laser) to reach a high energy state, releasing this energy in the form of photons. The photons collide within the laser chamber between mirrors creating more energy that then escapes in a controlled manner as the laser beam. This beam is collimated, maintaining a constant diameter for great distances (unlike an ordinary light beam, which expands). This beam is monochromatic and of a single optical frequency, and the energy particles (photons) travel in a coordinated fashion, in phase with each other (coherent). These properties allow the laser beam to travel over great distances with extremely concentrated energy. Each individually stimulated substance emits energy of a different wavelength, which influences the absorption of this energy in a selective manner.

Body tissues are affected by the laser beam as the light energy is converted to heat resulting in the coagulation, cutting, and vaporization (or "welding") of these tissues. The level of the power setting (wattage), the duration of the contact time with the target tissues, the use of continuous or pulsed mode, and the cooling action of the local blood flow will determine the effect of the laser beam on tissues.

Three laser types are in common use in the operating room. The *carbon dioxide (CO₂) laser* is used for cutting and vaporization of tissues (and welding of certain tissues, for example, vascular anastomoses). Because of its longer wavelength the CO_2 laser beam cannot be transmitted by lengthy fiber delivery systems. The *neodymium:yttrium aluminum garnet (Nd:YAG) laser* is used for deeper coagulation, or it can be transmitted by a flexible probe through an endoscope for coagulation of gastrointestinal, urinary, and respiratory tract tissues. The *argon laser* is used in ophthalmology (e.g., photocoagulation of retinal tears and bleeding points) and in plastic surgery to ablate cutaneous hemangiomata. The *krypton laser* can also be used for photocoagulation of the retina. The *excimer laser* system is incorporated in a fine catheter that includes a video system and irrigating mechanism and is used to open occluded coronary arteries. An additional technique is *photodynamic therapy*, which involves the injection of a photosensitive dye (such as modified porphyrin), which is selectively retained by malignant tissues. These tissues (e.g., breast, retina, maxillary sinus) are then exposed to laser light of appropriate wavelength to produce a photochemical reaction resulting in tumor destruction. A tunable dye, adjusted (tuned) by prism to emit a red light (wavelength 630 nm), is used in conjunction with the porphyrin derivative. The laser does not, however, produce ionizing radiation and is not hazardous in that sense as are radioactive substances or x-rays.

Adapted to use with the operating microscope, the laser is invaluable in microlaryngeal and ophthalmologic procedures. Many laser procedures can be performed in outpatient surgery or special procedure units (e.g., the eye laboratory) with reduced operating room and anesthesia time. In many of its applications the laser permits minimal tissue trauma with reduced injury to adjacent structures and a relatively dry field with reduced blood loss. Direct tissue contact is not necessary and otherwise inaccessible areas may be treated. Faster wound healing with less pain, edema, scarring, etc., are often attributed to laser surgery. However, the laser and its obligate special equipment, complex maintenance, and evolving technologic advances with continuously upgraded instrumentation make laser surgery costly. More significant is that laser procedures are potentially hazardous to patients and operating room personnel.

Safety Precautions

Strict safety precautions must be enforced. Signs posted on the operating room doors warn of laser use. All equipment must be checked prior to the procedure, not limiting equipment checking to testing beam focus, electrical connections, suction apparatus, etc. Only personnel trained in laser safety and technique should participate. A master key enabling operation of the laser must be obtained and then returned at the completion of the procedure. The laser is set at "standby" or "stop" mode during significant interruptions in its use. Eye protection for patients and all personnel is mandatory. For the CO_2 laser clear glasses with side wings are used (including the patient, if awake). Under general anesthesia the patient's eyes are taped shut and covered with wet pads and the face is covered with a wet towel (unless of course the procedure involves this area). The Nd:YAG laser requires blue-green safety goggles and the argon laser, orange goggles. Fire is a realistic potential hazard, particularly when the CO_2 laser is used near the airway (as in laryngeal procedures). Only nonflammable anesthetics are used. Conventional endotracheal tubes must be wrapped with aluminum foil tape. Flexible metallic (matte-finished to reduce deflection of the laser beam) and insulated silicone endotracheal tubes are available. A protocol for endotracheal tube fire must be rehearsed to minimize any untoward effects. Nonreflective instruments that defocus and disperse the laser energy are used. Wet towels or sponges surround the operating field, but precautions are taken to prevent strike-through contamination. A saline-filled irrigating syringe is available to cool local tissues or extinguish a flash fire. The skin preparation solution must contain no combustible agents (i.e., no alcohol or ether). The laser activation switch or pedal must be controlled only by the surgeon; other controls (e.g., for the electrosurgical unit) may be delegated to the assistant. A satisfactory smoke evacuator to remove noxious smoke (plume) is necessary. Movement of the patient is limited by restraints if the patient is awake, and for delicate microscopic surgery general anesthesia with muscle paralysis is used. The circulator enforces these precautions, provides support to the patient, and documents the procedure. The scrub person keeps the immediate field surrounded by wet towels or sponges while guarding against contamination, assists in suctioning the plume, and anticipates the need for special instruments and supplies.

The Joint Commission on Accreditation of Health Care Organizations (JC) recommends (mandates) that physicians employing the laser are credentialed, that operating room personnel are instructed in laser use and safety including hands-on training, and that quality maintenance of equipment is observed. Documentation of laser procedures becomes part of the patient's operating room record. Data includes type of procedure, type of laser, duration of use, wattage settings, and documentation that the safety protocol was observed, and if necessary, additional documentation of untoward occurrences and measures taken to minimize them.

BIBLIOGRAPHY

Adams, GL, Lawrence, RB, and Paparella, MM: Boies' Fundamentals of Otolaryngology: A Text of Ear, Nose, and Throat Diseases, ed 5. WB Saunders, Philadelphia, 1978.

Aimino, PA: Perioperative nursing documentation: Developing the record and using care plans. AORN J 46:73, 1987.

Aronoff, BL: The star wars revolution: Lasers in cancer surgery. Bull Am Coll Surg 72:8, 1987.

Atkinson, LJ and Kohn, ML: Berry and Kohn's Introduction to Operating Room Technique, ed 6. McGraw-Hill, New York, 1986.

Ball, KA: Controlling smoke evacuation and odor during laser surgery. Todays OR Nurse 8:4, 1986.

Ball, KA: Developing a laser program. Todays OR Nurse 8:16, 1986.

Ball, KA: Laser safety. Todays OR Nurse 8:10, 1986.

Ballenger, JJ: Diseases of the Nose, Throat and Ear, ed 12. Lea & Febiger, Philadelphia, 1977.

Bendick, PJ: Laser safety in the operating room. Bull Am Coll Surg 71:10, 1987.

Bennett, CN (ed): Lasers. Humana Technos 1:1, 1982.

Benson, CD, et al.: Pediatric Surgery. Year Book Medical Publishers, Chicago, 1962.

Bigos, DM and Davis, JL: Idiopathic radial tunnel syndrome: Surgical treatment and nursing care. AORN J 46:255, 1987.

Brooks, SM: Instrumentation for the Operating Room, ed 2. CV Mosby, St. Louis, 1983.

Canala, LS: Advancements in internal surgical stapling. Todays OR Nurse 8:11, 1986.

Churchill-Davidson, H: Wylie and Churchill-Davidson's A Practice of Anesthesia. Year Book Medical Publishers, Chicago, 1984.

Cowden, JW, et al: Repeated radial keratotomy in the prospective evaluation of radial keratotomy study. Am J Ophthalmol 103:423, 1987.

Crenshaw, AH (ed): Campbell's Operative Orthopedics, ed 7. CV Mosby, St. Louis, 1987.

Danforth, DN (ed): Obstetrics and Gynecology, ed 4. Harper & Row, Philadelphia, 1982.

Deitz, MR, Sanders, RR, and Raanan, MG: A consecutive series of radial keratotomies performed with a diamond blade. Am J Ophthalmol 103:417, 1987.

De Weese, DD and Saunders, WH: Otolaryngology, ed 5. CV Mosby, St. Louis, 1977.

Dienno, ME: Esophageal atresia: Corrective procedures and nursing care. AORN J 45:1356, 1987.

Dixon, JA: Surgical Application of Lasers. Year Book Medical Publishers, Chicago, 1983.

Donnelly, J and Livacz, L: New instruments in ophthalmic surgery. Todays OR Nurse 8:8, 1986.

Dornier Medical Systems, Inc.: Instructional films, and personal communication. Marietta, Georgia, 1987.

Drucker, MD: Arthroscopic surgery of the knee joint. AORN J 36:585, 1982.

Feldman, ST and Brown, SI: Reduction of astigmatism after keratoplasty. Am J Surg 103:477, 1987.

Fezer, SJ: Cricoid pressure: How, when, and why. AORN J 45:1374, 1987.

Friel JP (ed): Dorland's Illustrated Medical Dictionary, ed. 26. WB Saunders, Philadelphia, 1981.

Fuller, JR: Surgical Technology Principles and Practice. WB Saunders, Philadelphia, 1986.

Goldberg, SM, Gordon, P, and Nivatvongs, S: Essentials of Anorectal Surgery. JB Lippincott, Philadelphia, 1980.

Greene, VW, Klapes, NA, and Langholz, AC: Interhospital transportation: Monitoring sterilty of instrument packs. AORN J 45:1420, 1987.

Gruendemann, BJ and Meeker, MH: Alexander's Care of the Patient in Surgery, ed 8. CV Mosby, St. Louis, 1987.

Huff, BB (ed): Physicians' Desk Reference, ed 41. Medical Economics, Oradell, NJ, 1987.

Jackson, EW (ed): Caring for Surgical Patients. Intermed Communications, Springhouse, PA, 1982.

Kaufman, HE: Refractive surgery (editorial). Am J Ophthalmol 103:355, 1987.

Krumeich, JH and Swinger, C: Non freeze epikeratophakia for the correction of Myopia. Am J Ophthalmol 103:397, 1987.

Kuhn, PA: Operating Room Procedure Manual. Reston Publishing Company, Reston, VA, 1981.

Lach, J: OR Nursing: Preoperative Care and Draping Technique. Kendall, Chicago, 1974.

Lambrix, K: Epikeratophakia: Correcting visual deficits with corneal tissue. AORN J 46:218, 1987.

Laskin, RS and Varrichio, DM: Total knee replacement. AORN J 36:577, 1982.

Le Maitre, G and Finnegan, J: The Patient in Surgery, ed 4. WB Saunders, Philadelphia, 1980.

LoCicero, J, Quebbeman, E, and Nichols, R: Health hazards in the operating room: An update. Bull Am Coll Surg 72(9):4, 1987.

Lore, JM: Atlas of Head and Neck Surgery, ed 2. WB Saunders, Philadelphia, 1973.

Madden, JL: Atlas of Techniques in Surgery, ed 2. Appleton-Century-Croft, New York, 1964.

Marshall, JG and Ross, JL: Hydrocephalus: Ventriculoperitoneal shunting in infants and children. AORN J 40:842, 1984.

Mattingly, RF and Thompson, JD: Te Linde's Operative Gynecology, ed 6. JB Lippincott, Philadelphia, 1985.

Miner, D: Patient positioning: Applying the nursing process. AORN J 45:1117, 1987.

Moore, DC: Regional Block, ed 3. Charles C Thomas, Springfield, IL, 1962.

Pack, GT and Oropeza, R: A technique for superficial and deep groin dissection surgical procedures. 3:2, 1966.

Podrasky, P and Rudzinski, HM: Percutaneous endoscopic gastrostomy: An alternative to laparotomy. AORN J 45:1403, 1987.

Quattro, LS: Spinal instrumentation: An introduction to Cotrel-DuBousset Instrumentation. AORN J 46:54, 1987.

Raffensperger, JG: Swenson's Pediatric Surgery, ed 4. Appleton-Century-Crofts, New York, 1980.

Sabiston, D (ed): (Christopher's) Textbook of Surgery, ed 13. WB Saunders, Philadelphia, 1986.

Smith, RR: Essentials of Neurosurgery. JB Lippincott, Philadelphia, 1980.

Spaeth, GL: Ophthalmic Surgery. WB Saunders, Philadelphia, 1982.

Torresyap, PM: Esophagogastrectomy for carcinoma of the esophagus. Todays OR Nurse 9:10, 1987.

Tupa, B: Alleviating the fears of pediatric patients. Todays OR Nurse 9:33, 1987.

Turek, S: Orthopaedics, ed 4, vol 2. JB Lippincott, Philadelphia, 1984.

Vaiden, RE and White, WR: Arteriovenous malformations of the brain. AORN J 46:37, 1987.

Vaughn, D and Ashbury, T: General Ophthalmology, ed 10. Lange Medical Publications, Los Altos, CA, 1983.

Walsh, PC, Gittes, RF, and Perlmutter, AD (eds): Campbell's Urology, ed 5. WB Saunders, Philadelphia, 1986.

Waughman, WR, Jordan, LM, and Norris, JL: Nurse anesthesia: Patient-centered nursing. Todays OR Nurse 8:16, 1986.

Wilson, JR, Beecham CT, and Carrington, ER: Obstetrics and Gynecology. CV Mosby, St. Louis, 1971.

Youmans, JR (ed): Neurological Surgery. WB Saunders, Philadelphia, 1982.

INDEX

A "t" following a page number indicates a table. An "f" following a page number indicates a figure.

579